Blaber's Foundations for Paramedic Practice

A theoretical perspective

Third Edition

Edited by Amanda Y. Blaber

D1334238

 Open University Press

Open University Press
McGraw-Hill Education
8th Floor, 338 Euston Road
London
England
NW1 3BH

email: enquiries@openup.co.uk
world wide web: www.openup.co.uk

and Two Penn Plaza, New York, NY 10121-2289, USA

First edition published 2008, second edition published 2012,
first published in this 3rd edition 2019.

Editorial Director: Teresa Massara
Commissioning Editor: Vivien Antwi
Editorial Assistant: Karen Harris
Content Product Manager: Ali Davis

A catalogue record of this book is available from the British Library

ISBN-13: 9780335243273
ISBN-10: 0335243274
eISBN: 9780335243280

Library of Congress Cataloging-in-Publication Data
CIP data applied for

Typeset by Transforma Pvt. Ltd., Chennai, India
Printed and bound by CPI Group (UK) Ltd, Croydon, CR0 4YY

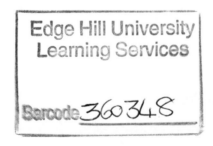

Contents

Handwritten annotation: Maybe Professional

mentioned CPD in Paragraph 5

Contributors

Amanda Y. Blaber has 17 years teaching in higher education institutes, with many years of emergency care experience. Amanda contributes to the Forum for Higher Education for Paramedics and the Council of Deans Paramedic Advisory group. Amanda is an Honorary Fellow of the College of Paramedics and is extremely proud of the literary contribution she and her colleagues have made to the education of paramedics in the UK. She has extensive knowledge and experience in curriculum design and validation processes and is a Senior Fellow of the Higher Education Academy.

Dave Blain is a dedicated professional for safeguarding adults, with 37 years in the ambulance sector as PTS, EMT, Paramedic and management roles. This included a period as a clinical tutor and safeguarding children and adults posts for seven years. He has been involved in over 100 safeguarding multi-agency reviews and 30 Domestic Homicide Reviews across the Yorkshire and Humber region and previously was involved in national safeguarding work, as national ambulance sector representative with the Department of Health and Department for Education for policy and guidance in safeguarding children. Dave established the National Ambulance Safeguarding Group (NASG) in 2009 and chaired this until 2014. Dave has a BA Hons in Teaching and Learning, a PGCE and currently is at NHS Hull Clinical Commissioning Group in the above role and also safeguarding advisor to the College of Paramedics.

Mike Brady is a paramedic by background, a lecturer in emergency and unscheduled care, a doctoral student (PhD), and a clinical team leader within an ambulance service clinical hub. Mike has contributed heavily to the paramedic literature in areas including end-of-life care, healthcare quality, death anxiety, as well as child safeguarding and remote clinical decision-making (RCDM). Paramedics have an underplayed but integral role in both child safeguarding and RCDM and Mike is keen to advertise and research these roles as much as possible, to inform future paramedic practice, policy, and education.

Gemma Chapman qualified as a paramedic in 2012, working on a double-crewed ambulance and rapid response vehicle for two years, during which time she completed a mentorship module and successfully mentored undergraduate student paramedics. Gemma became an Operations Officer in 2014, providing day-to-day leadership, management and incident command cover at incidents and various public events.

Gemma completed the CMI leadership and management programme before embarking on an MSc Healthcare Management programme. She contributed to the *Student Paramedic Survival Guide* in 2015. She is currently seconded to an Operational Support Officer role within the clinical hub, looking at reducing the unavailability of resources as part of a Trust-wide Quality Performance Improvement Plan. Gemma feels passionately that students should develop both the clinical skills required and possess the knowledge in other areas where they can make a difference, such as public health.

Vince Clarke is a Senior Lecturer in Paramedic Science at the University of Hertfordshire, where he has been employed since 2016. Vince joined the London Ambulance Service in 1996, qualified as a paramedic in 1998 and entered the Education and Development Department in 2001. He worked as part of the Higher Education team and developed in-house paramedic programmes, as well as working closely with higher education partner institutions. A Health & Care Professions Council partner since 2006, he has been involved in the approval of a wide range of paramedic educational programmes across the country as well as assessing Continuing Professional Development (CPD) submissions and sitting on Conduct and Competence Fitness to Practise panel hearings. Vince also works as an independent paramedic expert witness for the Court and prepares reports on breach of duty for both claimants and defendants.

Alison Cork qualified as a nurse in 1989 and worked in emergency care for 15 years. Alison then chose a career in education and teaches student paramedics and nurses at the University of Greenwich. Alison has a particular interest in leadership and clinical decision-making.

Steve Cowland joined the London Ambulance Service in 1984. He has been a paramedic since 1991. He has been involved with education programmes for a number of years in his role as ambulance tutor and now works at Kingston St. George's, London, and continues to be a paramedic educator.

Bob Fellows has been in and around the ambulance world as a paramedic (working for the London Ambulance Service), clinical tutor and leader for close on 40 years and continues in his role on the executive of the paramedic professional body, the College of Paramedics, as Head of Professional Development. He continues to be active in clinical teaching and writing as a pioneer in several fields of education. In addition, his passion for life-long learning has led to many productive years as a CPD assessor for the regulatory body, the HCPC.

Rachael T. Fothergill has worked for the London Ambulance Service for the past 17 years, and as Head of Clinical Audit and Research is considered to be one of the national leaders in this field. Rachael is also an Honorary Research Fellow at the University of Warwick's Clinical Trials Unit. She has a long track record in managing large-scale clinical research trials and health-related projects. Her involvement in research and clinical audit, both within the UK and internationally, has led to changes in clinical practice and patient care and influenced pre-hospital clinical guidelines.

Ann French qualified as a Registered Nurse in 1988 and worked as a Staff Nurse in Neurosciences. In 1994, Teesside Hospice opened and Ann became the Sister in the in-patient unit providing specialist palliative care for patients with life-limiting illnesses. Following this, she became a Macmillan Clinical Nurse Specialist working in the community. Ann is now a Principal Lecturer at Teesside University and is involved in a variety of palliative care modules. She has recently completed a PhD in Palliative Care at the International Observatory on End of Life Care, Lancaster University. Her research focused on how people with a life-threatening illness cope at the end of life.

Graham Harris has a 46-year history in pre- and out-of-hospital care which covers working in the military, in the NHS, in higher education, and the professional body for UK paramedics. He co-edited with Amanda Blaber the first and second editions of *Assessment Skills for Paramedics*, and *Clinical Leadership for Paramedics*, and co-authored chapters in all three editions. He has held Council, Executive and Board positions in the College of Paramedics, and for the past two years has been employed as the National Education Lead, developing pre-registration and post-graduate curriculums, and other national standards for the paramedic profession.

Kath Jennings, Senior Lecturer in the Faculty of Education and Health, University of Greenwich, is programme leader for the BSc (Hons) Paramedic Science (LONDON) programme. Kath believes that paramedics have always had to be leaders. By studying how leadership has evolved we can better relate theory to the development of our own leadership practice. Her research interests cover a wide range of paramedic practice and she currently has a number of funded research projects underway, including paramedic management of pelvic injuries, palliative and end-of-life care, as well as leadership in paramedic practice.

John Krohne has clinical experience in a variety of mental health settings including psychiatric intensive care and working-age/older adult in-patient services. Since 2003, he has worked in education roles supporting nurse mentors and students in clinical practice across adult, child and mental health fields. John was the Education Lead for a Community NHS Trust before joining the University of Brighton as a Senior Lecturer in 2016. This role contributes to dementia, ethics, psychosocial studies and leadership teaching for pre-registration nursing and Foundation Degree programmes. John also teaches new paramedic and nurse mentors on the Mentorship module.

Christopher Matthews is a Fellow of the Higher Education Academy, Critical Care Paramedic Practice Lead and a Senior Lecturer at the University of Brighton. Chris started his ambulance career after being medically discharged as a Commissioned Officer, after a varied and exciting career in the Royal Marine Commandos. On joining the Ambulance Service, he quickly progressed to become a paramedic after completing a three-year course at St. George's Hospital Medical School. Keen to develop his interest in the management of high acuity patients, he completed a post-graduate course at the University of Hertfordshire to become a Critical Care Paramedic. He is now a Critical Care Paramedic Practice Lead (CCPPL) and passionately believes that expert pre-hospital critical care must become an integral component within all ambulance services. Alongside his role as a CCPPL, Chris also works as a Senior Lecturer on a BSc (Hons) Paramedic course. His time in the military and in pre-hospital critical care has led him to realise the importance of human factors within paramedicine. He developed a university module integrating human factors and leadership skills into the BSc (Hons) course. He hopes all paramedic courses will embrace teaching in this field. He is currently in the process of completing his MSc.

Vicky Milburn is a specialist paramedic in urgent and emergency care. Her interest in dementia stems from years of experience attending patients with dementia in both an emergency situation when working for an ambulance service and more recently in an urgent care setting, being based in a GP surgery. Vicky found assessing pain challenging in cognitively impaired patients; this has fuelled her interest in this group of patients. She has been lecturing on the BSc (Hons) Paramedic Practice programme at the University of Brighton for over two years.

Chris Preston is an Advanced Paramedic Practitioner, North West Ambulance Service. Chris has 15 years paramedic experience, the last five years in an advanced practice role. He leads on all aspects of paediatric practice at North West Ambulance Service as well as undertaking shifts at a Children's Emergency Department. He completed an advanced practice MSc in 2014 and undertook additional MSc level study to specialise in advanced paediatrics and is currently in his fourth year of a PhD exploring paramedic clinical reasoning during non-time critical clinical interactions with children. Chris is also a fitness to practise panel member for the Health and Care Professions Council and a member of the College of Paramedics.

David Rea is Head of the Department of Public Health, Policy, and Social Sciences at Swansea University, where he leads a multi-disciplinary team whose work contributes to increasing the health and social care workforce and fostering academic expertise. David has a PhD in Social Policy and Administration (Kent 1988). He has taught healthcare management in a number of countries, is an experienced qualitative researcher, and regularly publishes on management and service improvement.

Marion Richardson is a Senior Lecturer, Paramedic Science. Marion joined the Ambulance Service in 1986 and qualified in 1992 as a paramedic. During her time in the Ambulance Service, she has held many posts, including Leading Ambulance Woman, Team Leader, Ambulance Tutor and Divisional Education Lead. As Divisional Education Lead it was Marion's responsibility to develop, coordinate and deliver educational programmes for all levels of staff within her division of the organisation. Marion now teaches at Teesside University.

Joanna Shaw is a Clinical Audit Manager. Since joining the London Ambulance Service (LAS) NHS Trust, Joanna has had responsibility for managing the Service's clinical audit programme, producing changes to LAS clinical practice and improving the care delivered to patients. She monitors clinical audit activities across the LAS, supporting and facilitating other staff undertaking clinical audit, both internally and externally, by providing individual tuition and running clinical audit training sessions. Joanna has accreditations as Advanced Clinical Audit, Trainer in Clinical Audit and Significant Event Audit.

Chris Storey graduated with a BSc (Hons) in Paramedic Practice from the University of Brighton, after a 15-year career as a church minister and five years working as a Teaching Assistant for young people with physical and sensory impairments. In 2015, he took up a position as a Senior Lecturer on the same Paramedic Practice course at the University of Brighton and now divides his time between the classroom and working as an A&E ambulance paramedic.

Paul Street is a Teaching Fellow and has a broad background in clinical practice, education and practice development. He started as an enrolled nurse in general surgery in 1982. Before becoming a Teaching Fellow and completing his Doctorate, he worked clinically in medical, surgical areas, ear and nose, HIV & AIDS areas and practice development. He has worked with practitioners from a wide range of disciplines in both practice and educational settings to develop practice initiatives. He passionately believes that communication and interpersonal skills lie at the heart of quality healthcare practice.

Gary Vale is Senior Lecturer, School of Health and Social Care, Teesside University. Gary joined the West Midland Ambulance Service in 1976, he gained his paramedic status in 1986, also becoming an IHCD clinical and driving instructor. He moved to North Yorkshire Ambulance Service in 1996 as an Executive Director, heavily involved with communication and the fast emerging unscheduled care agenda. In 2004, Gary became part of a partnership arrangement with Teesside University to develop a Foundation Degree programme for paramedics. In 2012, he left the Ambulance Service to join the academic team at Teesside University full-time to help develop the BSc (Hons) Paramedic Practice programme. He is committed to the increasing trend of the profession extending beyond its birthplace of the Ambulance Service.

Jackie Whitnell worked in the NHS for 28 years. Her career spans theatre and intensive care nursing, plus she worked for 18 years in Children's Services as a children's nurse and Health Visitor. Jackie has a MA in sociology and BSc (Hons) in psychology. She has worked as a Senior Lecturer since 2002 in Hertfordshire, Greenwich and Chichester universities. She has taught abnormal and developmental psychology and aspects of child health to students studying paramedic science, nursing, midwifery and childhood studies. Jackie continues to work as an Associate Lecturer in her chosen topic areas and prides herself on the professional and fun way in which she delivers her teaching sessions.

Julia Williams is Professor of Paramedic Science at the University of Hertfordshire. Julia has been involved in the development and delivery of higher education programmes for both already qualified paramedics and also for students on pre-registration Paramedic Science programmes since 1996. As Head of Research for the College of Paramedics, she is committed to increasing the capacity and capability of paramedics within clinical research, and she takes every opportunity to inform other agencies about the rich talent that exists within the paramedic profession in relation to clinical research, highlighting the positive contribution paramedics can make to the healthcare research agenda. Over the years, she has been involved in a variety of qualitative, quantitative and mixed methods research studies related to different aspects of paramedic practice and unscheduled emergency healthcare provision. Julia describes herself as having an 'amazing job' as her primary role is at the University of Hertfordshire teaching undergraduate students and supervising Paramedic post-graduate research studies, but, at the same time, she has a secondment to an ambulance Trust for part of the week where she undertakes research and clinical practice. A perfect combination!

Acknowledgements

I am grateful to many colleagues I have met throughout my career who influenced me both as a professional and a person. My thanks to all students who have read and commented on previous editions of *Foundations*, it has helped shape this third edition. I would like to say a special thank you to all the students I have had the pleasure of teaching; I too have learnt from you and have enjoyed sharing your journey.

My warmest thanks to all my colleagues who have shared this third edition journey (and previous editions); for their due diligence and commitment to a book that we hope will help enlighten and educate a generation of future paramedics.

Thank you, Jackie (co-editor in all but name), for your innovative and unique thinking; being my 'sounding board' for new ideas; for the hours of proof-reading and encouragement, plus being involved from the very inception of the first *Foundations*.

Thank you to all of the contributors and their significant others (past and present) for their unwavering support.

Introduction
Amanda Y. Blaber

This book should be the start of your reading, investigation and research. Some of the chapters have been written by paramedics, some written by a non-paramedic subject experts and many jointly written by subject experts and paramedics. This provides a strong contemporaneous academic focus together with application to the reality of paramedic practice.

If you look through the chapter content of each of the three *Foundations for Paramedic Practice* texts (2008, 2012 and 2018) some chapters have been removed, some updated and many replaced. Together with the first and second editions, this text reflects a historical journey of the paramedic role in the UK and the changing face of society and expectations.

 Throughout the chapters there is a symbol which serves as a prompt to the reader to 'link to' other chapters or specific pages, where you can read more on a specific subject. There are also 'Reflection: points to consider' boxes where you are invited to consider what you have just read and apply it to your own life experience and/or practice. There are many case studies for you to consider and think about applying the theory to the cases presented and the questions the contributors pose for the reader. It is hoped that these features bring the book to life for the reader and help make links to practice more explicit and encourage additional critical thinking.

1 Interpersonal communication: a foundation of practice

Paul Street

In this chapter:

INTRODUCTION

Communication is one of the most fundamental elements of human existence and is integral to our lives from birth. It involves the transfer of information between people and it is difficult to think of any situation when a person is not communicating in some way, because even when you are not speaking, your body is constantly presenting a stream of non-verbal messages to those around you (Gamble and Gamble 2017). Outwardly, communication appears normal and straightforward, but actually it is complex and open to many influences, which can lead to being misunderstood, if the meaning within the communication is not clear and consistent in all the forms that the information is being sent, received and understood (Pavord and Donnelly 2015).

WHY IS THIS RELEVANT?

Vermier et al. (2015: 1257) state, 'Effective communication is crucial to healthcare.' Further, Hayley (2014) argues that communication is one of the most important skills needed by a paramedic. Without interpersonal communication, paramedics would not be able to talk to patients, know the location of their next call, hand over a patient to the staff in an emergency department or really undertake most of their clinical skills safely. Hence, the ability to communicate with patients, relatives, colleagues and the public is seen as an essential skill required by ambulance clinicians and all health-care practitioners (Pavord and Donnelly 2015; HCPC 2016). Despite the importance of communication, it has often been seen as a soft skill and not as important as the technical skills, such as cannulation and intubation, for example. However, Lucas et al. (2015) are critical of this view, suggesting communication should be considered along-side, and equal to, those technical skills, because they often cannot occur without it. Despite communication being such a fundamental part of professional practice, over 13 per cent of written complaints received by the National Health Service are concerned with communication issues alone (Health and Social Care Information Centre 2016). It seems evident, then, that all health practitioners should be constantly aware of 'what and how they communicate', because the results of this could have either a positive or negative effect on every aspect of their relationships with patients, relatives and colleagues. So, communication warrants a place at the heart of practice.

THE BASICS OF COMMUNICATION

Communication is a two-way process that includes the exchange of information, thoughts and feelings by speaking, body language, or writing of some sort, according to the *Oxford English Dictionary* (2017). It has been established for some time that only 7 per cent of communication is attributed to the words used, while 38 per cent is derived from the tone of voice and a further 55 per cent from non-verbal cues used (Mehrabian 1981).

The most common model of interpersonal communication proposes that one person is 'the sender' who will formulate a message and send it verbally, non-verbally, or in a combination of both, to another person, 'the receiver'. Once a message has been sent, the receiver uses their senses (hearing, sight, etc.) to receive it. The receiver then interprets that message and responds verbally or non-verbally or both, with what they think is appropriate feedback to the sender, based on the receiver's interpretation. The original sender, then, in turn, interprets that feedback and responds, based on what they think the feedback was (Shannon and Weaver 1949). If any messages con-tain conflicting verbal and non-verbal cues within the same messages, these so-called mix messages can easily be misunderstood and misinterpretations result. Hence, all practitioners need to send clear messages where there is no inconsistency between the verbal and non-verbal features they use to minimise any potential misunderstandings (College of Paramedics and American Academy of Orthopedic Surgeons 2016).

However, communication is open to a range of factors that influence the way we formu-late and send messages (encoding) and interpret messages (decoding). Both the sender and receiver encode and decode the meaning of the message through the verbal and non-verbal features of communication alongside their senses (Argyle 1988). This pro-cess is influenced by many other factors within us – our social identity, personality, values, beliefs, gender, culture, status, to name just a few (see Figure 1.1) (Hartley 1999). So all healthcare practitioners should consider how these factors may influence what they communicate and how the patient's sociocultural factors may influence its

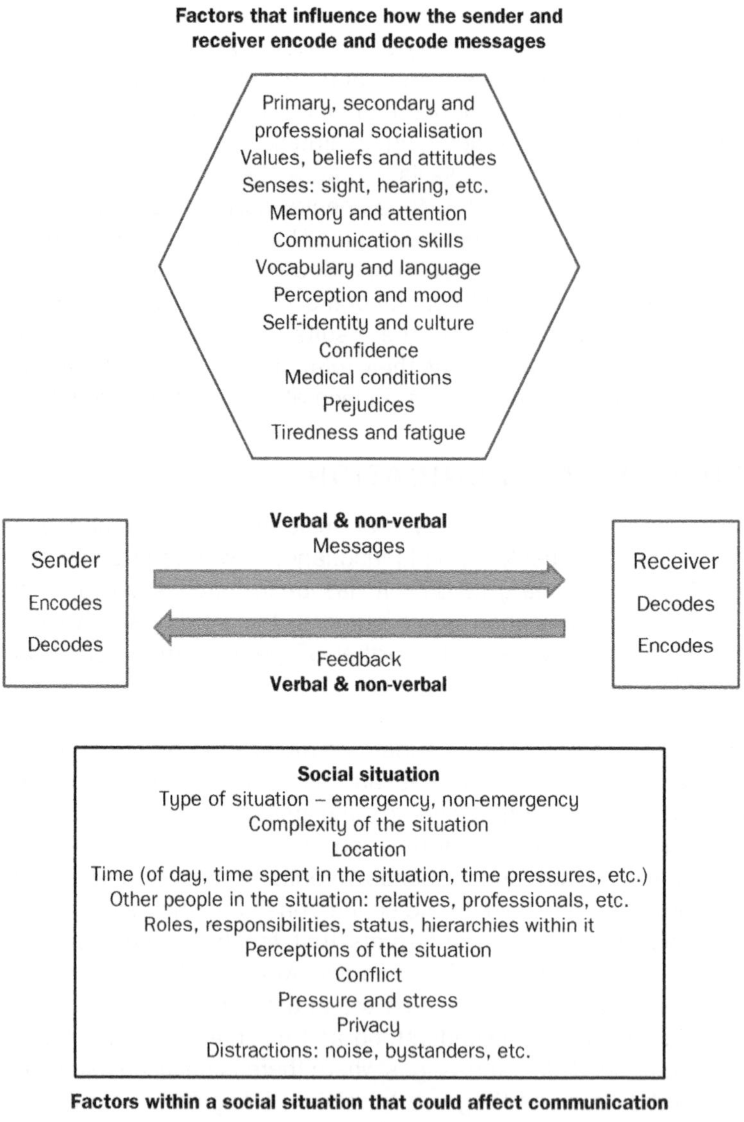

**Factors that influence how the sender and
receiver encode and decode messages**

Primary, secondary and
professional socialisation
Values, beliefs and attitudes
Senses: sight, hearing, etc.
Memory and attention
Communication skills
Vocabulary and language
Perception and mood
Self-identity and culture
Confidence
Medical conditions
Prejudices
Tiredness and fatigue

Sender	**Verbal & non-verbal** Messages ⟶	Receiver
Encodes		Decodes
Decodes	⟵ Feedback **Verbal & non-verbal**	Encodes

Social situation
Type of situation – emergency, non-emergency
Complexity of the situation
Location
Time (of day, time spent in the situation, time pressures, etc.)
Other people in the situation: relatives, professionals, etc.
Roles, responsibilities, status, hierarchies within it
Perceptions of the situation
Conflict
Pressure and stress
Privacy
Distractions: noise, bystanders, etc.

Factors within a social situation that could affect communication

Figure 1.1 A model of communication

Source: Adapted from Shannon and Weaver (1949), Hartley (1999), Pavord and
Donnelly (2015).

interpretation, particularly in the context of multicultural societies, where cultural differences in values, beliefs and behaviours need to be respected to enable paramedics to provide good quality care to a diverse patient group and prevent inadvertent offence being caused (Pavord and Donnelly 2015; HCPC 2016). In addition to this, the social situation in which the communication occurs can positively or negatively influence the effectiveness of communication within it (see Figure 1.1). If the situation was time-critical or complex, for example, this may influence how someone communicates, requiring very clear direct communication.

VERBAL FEATURES OF COMMUNICATION

Verbal communication is, in essence, a deliberate conscious process, because people select the words from their vocabulary that they want to use in order to communicate (Gamble and Gamble 2017). The meaning of the messages we communicate may change depending on the paralinguistic features used to convey them (Hogg and Vaughan 2013). The paralinguistic features contributing to paralanguage outlined in Figure 1.2 are used to emphasise the meaning of the message the sender wishes to place on it.

Paramedics would be expected to use professional level vocabulary with colleagues and other professionals who may have various levels of understanding of that terminology, yet also be able to translate that communication to meet the needs of patients and relatives who may have different levels of cognitive development and varied communication abilities. The optimum level of communication is one which is clear, understandable and appropriate to the situation and people in it.

Evidently when the sender speaks in order to send a verbal message, it needs to be sent at a volume that the receiver can hear (Pavord and Donnelly 2015). The volume used to send a message may vary depending on the situation, for example, two paramedics talking at a busy roadside would need a louder volume than those talking to a patient in their home. Further, ensuring an appropriate volume level is important in terms of the effectiveness of the communication – too loud and a patient may think you are shouting at them, too soft and they may not hear you at all. Both these forms could limit the patient's ability to interpret the correct meaning of the message, let alone having the potential to leave the patient with a lasting negative impression of how health practitioners communicate.

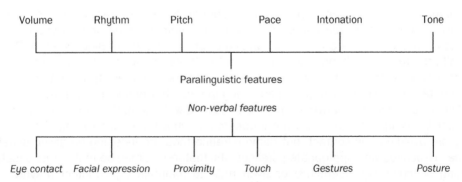

Figure 1.2 Paralinguistic and non-verbal features of communication

Closely linked to volume is pitch – usually the louder the volume, the higher the pitch of voice. If these two elements are then linked to a fast pace and rhythm of speaking, these could then paralinguistically communicate a sense of urgency (Hogg and Vaughan 2013), but if taken further, they could be interpreted as a sign of stress or panic. Thus, the possible consequences for health practitioners using a raised volume, pitch, pace and rhythm are that the people receiving the message may potentially think the situation is serious, or perhaps that the practitioner may be unsure of what they are doing. These changes may be, in part, due to alterations in the practitioner's anxiety levels during any patient interaction, particularly if it is a stressful one. Additionally, the more the practitioner feels under pressure, the more these features may appear in the voice.

Intonation is the emphasis placed on the voice to communicate a particular tone or mood and the paralinguistic features are used to do this (Gault et al. 2016). Hence, controlling the intonation of the voice by having a calm pace, rhythm and tone at an appropriate volume may then communicate confidence, caring and trustworthiness. Tonal qualities inferring sarcasm, for example, should be avoided (Bledsoe et al. 2014).

NON-VERBAL COMMUNICATION

Communication not only occurs verbally, people instinctively use their bodies to communicate non-verbally. Further, non-verbal communication, in a similar way to the paralinguistic features, can replace, supplement or contradict the meaning of the verbal message being sent (Gamble and Gamble 2017). Many non-verbal cues are unconscious manifestations of thoughts and feelings. Consequently, it is difficult for an individual to have total conscious control over their non-verbal cues and to some degree they will always communicate non-verbal messages they are unaware of, even if they are acutely aware of their own body language, and this may lead to unintentional miscommunication (Hartley 1999).

Eye contact

Eye contact is a significant form of non-verbal communication (Argyle 1988). It is an important way that people initiate and maintain communication and its use by paramedics can show they are interested and care for their patients (Bledsoe et al. 2014). Usually the receiver will maintain eye contact with the sender for the main part of the message, while the sender will have periods when they look away and return to have eye contact with the receiver (Hogg and Vaughan 2013). Consequently, if you were not looking at a patient or relative when communicating with them, this could be a sign you are not listening to them or are not interested in what they have to say. Although, if they are avoiding eye contact, but demonstrating they are listening by giving suitable verbal responses with appropriate paralinguistic features, it may be that in this situation it may be culturally insensitive or even rude to maintain eye contact (Pavord and Donnelly 2015).

Facial expression

In conjunction with eye contact, the face is one of the most expressive parts of a human body (Gamble and Gamble 2017) and feelings such as anger, joy and surprise are quite often easy to identify non-verbally through facial expressions. It is evident that paramedics will encounter situations that they find shocking, fearful or surprising and there is a strong likelihood that they may display those emotions through their facial expressions. It is noticeable that patients can recognise the emotions and mood states displayed by the paramedics when caring for them (College of Paramedics and American Academy of Orthopedic Surgeons 2016). Again, the implications are that health practitioners need to have the self-awareness to understand the non-verbal cues they may exhibit and the effect they may have on the person they are communicating with (Pavord and Donnelly 2015).

 Reflection: points to consider

Consider the importance of reflecting on the reactions that patients and family members have demonstrated or expressed as a result of your facial expressions during certain types of calls. Have you observed a colleague make unprofessional and inappropriate facial expressions? If so, how did this make you feel? How might you 'tackle' this, if it happened again?

 Chapter 6 for more on communication and human factors and **Chapter 17** for discussion on how we make decisions. For specific discussion on conflict resolution, read **Chapter 9** in Blaber and Harris (2014).

Gestures and posture

Alongside facial expressions, both gestures and posture can emphasise and clarify the meaning of the spoken message (Gamble and Gamble 2017). People often use their hands to gesture when they are speaking. Some gestures like pointing can be problematic, depending on the context in which they have been used; pointing to a piece of equipment can be appropriate but pointing at a patient may not be. Equally, using large gestures may convey enthusiasm, but used extensively in a patient interaction can move the focus of the situation away from the patient to the ambulance clinician which may or may not be helpful in some situations.

Posture includes the way you stand, sit and position your body (Gamble and Gamble 2017). It is generally accepted that, if possible, when talking to patients, paramedics should use an open posture, i.e. not having your arms or legs crossed, because often standing with your arms crossed in front of a patient or relative can be seen as confrontational and uncaring (College of Paramedics and American Academy of Orthopaedic Surgeons 2016). Thus, an open posture suggests you are willing to communicate with the other person, as would positioning yourself at the same level as the patient to maintain eye contact on an equal level (Bledsoe et al. 2014). Nevertheless, using this posture may not always be particularly appropriate at the scene of a road traffic accident, but the principles can be applied to many other situations in which paramedics communicate with patients and relatives.

Both posture and gestures can have a positive effect on establishing and maintaining good communication, especially if used in combination with eye contact. If these are used appropriately, they can suggest you are concerned for the patient, are willing to listen to them, and are paying attention to what they say. But if posture and gestures are used unwisely, they can also alienate a patient or relative too because they can suggest you could be uncaring and unwilling to listen and are uncompassionate (Pavord and Donnelly 2015).

Proximity

People also communicate by how closely they stand or sit next to another person. This is referred to as personal space or proximity (Hogg and Vaughan 2013). Generally during social interaction, people who do not know each other tend to stand approximately at an arm's length away from each other (Bledsoe et al. 2014). This distance is often reduced when the people know each other, or when one person gives permission directly or indirectly for someone to enter their personal space and touch them. Being too close can cause discomfort and unease and be perceived as threatening, even if touch is not involved.

Additionally, touch is another significant element of non-verbal communication for ambulance clinicians (College of Paramedics and American Academy of Orthopaedic Surgeons 2016), because much of the care given requires touch, such as placing a blood pressure cuff, stabilising a C-spine, and so on. Although touch is an instinctive form of communication, it can be misinterpreted and become problematic, therefore, be sure to touch patients in socially acceptable parts of the body, the hands, for example, if that is clinically appropriate, until you have direct or implied consent to touch them elsewhere to undertake a procedure (Bledsoe et al. 2014).

 Reflection: points to consider

Thinking about these non-verbal cues, how else might you be able to identify the following?:

- Someone was not listening to you.
- A colleague was interested in what you were saying.
- The person you were talking to was worried.
- A colleague tells you to do something quickly.

Case study I.I

An ambulance was called to an urgent care centre, by a doctor who had assessed a 56-year-old patient. The patient had suspected pneumonia and was breathless, with low oxygen saturations, low blood pressure, a raised pulse and pyrexia. Two paramedics arrived at the reception desk. The first paramedic called the patient's name across the crowded waiting room. The patient identified themselves by raising their hand and saying 'yes'. The paramedic did not move from the desk and responded loudly with 'Do you want to do this here or in the back of the ambulance?'

Instantly, the second paramedic established eye contact with the patient, smiled, crossed the waiting room and sat on a chair next to them. They introduced themselves, and explained they needed to undertake an assessment and that they could either try to find somewhere in the centre to do it, or they could undertake it in the ambulance. The patient agreed to the latter. This paramedic then asked if the patient could walk and if they needed any assistance to get to the ambulance. This paramedic walked alongside the patient while reassuring them with touch and calm conversation. Once in the ambulance, the first paramedic sat diagonally across from the patient and asked a range of questions and recorded the answers on their documentation. During this they did not have any eye contact or look at the patient at all and used a very 'matter of fact' tone of voice. In a similar tone, they also asked the second paramedic to undertake a range of clinical observations and administer some oxygen, which they did. During this, the second paramedic explained to the patient what was happening, engaged in some conversation, maintained eye contact and used positive non-verbal communication. The second paramedic then left the patient, explaining they were going to drive them to the local hospital. The first paramedic remained with the patient, in the same seating position, but did not speak or look at the patient during the journey. On arrival the first paramedic left the ambulance and went into the Emergency Department, while the second paramedic helped the patient out of the ambulance and into a wheelchair and took them into the department.

- How appropriate were the features of communication used in this case study?
- What impact might they have on the potential public view of the paramedic profession?
- If you were a patient, which of these paramedics would you like to care for you and why?

COMMUNICATING WITH PATIENTS: EXPLORING THE CASE STUDY

In Case study 1.1, different levels of therapeutic communication were evident, some positive and others less so. Effective communication with patients, relatives and the public is an essential and integral part of the role of the paramedic from the very outset of a patient interaction (Hayley 2014; HCPC 2016). The main concern in this case study is that it is a real situation and has happened to a patient. It demonstrates very different first impressions of the paramedic profession to the patient and the other people in the waiting room.

When entering a situation, first impressions are important and can significantly influence how a patient interaction unfolds. First impressions are made up of both verbal and non-verbal features. So, having a clean smart uniform, establishing eye and verbal contact and introducing yourself, are all key elements (College of Paramedics and American Academy of Orthopaedic Surgeons 2016). According to Turner and Sefika (2016), from the start, effective communication should incorporate:

- beginning with a smile not a bias;
- having self-awareness and respect;
- listening, with care, compassion and appreciation;
- answering with understanding and empathy;
- explaining professionally with compassion.

If these are present, then the potential for the development of a compassionate relationship is increased, allowing the practitioner and patient to feel a personal connection with each other. Therefore, it is thought this would foster a deeper level of care and support and would increase the potential for the patient to feel they have been cared for with dignity and respect (Windover et al. 2014).

In the case study, the second paramedic did demonstrate positive elements of communication, they used both verbal and non-verbal communication to demonstrate the elements proposed by Turner and Sefika (2016). The positive elements of their initial communication style were that they established eye contact, smiled, moved towards the patient, sat at their level and introduced themselves. In contrast, the first paramedic did none of this; indeed their communication style perhaps was one of power, or perhaps they were just tired or fatigued. But if the latter were the case, it is questionable whether they should demonstrate this to this degree, and they should at least try to appear caring and professional (HCPC 2016), but this could also demonstrate the level of stress and pressure paramedics face in their role and the emotional demands of their work. It was clear if the patient wanted care, they would have to go to the first paramedic and not the other way around. If the second paramedic had not gone over to the patient, the outcome of the situation could have been different; the patient might have felt vulnerable and perhaps under pressure to comply with the first paramedic's wishes. This could have resulted in the patient feeling under-valued and pressured, potentially setting the scene for frustration and confrontation or even the patient at a later point making a complaint.

 Chapter 4 for ethical considerations, **Chapter 9** for power of the professions and **Chapter 10** for factors affecting patients' decision to access healthcare.

Reflection: points to consider

Go to the following website: www.hellomynameis.org.uk and find out who started this campaign and why they did so. Play some of the video clips on this site to help you.

Throughout case study 1.1 the second paramedic maintained good eye contact, used a supportive tone of voice and listened to the patient. Initially, both paramedics gave the patient some degree of choice in terms of where they should examine the patient. The first paramedic addressed the situation in such a way that the patient might have felt they had no option but to go with the paramedic to the ambulance. Or if the patient wanted to express any concerns, they would have no choice but to have done so across the waiting room, or asked the paramedic to come over to them. The patient might not have felt comfortable with either of these options. Therefore, the first impression made by this paramedic was not one of wanting to listen, but one of just wanting to get the 'job done'. Meanwhile the second paramedic did show they were listening and respecting the patient as an individual. They gave the patient some choice, discussed it in a sensitive way, and tried to protect the patient's privacy and dignity by discussing it next to them, even though it was in a crowded waiting room. Throughout the incident, the two paramedics maintained very different communication skills, one professional, compassionate and respectful, the other not, so demonstrating a contradiction in the standards of conduct and performance recommended for practice (HCPC 2016).

Effective communication is an essential part of patient-centred care and is essential to professional practice (HCPC 2016). If used correctly, it can significantly help a patient feel they have been treated and respected as an individual (Turner and Sefika 2016; Ayud et al. 2017). If effective communication was used by other professionals with paramedics, it would make the paramedic feel valued and respected too. The significance is that communication is not just about ensuring people receive the correct information and that the correct information is collected, it is about making sure that patients and staff feel valued, trusted and respected through the way they are communicated with. The clinical outcome of a situation should be significantly improved because there is an effective exchange of information. Communication can also affect the way a patient perceives a situation and potentially can make the difference between a positive or negative clinical outcome (Vermier et al. 2015). In the case study it was fortunate that the clinical outcome was not affected, but the impact the two paramedics had on the patient was significantly different, one appearing kind, compassionate and caring, the other not. One making the patient feel like a respected individual, with time for the patient, the other not. Hence, all health practitioners need to consider which words they use and how they emphasise them to give clear, caring, empathetic and assertive messages to patients and not ones that indicate the clinician's frustrations, attitudes or assumptions. But it is clear that in any one situation all the elements in the model outlined in Figure 1.1 clearly do contribute to effective communication.

INTER-PROFESSIONAL COMMUNICATION TOOLS

Much of the communication that paramedics are involved in requires information to be transmitted quickly, accurately and effectively about the specifics of any given situation, either at the scene or in a handover situation (College of Paramedics and American Academy of Orthopaedic Surgeons 2016). Hence, the need for effective inter-professional communication is a key element of paramedic practice (HCPC 2016). Standardised handover frameworks provide a systematic way of promoting the effective and comprehensive transfer of key clinical information from one practitioner to another, thus reducing the risk of information being forgotten or overlooked within the handover (Rosenberg et al. 2009; Murray et al. 2012; Flynn et al. 2017). These frameworks provide paramedics with a structured format by which to hand over key information about the patient and the situation. But this also means that the practitioner receiving the information knows the broad areas of information to expect within the handover, and therefore what to ask for if there appears to be any gaps in the information provided.

The research evaluating these tools suggests they are useful and can enhance communication and handover, however, it has also been established that their effectiveness can be influenced by a range of communication factors like, time, status, busyness, and the relationships of the people involved in the handover (Bost et al. 2012; Flynn et al. 2017). These factors are highlighted in the model of communication outlined in Figure 1.1. Therefore, to use these tools effectively, the aforementioned issues also have to be addressed. For example, the information and communication provided by any practitioner has to be valued by the other practitioners involved in that communication situation, and issues like status, hierarchy and time have to be overcome to ensure that the relevant information in that situation is handed over and clearly understood. Hence, the models of communication and theories that support them have a direct link to underpinning communication in practice.

Therefore, all the issues discussed so far concerning clear verbal and non-verbal communication are relevant here, as the information gained through these processes at some point will be recorded in written documentation (Vermier et al. 2015).

 Reflection: points to consider

Look at Figure 1.3. Think back to a recent situation when you handed over patient information to another practitioner. Write down what you remember you said about the patient and their condition. Now put the information under the headings (SBAR, ATMIST, ASHICE) in each of the frameworks.

- Did you have something in every area for each?
- Would using one of these frameworks help you structure your handovers in future?

(1) SBAR	(2) ATMIST	(3) ASHICE
(S) Situation • Identify yourself • Identify the patient by name • Give details about the situation, e.g. patient involved in a road traffic collision • Give any details of initial vital signs, oxygen given, level of consciousness, etc. • Describe your concerns **(B) Background** • Give the patient's reason for admission • Explain significant medical history • Current medication and allergies • Procedures you have undertaken • Medications given by you and those normally taken by the patient • Treatments/procedures you have undertaken **(A) Assessment** • Vital signs • Contraction pattern • Clinical impression and concerns **(R) Recommendations** • Explain what you think the patient needs now • Make suggestions • Clarify expectations	**(A) Age** Age and sex of casualty **(T) Time** Estimated time of arrival and time incident occurred **(M) Mechanism of injury** • The gross mechanism of injury, e.g. motor vehicle collision, stab wound to chest • Details of other factors known to be associated with major injuries, e.g. entrapment, vehicle rollover, occupant ejected from vehicle **(I) Injury** What can be seen or suspected **(S) Signs** Vital signs including heart rate, blood pressure, respiratory rate, oxygen saturation, Glasgow Coma Score **(T) Treatment** Treatment given to the patient	**(A) Age** What is the patient's age? **(S) Sex** Is the patient male or female? **(H) History** What happened to the patient, e.g. road traffic collision, etc. **(I) Injuries sustained** Stab wound to the chest, fractured femur, etc. **(C) Condition** Patient's vital signs, including heart rate, blood pressure, respiratory rate, oxygen saturation, Glasgow Coma Score **(E) Estimated time of arrival** Time of arrival at the receiving hospital

Figure 1.3 Examples of frameworks to support handover

Source: Collated from: NHS Institute for Innovation and Improvement (2008); Brown et al. (2016) – Republished with kind permission of Class Professional Publishing.

CONCLUSION

Inter-personal communication is a complex exchange of information between people who constantly send and receive messages to each other and is a fundamental element of a paramedic's practice. The way a paramedic encodes and sends their message will affect the way the patient or colleague decodes and interprets that message. This may lead to clear accurate communication or miscommunication, depending on the factors that are influencing the way the paramedic and the patient or colleague are sending and receiving messages in that situation. It is important to remember, therefore, that both verbal and non-verbal communication are inextricably linked and it is the way a person uses them in combination that impacts on their interactions with their patients and colleagues and can positively or negatively affect the outcome of any situation. It is this combination that allows paramedics to effectively communicate a range of messages from the very subtle to the blatantly obvious. The social situation in which communication occurs will also affect the sending, receiving and interpretation of any particular message whether that is by the paramedic, the patient or colleague, whether it occurs at an accident scene, in an ambulance, in a patient's home or an emergency department. It is of vital importance that our communication is effective and sensitive to the situation and the people involved within it. All healthcare practitioners need to be constantly aware not only of what they say, but also how they say it. Our interactions with patients and families require thought (prior to and during our communications) and are deserving of reflection afterwards. Communication is at the forefront of our practice and is an essential fundamental skill that we can strive to improve throughout our careers. Further, when communicating about patients to other healthcare professionals, there is a need to ensure that all information is accurate and often it is required to be given quickly. Hence, handover frameworks could provide a systematic framework to facilitate the effectiveness of communication between ambulance clinicians and other members of the inter-professional team, thus promoting quality care through skilled communication.

Chapter key points:

- We are always in a state of communicating something to someone.
- Communication is a mix of verbal and non-verbal elements. Both these elements act as carriers of the messages we send and receive.
- The way we formulate, send, receive and interpret messages is influenced by our values, beliefs, social identity, perceptions and the context in which the communication occurs.
- Communication is a fundamental and vital part of all healthcare practitioners' practice, because care and treatment cannot effectively occur without communication of some kind.
- Communication is a central component in providing compassionate patient-centred care in a multicultural society.
- Communicating patient information to other professionals needs to be accurate and undertaken quickly and effectively, to promote quality care.

REFERENCES AND SUGGESTED READING

Argyle, M. (1988) *Bodily Communication*, 2nd edn. London: Routledge.

Ayud, E.M., Sampayo, E.M., Shah, M.I. and Doughty, C.B. (2017) Prehospital providers' perceptions on providing patient and family centred care. *Prehospital Emergency Care*, 21(2): 233–41.

Blaber, A. and Harris, G. (eds) (2014) *Clinical Leadership for Paramedics*. Maidenhead: Open University Press.

Bledsoe, B.E., Porter, R.S. and Cherry, R.A. (2014) *Essentials of Ambulance Clinician Care Update*. Edinburgh: Pearson Education (Kindle edition).

Bost, N., Crilly, J., Patterson, E. and Chaboyer, W. (2012) Clinical handover of patients arriving by ambulance to a hospital emergency department: a qualitative study. *International Emergency Nursing*, 20(3): 133–41.

Brown, S.N., Kumar, D. and Millins, M. (eds for JRCALC and AACE) (2016) *UK Ambulance Service Clinical Practice Guidelines*. Bridgwater: Class Professional Publishing.

College of Paramedics and American Academy of Orthopedic Surgeons (2016) *Nancy Caroline's Emergency Medicine on the Street, United Kingdom,* 7th edn. Burlington, VA: Jones and Bartlett Learning.

Eggins, S. and Slade, D. (2015) Communication in clinical handover: improving the safety and quality of the patient experience. *Journal of Public Health Research*, 4(666): 197–9.

Flynn, D., Francis, S., Robalino, S., Lally, J., et al. (2017) A review of enhanced paramedic roles during and after hospital handover of stroke, myocardial infarction and trauma patients. *BMC Emergency Medicine*, 17(5): 1–13.

Gamble, T.K. and Gamble, M. (2017) *Nonverbal Messages Tell More: A Practical Guide to Nonverbal Communication*. New York: Routledge.

Gault, I., Shapcott, J., Luthi, A. and Reid, G. (2016) *Communication in Nursing and Healthcare*. Los Angeles: Sage.

Hartley, P. (1999) *Interpersonal Communication*, 2nd edn. London: Routledge.

Hayley, A. (2014) *Paramedic Communication, Influence and Decision Making: A Guide for EMS Professionals*. Amazon Media. Kindle edition.

HCPC (Health and Care Professions Council) (2016) *Standards of Conduct, Performance and Ethics*. London: HCPC.

Health and Social Care Information Centre (2016) *Data on Written Complaints in the NHS 2015–16: Provisional Experimental Statistics*. Available at: http://content.digital.nhs.uk/catalogue/PUB20940/data-writ-comp-nhs-2015-2016-Q4-rep.pdf (accessed 3 September 2017).

Hendrickson, S.W. (2008) *SBAR Basics: A Resource Guide for Healthcare Managers*. Marblehead, MA: HCP Pro Inc.

Hogg, M.A. and Vaughan, G.M. (2013) *Social Psychology*, 7th edn. Harlow: Pearson.

Loseby, J. and Lyon, R. (2013) Clinical handover of the trauma and medical patient: a structured approach. *Journal of Paramedic Practice*, 5(10): 563–7.

Lucas, P.V., McCall, M., Eccleston, C., Lee, E., et al. (2015) Prioritising the development of paramedic students' interpersonal skills. *Journal of Paramedic Practice*, 7(5): 242–8.

Mehrabian, A. (1981) *Silent Messages: Implicit Communication of Emotions and Attitudes*, 2nd edn. Belmont, CA: Wadsworth.

Murray, S.L., Crouch, R. and Ainsworth-Smith, M. (2012) Quality of the handover of patient care: a comparison of pre-hospital and emergency department notes. *International Emergency Nursing*, 20(1): 24–7.

National Health Service Institute for Innovation and Improvement (2008) *Quality and Service Improvement Tools: SBAR Situation – Background – Assessment – Recommendation*. Available at: http://www.institute.nhs.uk/quality_and_service_improvement_tools/quality (accessed 7 September 2017).

Pavord, E. and Donnelly, E. (2015) *Communication and Interpersonal Skills*, 2nd edn. Banbury: Lantern.

Rosenberg, L.A., Leitzsch, J. and Little, B.W. (2009) Systematic review of handoff mnemonics literature. *American Journal of Medical Quality*, 24(3): 196–204.

Shannon, C.E. and Weaver, W. (1949) *The Mathematical Theory of Communication*. Urbana, IL: University of Illinois Press.

South Western Ambulance Service (2016) *ATMIST patient pre-alert and hand over system*. Available at:https://www.swast.nhs.uk/Downloads/Clinical%20Guidelines%20SWASFT%20staff/CG05_ATMIST_Patient_Pre-Alert.pdf (accessed 1 September 2017)

The Oxford English Dictionary (2017) Communication. Oxford: Oxford University Press. Available at: https://www.oxforddictionaries.com/oed (accessed 7 September 2017).

Turner, S.Y. and Sefika, K. (2016) *The Three Fundamental Principles of Effective Communication in Healthcare Settings.* Amazon Media. Kindle edition.

Vermier, P., Vandijck, D., Degroote, S., Peleman, R., et al. (2015) Communication in healthcare: a narrative review of the literature and practical recommendations. *International Journal of Clinical Practice*, 69(11): 1257–67.

Windover, A.K., Isaacson, J.H., Pien, L.C., Merrell, J. and Slugg Moore, A. (2014) *Relationship-Centred Healthcare Communication. An Advanced Topic Guide.* North Charleston, SC: Create Space.

Reflective practice in relation to out-of-hospital care

Marion Richardson

In this chapter:

- Introduction
- Why is this relevant?
- What are reflection, critical reflection and reflective practice?
- What should I reflect upon?
- Structuring reflection
- Depth of reflection
- When to reflect
- Skills needed for reflective practice
- Reflective practice and evidence-based practice
- Reflective practice and continuing professional development
- Conclusion
- Chapter key points
- References and suggested reading

INTRODUCTION

Making safe and ethical decisions for patient care in the complex, dynamic and unpredictable nature of paramedic practice can be challenging. Everyday experiences in paramedic practice provide opportunities to enhance practice through reflection. Reflective practice allows you to transform basic knowledge and skills into expert knowledge and skills and it enables you to learn outside of formal learning environments throughout your working life (Jasper 2013). This chapter will discuss strategies to make reflection purposeful and demonstrate how reflective practice can improve your professional practice, and help meet the Health and Care Professions Council's (HCPC) Standards of Proficiency and standards of continuing professional development (CPD).

WHY IS THIS RELEVANT?

Reflection plays a central part in the education of paramedics from pre-registration to continuing professional development and facilitates the progression from a novice practitioner to expert practitioner (Tarrant 2013). As a responsible and accountable paramedic, you need to have a good understanding of the research, knowledge base and working context that underpin your practice.

 Chapter 5 Reflection is a way for you to integrate theoretical and experiential learning into your practice (Jasper 2013; Knott and Scragg 2016). It also plays a key role in delivering evidence-based practice. Many additional benefits are detailed in Box 2.1.

Box 2.I Benefits of reflection

- Reflection enables you to understand your personal beliefs, attitudes, assumptions and values and analyse how these may influence your professional practice as these form your frame of reference (Knott and Scragg 2016; Pretorius and Ford 2016).
- Reflective practice will enable you to become more self-aware and as such be able to monitor and improve your professional practice (Pretorius and Ford 2016; Cottrell 2017) and can be used as a means of professional supervision (Johns 2010), which is essential in a profession where you work largely unsupervised with little opportunity to discuss at length incidents with peers (Turner 2015).
- As a result of critical reflection on your experiences, you may identify educational needs which you will need to address which can be the focus of your CPD activities (Pretorius and Ford 2016).
- The HCPC (2017) view reflection as practice-based learning that contributes towards CPD. The need to demonstrate CPD for HCPC registration provides a useful external incentive to routinely adopt critical reflection (Cottrell 2017). As we explore reflection further, we can see how reflection helps us maintain the HCPC's Standards of Proficiency and is a way of maintaining currency in a dynamic and ever-changing profession. Reflective practice therefore can be a key way of providing evidence of your continued professional development.
- As a healthcare professional, maintaining your mental well-being is important and reflecting on your critical incidents may prevent issues from 'playing on your mind' or from having sleepless nights and, as a result, reflection is a means to maintain positive mental health (Blaber 2008).
- Critical reflection is informed by external sources, theories and research which enables you to integrate theoretical knowledge into your practice and enhances traditional forms of knowledge (Oko and Reid 2012; Knott and Scragg 2016).
- Reflective practice promotes patient safety by analysing the causes of errors, near misses and complaints as recommended in the Francis Report (2013) (Howatson-Jones 2016).

- Learning can be classified in many ways, one of which is 'superficial vs deep learning'. Superficial learning could be described as surface learning, merely memorising facts with no real understanding (rote learning). Conversely, deep learning builds on existing knowledge and seeks to understand underpinning theories and concepts. Reflection is an essential skill for the development of a deep approach to learning.
- Reflection helps to develop understanding of challenging or difficult situations, enabling improved professional practice (Cottrell 2017) and generates practice-based knowledge based on real practice experience.

WHAT ARE REFLECTION, CRITICAL REFLECTION AND REFLECTIVE PRACTICE?

Reflection, critical reflection and reflective practice, along with their numerous definitions, are frequently encountered in healthcare literature. In professional practice we are no doubt familiar with the term 'reflection' and it is clear from the numerous definitions that it is a more complicated and thought-provoking process than the common understanding of reflection as simply recalling an event. Reflection can be viewed as a transformative process of looking back on your experience using a structured approach which ultimately transforms your experience into new knowledge, including an understanding of the consequences of your actions that can inform your future practice (Oko and Reid 2012; Howatson-Jones 2016). Reflection is a key strategy to transform your experiences into knowledge, which, when applied, will develop your professional practice (Oko and Reid 2012).

The term 'critical reflection' is increasingly used for professional and academic purposes. In this context, 'critical' refers to the ability to analyse and evaluate both positive and negative aspects of an experience that moves beyond simply identifying what was good or bad but more importantly to evaluate why something was good or bad (Oko and Reid 2012). In order for you to evaluate and justify your actions, these should be examined in light of what you have read and been taught, e.g. external sources such as theories and research. In this way you will challenge your previous understanding and increase your awareness of the assumptions that underpin your practice. The aim of critical reflection is to facilitate change that benefits you or others, no matter how small (Cottrell 2017).

It should be noted that reflection alone is not reflective practice unless it results in action. Reflective practice uses our experiences in practice as a catalyst for purposeful reflection from which we seek to fully understand the learning gained from our experiences and take action as a result (Jasper 2013). As such, the three main components of reflective practice can be viewed as: (1) having an experience; (2) engaging in reflective processes; and (3) taking action (Jasper 2013). In line with many professions, action resulting from reflection is central to good paramedic practice. The importance of reflection and reflective practice cannot be underestimated and as a result it underpins many pre-registration and post-registration professional courses and supports continuous professional development (Knott and Scragg 2016).

WHAT SHOULD I REFLECT UPON?

It takes time to purposefully reflect and would be impractical to reflect on everything that you do as a paramedic, so you need to have a reason for deciding which experiences to reflect upon – usually these will be significant events that have had an impact on you (Ghaye 2000; Oko and Reid 2012). Such experiences are often referred to as 'critical incidents', i.e. events that stand out in your mind and contribute directly to your development as a practitioner (Ghaye 2000; Jasper 2013). It is important therefore to identify what you want to achieve from the reflection in terms of knowledge, understanding or performance, and what is the most useful form for the conclusions of your reflection to be presented, e.g. learning contracts, action plans, or an academic piece of work (Cottrell 2017).

Case study 2.1

Claire, a newly qualified paramedic attended a cardiac arrest which was unsuccessful and, for the first time as lead clinician, had to deliver the news that the patient had died to distraught relatives. She felt overwhelmed, sad and did not feel prepared for this and struggled to know what to say. Throughout the day she could not stop thinking about the incident; she worried that her communication with the relatives might have led to heightened distress and that her colleague would have a negative view of her competence. Claire decided in order to make sense of the situation, she needed to reflect on the incident. She questioned the event from different perspectives and explored current subject knowledge and research to enhance her interpretation of the event. Following the reflective process, Claire identified her educational needs and created a learning contract to address them.

A difficult incident triggered Claire to reflect. As an outcome, she wished to develop her knowledge, understanding and communication skills, develop her self-awareness to manage unfamiliar and unpredictable contexts better and ultimately develop her confidence when delivering bad news. The outcomes of her reflection were captured in a learning contract and written reflection that would form part of her CPD portfolio. In this case it was a difficult event that in Claire's view did not go well, however, it should be noted that knowledge, understanding and performance can equally be developed by reflecting on incidents that did go well; where there was an unexpected turn of events or where you reacted in a particular way and wish to explore why (Cottrell 2017). It is a popular misconception by health professionals that the term 'critical incident' relates specifically to large and highly dramatic incidents (Blaber 2008). However, 'ordinary' incidents may also be a rich source for reflection and warrant attention (Ghaye 2000), and thus the choice of experience should not be restricted to the 'extraordinary'.

STRUCTURING REFLECTION

It is important that you adopt a structured approach to your reflection that prompts you to consider key aspects of your critical incident, especially if you are new to reflection. Your reflective thoughts and discussions may not reach a conclusion or be evaluated if your approach lacks structure (Blaber 2008).

There are many reflective frameworks available that can be used to assist with the structure of your reflection. Several well-known frameworks are Gibbs (1998) and Johns (2010). Gibbs (1988) is a relatively simple framework that guides the reflector through six distinct stages: (1) description of the critical incident; (2) exploration of feelings; (3) evaluation; (4) analysis of the experience; (5) drawing conclusions; and, finally, (6) create an action plan. Gibbs' simple approach influenced many subsequent reflective frameworks (Jasper 2013). Johns' (2010) framework consists of a set of five categories with associated questions to guide the reflector: (1) you are prompted to describe the critical incident and identify essential factors, key people involved and the context of the event; (2) you reflect on your goals, interventions, consequences and feelings; (3) you consider internal and external influencing factors, knowledge and skills; (4) you consider alternatives and their consequences; and, finally, (5) you consider what learning and understanding have taken place, your feelings about the event now, and what actions and support are required. Other frameworks, including Borton's and Driscoll's, are commonly used (Cottrell 2017). It is worth noting, however, that they are all guides and not intended to be rigidly prescriptive and you can adjust them to suit your purpose so that they can be used effectively for the task at hand.

More recently, as reflection has been embraced by the paramedic profession, new reflective frameworks have emerged, such as those developed by Willis (2010), Wade (2011) and Smart (2011), that more explicitly guide the reflector to evaluate their practice against published knowledge and evidence, to provide an opportunity to embrace evidence-based practice (Turner 2015). Having a good understanding of the knowledge base and procedures that underpin everyday paramedic practice will stand you in good stead to make sound decisions when difficult situations arise, e.g. when it would be inappropriate to follow the normal procedures or where procedures do not exist.

Despite the differences in format and structure all frameworks share many features, which are summarised in Box 2.2.

Assuming that you are not required to use a particular reflective framework for an academic course, you can choose to use existing frameworks to provide structure and direction to your reflection. Otherwise you may wish to adapt an existing framework or develop your own reflective framework. When developing your own framework, consideration should be given to the key features outlined in Box 2.2. What is important is that you choose a framework that you can work with and achieve your intended outcomes.

> **Box 2.2 Common features of reflective frameworks**
>
> - A significant event (critical incident) should be selected and described upon which you can purposefully reflect (Oko and Reid 2012).
> - A re-examination of the critical incident should be undertaken in detail from a variety of perspectives.
> - Findings should be analysed to enhance your understanding and make sense of the event, your emotions and develop your self-awareness.
> - External sources of knowledge, theory and research need to be considered to enhance your understanding and enable you to evaluate your experiences. This will enable you to make informed judgements and justify your reasoning by reflecting critically on the evidence base that underpinned your actions.
> - Action – identify how new knowledge and understanding can be applied to your practice.

 Reflection: points to consider

Identify a recent critical incident that had significance for you, then review some of the reflective frameworks that are available. Identify which frameworks you think would work well for you and why.

DEPTH OF REFLECTION

As well as using a framework to structure your reflection, consideration should be given to the depth of reflection. If learning is to be maximised, it is important that your reflective skills move beyond a descriptive and superficial level. It is suggested that a hierarchy of reflection exists similar to the academic levels encountered in paramedic education that mirrors the depth and breadth of reflection (Knott and Scragg 2016).

At level one, reflection is largely a descriptive account that identifies what happened, including the main features of the incident; it should demonstrate that the practitioner had some awareness of what was going on at the time and that something had been learned as a result.

At level two, reflection is more analytical than level one and should identify and challenge the validity of the assumptions that lie behind our thoughts and actions, such as the theory or knowledge we take for granted, rules of thumb and common practice (Jasper 2013). Level two reflection should explore the incident, apply theory to practice and make explicit the rationale and evidence-base for any actions taken (Burns 1994; Jasper 2013). You should identify your learning and come to conclusions as to how this learning is transferable to other situations in order to improve your practice (Oelofsen 2012; Jasper 2013).

Reflection at level three will acknowledge how wider influences such as ethical and social factors impact on your practice. It will critically analyse your delivery of care in relation to health policy, economics and available resources (Jasper 2013).

WHEN TO REFLECT

In the second edition (Blaber 2012) of this textbook, we explored how our practice might be improved by considering Schön's (1983) concepts of reflection *in* action and reflection *on* action. Reflection in action is thinking about what you are doing while you are doing it, in other words, 'thinking on your feet' where we use our existing knowledge and skills to modify our response to a situation (Oelofsen 2012), and reflection on action is a retrospective activity that evaluates our current knowledge, skills, competence and professional practice and actively seeks out new knowledge from theories, evidence, guidelines and clinical experience to inform and enhance our understanding. Thompson and Pascal (2012) suggest that we should also 'reflect for action'. By planning and thinking ahead, we can draw on our experience and professional knowledge to make effective use of the time and resources available to us.

For paramedic practice, reflection for action could involve the gathering and appraisal of what information is made available before the initial contact with the patient and identifying the theories, evidence and professional knowledge associated with the case. Thinking about what needs to be done and why. During the treatment of our patient we are reflecting in action, by keeping the situation under review and adapting our practice as a result of these reflections as the situation unfolds. Finally, in order to uncover new learning from the situation as a whole that can be applied to future practice. we may engage in 'reflection on action' (Knott and Scragg 2016).

SKILLS NEEDED FOR REFLECTIVE PRACTICE

As we have seen, reflective practice is a more complicated and thought-provoking process than merely recalling an event. It is evident from reviewing various reflective frameworks that there are many skills that underlie reflective practice. Fortunately, with the exception of self-awareness, many of these skills are the same as those used in academic study (Atkins and Schutz 2013).

Self-awareness is an important skill for reflective practice and it is this self-awareness and personal knowledge that distinguishes reflective learning from other types of learning. Many things influence our character, beliefs and values throughout our lives, such as family, experience, culture and socialisation. Self-analysis of our behaviour, thoughts, emotions, mental state, assumptions and motives and the impact that these have on a given situation, and indeed the impact that the situation has on us, is an important part of reflective practice (Atkins and Schutz 2013; Howatson-Jones 2016).

See also **Chapter 1** for communication theories and strategies and **Chapter 9** for some relevant sociological theories.

Arguably, all reflective frameworks require you to describe your experience, therefore, the ability to provide a concise account of the context of the experience, what happened, what your thoughts and feelings were and the eventual outcome is important, so that the essence of the experience from your perspective is captured and can be readily understood by someone else (Atkins and Schutz 2013).

Critical analysis involves breaking down the component parts of an experience and subjecting it to scrutiny. An analogy could be that of a blood test, each component of the blood is looked at individually for abnormalities to gain a better understanding of what is happening. Critical analysis stops us taking things on face value. It should challenge our assumptions, for example, our knowledge – what do we know about this situation?, how do we know it?, is our knowledge based on experience or current research or both?, and how does it apply to this situation? What other alternatives are available? To what extent have our feelings, values and beliefs influenced the situation (Atkins and Schutz 2013)?

After having broken down the component parts of the experience and identified learning, it is important that you have the skill to integrate any new knowledge, feelings or attitudes into your existing knowledge, feelings and attitudes. This is known as synthesis (Atkins and Schutz 2013).

The final skill for reflective practice is the ability to evaluate your practice against public knowledge and empirical evidence (Turner 2015). Judgements of practice are often made against pre-determined standards, patient outcomes and key performance indicators, for example.

REFLECTIVE PRACTICE AND EVIDENCE-BASED PRACTICE

As you review the literature you will discover that 'evidence-based practice' and 'reflective practice' are frameworks that can guide clinical practice. They, however, represent two very distinct epistemologies in the ways in which they develop and use theory in practice (Mantzoukas and Watkinson 2008; Knott and Scragg 2016).

Evidence-based practice is often portrayed as a rational, moral and a superior decision-making framework that prevents clinical errors and suboptimal care. Knowledge is created that is acontextual, generalised, unbiased and predictive. The core concept is 'evidence' that has been tested through scientific research methods (Mantzoukas and Watkinson 2008; Knott and Scragg 2016). Reflective practice, on the other hand, produces knowledge that results 'from the lived experience', it is contextual, subjective and explanatory.

On the surface, these two approaches seem incompatible, which stems from the language used within each discourse, i.e. how both are described as opposites, e.g. objective vs subjective; rational vs intuitive. It is suggested, however, that this perceived incompatibility can be overcome by viewing the knowledge produced by both approaches as complementary or at either end of a continuum and that the paramedic can move between the two sources of knowledge as necessary to inform their practice (Mantzoukas and Watkinson 2008). Paramedics need to be aware of where the knowledge they are using is coming from to ensure that it is not solely based on reflection or evidence alone. They should be able to provide a critical and coherent argument as to why they are using a specific type of knowledge in their care of a patient.

If evidence-based practice and reflective practice are viewed as complementary 'ways of knowing', then these need to be part of a paramedic's repertoire of skills. Critical reflection is viewed as an efficient way that a paramedic can move between the different types of knowledge (Mantzoukas and Watkinson 2008). Paramedic practice is based on theories, research and established professional knowledge and these should be drawn upon when critically reflecting on practice to enhance your learning and understanding. When critically reflecting on practice, you should consider whether your experiences support theory and research and to what extent; also whether the theories and research support or contradict your findings (Cottrell 2017).

See also **Chapter 5** on evidence-based practice.

REFLECTIVE PRACTICE AND CONTINUING PROFESSIONAL DEVELOPMENT

In order to remain registered as a paramedic with the HCPC you must be able to demonstrate how you continue to meet the Paramedic Standards of Proficiency (2014), Standards of Continuing Professional Development and your fitness to practice (HCPC 2017). To do this you must undertake continuing professional development (CPD) using a variety of activities that are relevant to your current or future practice (HCPC 2017). Critical reflection on practice by its very nature is relevant to your current and future practice, contributes to the quality of your practice, which in turn benefits service users and is therefore an excellent CPD strategy. Reflective practice, in addition to enhancing your practice, can be a source of evidence of how you meet the standards in the event that you are audited by the HCPC. Box 2.3 identifies aspects of the standards that critical reflection will enable you to demonstrate.

Box 2.3 HCPC's (2014) Standards of Proficiency that critical reflection will enable you to demonstrate

- Self-awareness.
- Professional effectiveness.
- Psychological self-awareness.
- Use of knowledge and skills to solve problems.
- Justifying decisions.
- Considering the impact of culture, equality and diversity on practice.
- Adapting practice to meet individual needs.
- Reflecting and reviewing practice.
- Engaging in evidence-based practice.
- Monitoring and evaluating practice.
- Evaluating research and other evidence to inform practice.

 Chapter 18 for more detail on continuing professional development (CPD).

 Reflection: points to consider

Review Case Study 2.1 and consider which HCPC's Standards of Proficiency and Standards of CPD Claire's reflection meets.

Barriers and limitations

As discussed earlier, reflective practice is more complicated than merely recalling events and requires a variety of skills to be effective. Several situations exist that can limit the effectiveness of reflection or cause a barrier, and these are listed in Box 2.4.

Box 2.4 Situations that may lead to ineffective reflection

- Poor reflection skills and/or poor academic skills may limit the quality of reflection.
- Motivation may be poor if there is a lack of understanding of the relevance of reflection in professional practice.
- Insufficient time, feeling tired and frequent distractions can all impact on the quality of reflection (Howatson-Jones 2016; Cottrell 2017).

- At times the consequences of reflection may be painful (Howatson-Jones 2016; Cottrell 2017) and emotional responses can impair our ability to think critically (Knott and Scragg 2016).
- Where thoughtfulness is mistaken for critical analysis, reflection will be superficial (Howatson-Jones 2016; Cottrell 2017). Superficial reflection also can occur when it is undertaken merely to fulfil requirements of a programme of study.
- Lack of current evidence-based knowledge.
- Practitioners may be caught up in routine and lose sight of reasoning behind actions.
- For reflection to take place honestly and openly, a supportive environment is essential. Reflection can uncover some deep-seated past traumas from childhood or relationships which may need referral to expert support (Knott and Scragg 2016).

CONCLUSION

The everyday experiences encountered by paramedics provide numerous opportunities to reflect on practice. To help you to reflect in a meaningful and structured manner, you can use one of the many reflective frameworks available. To maximise your learning potential further, you should aim to develop the depth of your reflection from largely descriptive accounts to ones that critically analyse your delivery of care in relation to the wider context, such as research, ethical and social factors and health policy. Critical reflection can enable you to provide a critical and coherent argument as to why you use specific types of knowledge that emerge from either evidence-based practice or reflective practice in the care of your patient.

Reflective practice is an important aspect of your continuing professional development and can provide valuable evidence to demonstrate that you continue to meet the HCPC's Standards of Proficiency and Standards of CPD. Learning needs uncovered through the process of reflection can inform the direction of your CPD and assist your journey from novice to expert. Through honest and open reflection, you will develop increased self-awareness and an enhanced sense of professionalism.

Chapter key points:

- Reflection is more than merely recalling an event.
- Critical incidents are events that stand out in your mind and contribute directly to your development as a paramedic; they can be positive or negative experiences.
- A structured approach to reflection prompts you to consider key aspects of your critical incident.

- It is important to choose a framework that you can work with and achieve your intended outcomes.
- If learning is to be maximised, reflection should move beyond a descriptive level.
- Reflection plays a role in maintaining your mental well-being as a professional.
- Skills for reflective practice are broadly the same as those used in academic study.
- Critical reflection is an important part of evidence-based practice.
- Reflection is an excellent CPD strategy to meet the HCPC Standards of Proficiency and Standards of CPD.
- Reflective practice is central to improving professional practice.

REFERENCES AND SUGGESTED READING

Alegado, E. (2017) Reflective practice. *Nursing Standard*, 31(29): 72.

Atkins, S. and Schutz, S. (2013) Developing skills for reflective practice, in C. Bulman and S. Schutz (eds) *Reflective Practice in Nursing*, 5th edn. Chichester: Wiley-Blackwell, pp. 23–52.

Blaber, A.Y. (2008) Reflective practice in relation to pre-hospital care, in A.Y. Blaber (ed.) *Foundations of Paramedic Practice: A Theoretical Perspective*. Maidenhead: Open University Press.

Blaber, A.Y. (ed.) (2012) *Foundations of Paramedic Practice: A Theoretical Perspective*. Maidenhead: McGraw-Hill.

Burns, S. (1994) Assessing reflective learning, in A. Palmer, S. Burns and C. Bulman (eds) *Reflective Practice in Nursing: The Growth of the Professional Practitioner*. London: Blackwell.

Cottrell, S. (2017) *Critical Thinking Skills: Effective Analysis, Argument and Reflection*, 3rd edn. London: Palgrave Macmillan.

Francis, R. (2013) *Report of the Mid-Staffordshire NHS Foundation Trust Public Inquiry: Executive Summary*. London: The Stationery Office.

Ghaye, T. (2000) *Reflection: Principles and Practice for Healthcare Professionals*. Wiltshire: Mark Allen Publishing Limited.

Gibbs, G. (1988) *Learning by Doing: A Guide to Teaching and Learning Methods*. Oxford: Further Education Unit: Oxford Polytechnic.

Health and Care Professions Council (2017) *Continuing Professional Development and your Registration*. Available at: http://www.hpc-uk.org/assets/documents/10001314CPD_and_your_registration.pdf (accessed 30 July 2017).

Howatson-Jones, L. (2016) *Reflective Practice in Nursing*, 3rd edn. London: Sage.

Jasper, M. (2013) *Beginning Reflective Practice*, 2nd edn. Andover: Cengage Learning.

Johns, C. (2010) *Guided Reflection: A Narrative Approach to Advancing Professional Practice*. London: Wiley-Blackwell.

Knott, C. and Scragg, T. (2016) *Reflective Practice in Social Work*, 4th edn. London: Sage.

Mantzoukas, S. and Watkinson, S. (2008) Re-describing reflective practice and evidence-based practice discourses. *International Journal of Nursing Practice*, 14: 129–34.

Oelofsen, N. (2012) *Developing Reflective Practice: A Guide for Students and Practitioners of Health and Social Care*. Banbury: Lantern.

Oko, J. and Reid, J. (2012) *Study Skills for Health and Social Care Students*. London: Sage.

Pretorius, L. and Ford, A. (2016) Reflection for learning: teaching reflective practice at the beginning of university study. *International Journal of Teaching and Learning in Higher Education*, 28(2): 241–53.

Schön, D.A. (1983) *The Reflective Practitioner: How Professionals Think in Action*. New York: Basic Books.

Smart, G. (2011) I.F.E.A.R. reflection: an easy to use adaptable template for paramedics. *Journal of Paramedic Practice*, 3(5): 255–7.

Tarrant, P. (2013) *Reflective Practice and Professional Development*. London: Sage.

Thompson, N. and Pascal, J. (2012) Developing critically reflective practice. *Reflective Practice*, 13(2): 311–25.

Turner, T. (2015) Reflective practice for paramedics: a new approach. *Journal of Paramedic Practice*, 7(3): 138–41.

Wade, C. (2011) Planning and writing an evidence-based critical reflection. *Journal of Paramedic Practice*, 3(4): 190–6.

Willis, S. (2010) Becoming a reflective practitioner: frameworks for the pre-hospital professional. *Journal of Paramedic Practice*, 2(5): 212–16.

Using clinical audit to improve patient care

Rachael T. Fothergill and Joanna Shaw

In this chapter:

- Introduction
- Why is this relevant?
- Clinical governance
- What is clinical audit?
- Peer review, critical incident analysis and deep dives
- What are the benefits of clinical audit?
- The role of the paramedic in clinical audit
- Conclusion
- Chapter key points
- References and suggested reading
- Useful websites

INTRODUCTION

This chapter is a very brief introduction to the concept of using clinical audit as a tool to improve clinical quality and patient care. The process of clinical audit dates back to the mid-nineteenth century and now has an important role in ensuring that a high standard of care is delivered to patients across the NHS today. This chapter outlines the process and importance of clinical audit, and briefly touches on other approaches to reviewing healthcare. An understanding of these approaches is the foundation not only of paramedic practice, but all other healthcare provider roles. Some definitions are included and sources of further reading provided.

WHY IS THIS RELEVANT?

Clinical audit has a direct effect on paramedic practice and is something that clinicians are involved with on a daily basis, even though they may not realise it. It can change practice by influencing protocols, policy development and treatments. Everything the paramedic does in practice is subject to the rigours of clinical audit. Clinical audit is reliant upon accurate clinical documentation and, as such, it is important that healthcare practitioners are aware of how their clinical records are used and how this influences future patient care.

CLINICAL GOVERNANCE

Clinical governance provides a mechanism for ensuring that quality is at the heart of the NHS. It is aimed at improving standards of clinical practice and ensuring that decisions are based on the most up-to-date evidence of what is clinically effective. Clinical governance is not simply concerned with achieving and maintaining high standards, but with continuously improving them to create an environment of clinical excellence. It has been defined as 'a mission not just to do well, but to do better' (Donaldson 2000: 7).

It is generally recognised that before the UK government introduced clinical governance into the NHS in 1997, there was a distinct lack of organisational responsibility for quality. Within a couple of years, the Health Act of June 1999 (Section 18) established a statutory duty of quality requiring NHS Trusts to monitor and improve the standards of care they provide.

It is helpful to view clinical governance as an 'umbrella' beneath which there are a number of key components that combine to make a quality organisation. Essentially clinical governance is about:

- clear lines of responsibility and accountability for the quality of clinical care;
- a comprehensive programme of quality improvement activities;
- clear policies for managing risks, and procedures for identifying and addressing poor performance.

Clinical audit is one of the principal methods for measuring clinical quality and identifying improvements in healthcare, and has been described as one of the cornerstones of clinical governance (Oyebode et al. 1999).

WHAT IS CLINICAL AUDIT?

Box 3.1 gives the NICE definition of clinical audit.

There are many definitions of clinical audit, but they generally all have the same key elements: the systematic evaluation of clinical practice against a set of criteria, and the implementation of change to improve care where indicated.

Box 3.1 Definition of clinical audit

'A quality improvement process that seeks to improve patient care and outcomes through systematic review of care against explicit criteria and the implementation of change' (National Institute for Clinical Excellence 2002: 1).

The emergence of clinical audit

The work of Florence Nightingale in the 1850s is widely considered to be one of the earliest examples of clinical audit. By monitoring medical practices during the Crimean War, she was able to identify a link between poor sanitation and high mortality rates.

Florence and her team of nurses methodically introduced strict sanitation procedures and were able to report a significant decrease in patient deaths.

Clinical audit (or 'medical audit' as it was once known) was not formally introduced into professional practice in the NHS until 1989 when the government published its White Paper *Working for Patients* (DH 1989: 3). It also set out the government's expectation that regular, systematic audit was something in which every doctor would participate. Just a few years later, it became clear that all healthcare professionals, not just hospital doctors, should play an active part in audit and so medical audit evolved into clinical audit. In 1997, along with the introduction of clinical governance, the government identified clinical audit as important to achieving a high-quality NHS (DH 1997; 1998). In 2000, clinical audit became further embedded when the *NHS Plan* (DH 2000) made it a requirement for all NHS organisations and a mandatory obligation for all doctors employed in, or under contract to, the NHS. Ten years later, in 2010, the government began linking NHS payment arrangements to quality measures reported in national clinical audits, solidifying a commitment to clinical audit.

The importance of the role of clinical audit in the NHS has been highlighted by a number of high profile public inquiries, including the inquiry into children's heart surgery at the Bristol Royal Infirmary where, during the 1990s, a higher number of deaths than expected occurred in babies following cardiac surgery. The inquiry's report (Bristol Royal Infirmary 2001) cited a 'lax approach to safety, secrecy about doctors' performance and a lack of monitoring' and recommended that clinical audit 'must be fully supported by Trusts', 'should be compulsory for all healthcare professionals providing clinical care' and the 'requirement to participate in it should be included as part of the contract of employment'. The value of clinical audit was further endorsed by the inquiry into the deaths of patients under the care of the General Practitioner, Dr Harold Shipman (DH 2004). The government's response to the Shipman Inquiry (DH 2007) acknowledged the progress made by the NHS in relation to clinical governance since the period covered by the Inquiry, and indicated that had such processes been in place at the time, 'it is highly unlikely that the abuses could have continued for such long periods without being detected'. This report also reiterated the importance of encouraging all clinicians to participate in clinical audit 'so that any problems are picked up by them and their peers at the earliest possible stage'.

Clinical audit clearly has an important and prominent role in the NHS, and all healthcare professionals need to have a basic understanding of its principles. This is something that is supported by a number of professional bodies including, but not limited to, the General Medical Council, the Royal College of Emergency Medicine and the Health and Care Professions Council. The Health and Care Professions Council's *Standards of Proficiency for Paramedics* (HCPC 2014) clearly identifies clinical audit as a key obligation and specifies that registrants 'must be able to assure the quality of their practice . . . be able to engage in evidence-based practice, evaluate practice systematically and participate in audit procedures'. Therefore, every paramedic has a role to play in clinical audit.

The clinical audit process

The clinical audit process consists of an iterative cycle of steps known as the audit cycle (see Figure 3.1). It involves selecting a topic, setting standards for clinical practice, and then measuring actual practice to determine whether the standards are being met. If practice is shown to deviate from the accepted standard, then reasons must be identified and improvements made. After a suitable time interval, clinical practice must be reassessed (re-audited) against the original criteria to confirm an improvement in healthcare delivery. The whole audit process should continue through as many cycles as necessary until there is evidence that improved standards of care are being delivered and maintained.

Topic selection

Practically any area of clinical care can be selected as a topic for clinical audit, as long as it is measurable. Topic selection will largely be determined at a local level (ideally with input from key stakeholders) and involve a variety of sources, including complaints, clinical incident reports and feedback from patient questionnaires or focus groups. The need for a particular clinical audit can also be triggered by the introduction of new drugs or interventions, new guidance or new care pathways. It is also common for topics to be specified at a national level through, for example, government-commissioned programmes and NICE guidance. As any audit project will inevitably involve a significant investment of resources, topic selection needs careful consideration and should link in with local and/or national priorities.

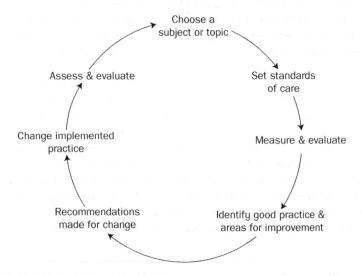

Figure 3.1 The audit cycle

Source: Contains public sector information licensed under the Open Government Licence v3.0. Adapted from DH (1997), based on information in NICE (2002).

Criteria, standards and exceptions

When a topic has been chosen, the criteria, expected standards of care and any exceptions to delivering that care must be established. Criteria are essentially explicit statements that describe the aspects of care being measured (for example, 'adequate analgesia must be given to patients in pain') and are used to assess the quality of care provided.

There are three types of criteria that can be measured:

- *Structure* – what was needed (e.g. the availability of resources and facilities)?
- *Process* – what was done/what action was taken (e.g. the treatment given)?
- *Outcome* – what was the clinical result (e.g. the patient's health status)?

Process criteria are generally considered to be the most sensitive measures of the quality of care, although within the NHS there is growing interest in the use of outcome measures. It is important to use outcome measures with caution as there are often many different factors that contribute to an outcome (such as other treatments and coexisting clinical conditions) and, as such, it is possible that patients who receive a good level of care may experience poor outcomes, and vice versa. Furthermore, some important outcomes occur long after care is provided, so it can be difficult to tease out the direct impact of a particular clinical intervention. This latter limitation is particularly pertinent to ambulance services where patients are frequently handed over to hospitals or other healthcare providers within a relatively short period of time. Outcome measures are also, in practice, often difficult to collect. When examining outcomes as part of ambulance service clinical audit, it is sometimes necessary to collect information not only from ambulance service clinical records, but from the records of other organisations that subsequently cared for the patient. With limited resources and authority, it is often a challenge for ambulance services to obtain data from these different organisations. Nonetheless, despite these limitations, outcome measures can be extremely powerful, particularly when used in conjunction with process measures.

When using outcome criteria, ambulance services may find it less problematic and more useful to select, where practical, outcomes that occur within a short period of time relative to the incident. These would be measured ideally at the point at which the patient is handed over to another healthcare professional and at most within a few days of such handover. In addition to collecting information from the patient care records, outcomes can be obtained directly from the patient via questionnaires and focus groups. For these techniques to be successful as tools within an audit, they must be well structured and the questions must clearly relate to the measures being examined. When using these methods, it is essential to consider ethical issues and confidentiality. In some cases, approval may be required from an NHS Research Ethics Committee.

 Turn to **Chapter 5** to read about the importance of research within the para-medic profession.

Standards are the expected levels of performance, that is, how often it is expected that the care given will comply with the criteria. Standards are usually expressed as percentage figures (e.g. 100 per cent of patients in pain should receive adequate analgesia).

Exceptions are valid clinical reasons why the standard of care could not be delivered (e.g. contraindication to analgesia). Exceptions do not include organisational issues, such as lack of equipment or lack of staff, as it is important for any clinical audit to be able to measure and highlight such issues with the ultimate aim of driving change.

Criteria, standards of care and exceptions within UK ambulance services are mainly derived from national ambulance clinical practice guidelines, other guidelines as appropriate (e.g. NICE), and local protocols.

Recommendations and actions

Once the data has been collected and practice measured, areas of care that do or do not meet the set standards are identified. Where care is found to meet the expected standard, it is important to communicate this and congratulate those involved, which may be at an individual, departmental or organisational level. When clinical practice does not meet the expected standard, recommendations for improving practice must be developed and an action plan devised. Once approved by the Trust's relevant executive committees, the recommended changes and actions are implemented in a systematic fashion.

A common criticism of the clinical audit process is that recommended changes are sometimes not fully or effectively implemented. For an audit to succeed in delivering change, it is important that there is strong clinical leadership and 'buy-in' at a senior level within the organisation. It is also crucial that key stakeholders, including relevant clinicians, patients or service users and staff whose support is necessary to implement changes, are involved from the outset. Key stakeholder involvement ensures that ownership of the project lies with those who are most likely to be affected by its findings. Their involvement also ensures commitment and increases the likelihood that changes to practice, and thus patient care, will be achieved.

 Chapter 16 for more detail on clinical leadership.

PEER REVIEW, CRITICAL INCIDENT ANALYSIS AND DEEP DIVES

There are a number of common methods of reviewing healthcare within the NHS that are often mistakenly considered to be clinical audit; these include peer review, critical incident analysis and deep dives. Peer review typically involves a group of clinicians randomly selecting a small sample of records for patients who were recently under their care and considering as a group whether the best care was provided. Critical incident analysis usually involves multidisciplinary teams reviewing cases that have caused concern or where there were unexpected, adverse outcomes. Deep dive reviews are increasingly being used by NHS Trusts to examine known or potential issues or concerning trends, and to provide assurance about the safety and quality of care. These approaches, when used on their own, are useful ways of assessing performance and highlighting areas of concern, but they do not constitute a clinical audit. Nonetheless, these methods can form a valuable part of a clinical audit project when incorporated as data collection tools during the measuring practice stage of the audit cycle.

WHAT ARE THE BENEFITS OF CLINICAL AUDIT?

Effective clinical audit is vital to the NHS; it brings many benefits to an organisation, healthcare professionals, patients and the public. Clinical audit enables organisations and practitioners to demonstrate to themselves and to others the effectiveness and quality of their service. It provides reassurance that patients are receiving the best pos-sible care and can increase confidence in the quality of the service as a whole. Where clinical audit identifies areas for improvement, it can aid practitioners and organisations by pinpointing where further education and training are needed, and so can provide opportunities for learning and development. It can also highlight to organisations areas where new investment and resources are needed to support clinical practice. Most importantly, clinical audit can reduce variability in practice and improve standards of clinical care.

For the participating paramedic, clinical audit can provide valuable, first-hand experience of using evidence as a tool for change, and enable the paramedic to be a direct part of that change and can be used to demonstrate a commitment to professional development. It can provide a different view of clinical practice, contributing to improved skills and confidence. In addition, by providing insight into how information from clinical records is used, it can enhance the paramedic's own documentation and record-keeping skills.

As clinical audit typically relies on extracting information from patient records, even if the standard of documentation is not itself the objective of the audit, levels of missing information and issues with documentation may be reported and action taken as a result to improve record keeping.

Clinical audit can also provide a valuable contribution to the existing medical evidence base. Using clinical audit findings to add to the evidence base is particu-larly important in the pre-hospital arena where research evidence for many interven-tions, although increasing, is currently lacking. Indeed, the findings from ambulance service clinical audits have been used to inform national ambulance clinical practice guidelines.

THE ROLE OF THE PARAMEDIC IN CLINICAL AUDIT

HCPC registrant paramedics are expected to meet specific Standards of Proficiency (Health and Care Professions Council 2014) in order to 'be able to assure the quality of their practice':

- 'be able to engage in evidence-based practice, evaluate practice and participate in audit procedures' (2014: 12.1);
- 'be aware of the role of audit and review in quality management, including quality control, quality assurance and the use of appropriate outcome measures' (2014: 12.3);
- 'be able to maintain an effective audit trail and work towards continual improvement' (2014: 12.4);
- 'be aware of, and be able to participate in, quality assurance programmes, where appropriate' (2014: 12.5);
- 'recognise the need to monitor and evaluate the quality of practice and the value of contributing to the generation of data for quality assurance and improvement programmes' (2014: 12.7).

As in other NHS organisations, ambulance service clinical audit is extremely dependent upon the information documented by the practitioner and the importance of high quality, complete documentation should not be underestimated. Full and accurate documentation allows those reviewing the records to gain a more comprehensive picture of the care that was delivered, which will in turn lead to accurate decisions about patient care. Ultimately, without a high standard of documentation, clinical audit cannot accurately assess the real clinical situation and deliver appropriate changes to practice and improvements for patients. Even if not directly involved in a clinical audit project, the paramedic still has a part to play by ensuring high quality, full and accurate documentation.

 Reflection: points to consider

How often are documentation audits carried out in your NHS Trust? Do you understand the importance of your documentation and the link to clinical audit?

CONCLUSION

This chapter has highlighted some important areas of practice that have their roots in providing a quality service. It is hoped that the various sections have improved your knowledge and understanding of the concepts of clinical audit and quality improvement, and the way in which systematically reviewing clinical practices can inform and improve patient care.

> ## Chapter key points:
> - Clinical audit is undertaken across all healthcare environments and the outcome can influence practice and provide real benefits for patients.
> - All paramedics have a key role to play in improving the care delivered by their organsation, whether directly or indirectly, and clinical audit is an intergral component of this.
> - Full and accurate documentation allows the systematic review of practices, which in turns leads to tangible actions to improve care.

REFERENCES AND SUGGESTED READING

Bristol Royal Infirmary (2001) *Learning from Bristol: The Report of the Public Inquiry into Children's Heart Surgery at the Bristol Royal Infirmary 1984–1995, Cm 5207(1)*. London: The Stationery Office. Available at: www.webarchive.nationalarchives.gov.uk/20090811143822/http://www.bristol-inquiry.org.uk/final_report/the_report.pdf (accessed 4 January 2018).

DH (Department of Health) (1989) *Working for Patients*, Cm 555. London: HMSO.

DH (Department of Health) (1997) *The New NHS: Modern, Dependable*, Cm 3807. London: HMSO.

DH (Department of Health) (1998) *A First Class Service: Quality in the NHS*. Available at: www.webarchive.nationalarchives.gov.uk/+/http://www.dh.gov.uk/en/Publicationsandstatistics/Publications/PublicationsPolicyAndGuidance/DH_4006902 (accessed 2 January 2018).

DH (Department of Health) (2000) *The NHS Plan: A Plan for Investment, a Plan for Reform*, Cm 4818-I. London: HMSO.

DH (Department of Health) (2004) *Safeguarding Patients: Lessons from the Past – Proposals for the Future*. Available at: www.the-shipmaninquiry.org.uk/images/fifthreport/SHIP05_COMPLETE_NO_APPS.pdf (accessed 2 January 2018).

DH (Department of Health) (2007) *Safeguarding Patients*. Available at: ww.dh.gov.uk/prod_consum_dh/groups/dh_digitalassets/@dh/@en/documents/digitalasset/dh_065954.pdf (accessed 1 January 2018).

Donaldson, L.J. (2000) Clinical governance: a mission to improve. *British Journal of Clinical Governance*, 5(1): 6–8.

Health and Care Professions Council (2014) *Standards of Proficiency: Paramedics*, 3rd edn. London: Health and Care Professions Council.

National Institute for Clinical Excellence (2002) *Principles for Best Practice in Clinical Audit*. London: Radcliffe Medical Press Ltd.

Oyebode, F., Brown, N. and Parry, E. (1999) Clinical governance: application to psychiatry. *Psychiatric Bulletin*, 23: 7–10.

USEFUL WEBSITES

NHS Evidence: www.evidence.nhs.uk/ (accessed 9 January 2018).

OpenGrey: www.opengrey.eu/ (accessed 4 January 2018).

PubMed: www.ncbi.nlm.nih.gov/pubmed/ (accessed 4 January 2018).

Ethics and law for the paramedic

Vince Clarke, Graham Harris and Steve Cowland

INTRODUCTION

The role of paramedics has undergone enormous development in the past three decades, with the term 'paramedic' now being synonymous with primary, acute, community, and urgent and emergency healthcare. As a protected title, anyone wishing to call themselves a 'paramedic' must first be registered with the Health and Care Professions Council (HCPC) and must adhere to the professional and ethical standards they prescribe.

In addition to adhering to the expectations of the HCPC, paramedics are also required to work within the legal parameters dictated by legislation. Readers are reminded to refer to the most up-to-date government documents and laws. All areas of paramedic practice, notably the gaining of consent, drug administration and issues of confidentiality, must be undertaken within the legal framework of the territory in which the paramedic practises.

WHY IS THIS RELEVANT?

Paramedics often meet people in extremely difficult and distressing personal circumstances and at critical times in their lives. Patients and families can be vulnerable during these moments, so it is crucial that paramedics understand the key legal and ethical issues that may impact on their decision-making. Without an understanding of the ethical principles, legislation or legal precedents that apply to their practice, paramedics may potentially be at risk of incurring fitness to practise investigations, civil litigation or, in extreme cases, criminal charges.

No text can prepare the reader for all eventualities, but a discussion of the key legal and ethical issues is vital for safe, competent and professional practice.

ETHICS

Ethics can be considered a 'moral code', and as such can be very subjective. There are many textbooks devoted to ethical principles and theories, including a number that focus specifically on medical ethics. Such texts often contain ethical scenarios for the reader to dissect, discuss and consider. Examples of subject matter for this type of scenario could include termination of pregnancy, resource allocation, assisted suicide, end-of-life issues, organ donation or 'saviour siblings', to name but a few. The difficulty with such ethical dilemmas from the perspective of the paramedic is that they tend to be focused on situations that occur in non-emergency environments within healthcare and can, therefore, be viewed as less relevant to the paramedic. However, with the expansion of the role of the paramedic to include alternative treatment pathways, and an increasing tendency to be able to treat at the point of contact, or refer patients to areas other than emergency departments (EDs), a deeper understanding of ethical decision-making should be considered a *must* for paramedics who are now at the front line of 'out-of-hospital' rather than 'pre-hospital' care.

The role of the paramedic often demands rapid decision-making capability where it could be argued that ethical considerations are put aside for clinical decisions to be made. There are generally very clear clinical guidelines for paramedics to follow, but there are rarely considered ethical decision-making processes that accompany them.

The principles of ethics proposed by Beauchamp and Childress (2013) are a good starting point for the paramedic (Box 4.1). Their 'four principles' approach provides paramedics with the basic tools that they need to enable them to consider ethics in their practice. By having some consideration to each of the four principles, paramedics can weigh up their decisions and ensure that they are in the best interests of the patient while being ethically sound.

The principles proposed by Beauchamp and Childress are just one approach to ethics and even these cannot be covered in great depth in an introductory text of this type. To give the paramedic an introduction to how these principles may be considered in practice, each of the principles will be discussed alongside the case studies presented later in this chapter.

Box 4.1 The 'four principles' approach to ethics

1. *Respect for autonomy – 'self-rule'*. Autonomy is the principle that allows an individual to have control over their being. This means that any decision that they make about their treatment must be respected.
2. *Non-maleficence – 'do no harm'*. This principle advocates not causing undue harm to the patient. Such harm may be considered direct physical harm, such as the insertion of an intravenous cannula, or harm brought about by failing to consider foreseeable outcomes of a proposed course of action, such as leaving a vulnerable patient at home when their presentation requires hospitalisation. The negative impact of any harm must be balanced against the potential benefit achieved.
3. *Beneficence – 'do good'*. This principle advocates maximising benefits and minimising harm to patients. Beneficence underlies all of the actions of the healthcare professional and can be allied with the term 'best interests'. It is important to note that a patient's perspective of what is in their best interests may not always be the same as that of the healthcarer dealing with them. In these cases, there may appear to the paramedic to be a conflict between beneficence, non-maleficence and autonomy.
4. *Justice – 'what is right?'* This principle looks at what is right or fair in any given situation. For example, patients who have mental health problems have the same right to appropriate treatment as those who do not. In the paramedic world situations such as availability of resources and time spent on scene with patients could be considered when looking at justice.

LAW

Law in the United Kingdom comes from several sources; legislation from Parliament, case law, books of authority, custom and law reform. For aspects of law, the UK is generally divided into three territories; Scotland, Northern Ireland, and England and Wales. The majority of legislation and case law is consistent between the territories, but there may be specific legislative requirements within each area, so the paramedic must be familiar with the peculiarities of the territory in which they practise.

The legal system in place within the UK can be broadly divided into two main branches: criminal law and civil law. Table 4.1 details the differences and similarities between these two areas.

Paramedics are subject to the same legislation as any other individual in the UK, and are specifically named in practice notes for particular legislation such as the Mental Capacity Act (MCA) 2005.

Table 4.1 Criminal law and civil law

	Criminal law	Civil law
Purpose	To protect society by maintaining law and order	To uphold the rights of individuals and to settle disputes
Participants	The case is brought by the Crown Prosecution Service on behalf of the State, and is represented as the crown versus the defendant, e.g. *R vs. Shipman*	The case is brought by one individual or organisation against another individual or organisation, *e.g. Griffiths vs. London Ambulance Service NHS Trust*
Standard of proof	To be found *guilty*, it has to be shown *beyond reasonable doubt* that the *defendant* committed the alleged crime	To be found *liable*, it has to be shown that, *on the balance of probabilities*, it is more likely than not that the *respondent* is responsible for the alleged act
Findings	The defendant can be found guilty or not guilty (or in Scotland a third possibility of 'not proven')	The respondent can be found liable or not liable
Outcomes	A guilty verdict will result in some sort of punishment, such as prison, a fine, or a community service order being imposed	A liable verdict should result in the situation being 'put right'. This may mean an apology, a change to policy or the awarding of compensation to the claimant

 Chapters 8 and **13** for practical application of the Mental Capacity Act.

In practice, the majority of legislation that impacts on the day-to-day work of the paramedic is dealt with by the paramedic's employing authority. Health and safety, data protection, drugs regulation, medical equipment safety, and human rights are all areas that are legislated and policies and systems are put in place by employers to ensure conformity. Individual paramedics, along with other employees, are required to conform to policies for which they have an individual responsibility, such as data protection and health and safety. This does not mean that all the policies and procedures produced by employers constitute 'the law' in themselves, rather that legislation has informed the development of such policies. Paramedics are more likely to encounter the civil branch of the law, as opposed to the criminal branch. For example, professional regulation follows the principles of civil law and will be discussed later.

A third branch of the legal system is that of the coroner's inquest. Threats of 'explain it to the coroner' have historically been used to encourage student paramedics to do the right thing when treating patients and when completing records, often portraying the coroner as someone to be feared. This is simply not the case. The role of the coroner in relation to deceased individuals is to establish facts. There are four main facts that the coroner must establish:

- the identity of the deceased;
- the place of death;
- the time of death;
- how the deceased came by their death.

Paramedics may be called upon to provide written witness statements of fact to the coroner and any patient report records that they have completed may also be subjected to scrutiny. In some cases where further clarification is needed, the paramedic may be required to give evidence at a coroner's inquest. Once the paramedic has answered any of the coroner's questions, the coroner may invite any interested parties to question the paramedic. This means that relatives of the deceased, or their representatives, may ask the paramedic questions. This can be a difficult and uncomfortable experience for the paramedic concerned, but it often goes a long way to giving bereaved relatives a greater understanding of what happened to their loved one. In order to make such experiences as pain-free as possible, it is vital that the paramedic thoroughly documents all details for all of the calls that they attend.

PROFESSIONAL REGULATION

The paramedic profession, together with certain other health professions, is regulated by the Health and Care Professions Council (HCPC). The HCPC was brought into existence by the Health and Social Work Professions Order 2001 (the Order) which sets out the roles and responsibilities of the HCPC.

The HCPC's overarching objective is the protection of the public, which it achieves in four main ways:

- maintaining a register of health professionals, including paramedics;
- the approval of education programmes leading to eligibility to apply for registration;
- the assessment of continuing professional development (CPD);
- the hearing of Fitness to Practise complaints.

The term 'paramedic' is a protected title, meaning that it can only be used by those whose name appears on the register maintained by the Health and Care Professions Council; there are over 24,000 registered paramedics in the United Kingdom. Use of the protected title by someone whose name does not appear on the HCPC register is a criminal offence. In order to gain entry to the HCPC register, an individual must demonstrate that they have achieved the threshold requirements of the profession – the HCPC *Standards of Proficiency – Paramedics* (HCPC 2014), generally by completing a programme of study approved by the Education and Training Committee (ETC) of the HCPC. To remain on the register, the paramedic must demonstrate CPD activities and adhere to the HCPC *Standards of Conduct, Performance and Ethics* (HCPC 2016a). The implications of failing to do so will be addressed later in this chapter.

 Chapter 18 for more detail on continuing professional development (CPD).

ACCOUNTABILITY AND CLINICAL NEGLIGENCE

Every paramedic applying to go on the register has to confirm that they have read and agree to adhere to the standards presented in the *Standards of Conduct, Performance and Ethics* (HCPC 2016a). The HCPC also publish *Guidance on Conduct and Ethics for Students* (HCPC 2016b) which outlines to students on pre-registration courses the expectations of the HCPC. The standards for registrants are outlined in Box 4.2 (adapted from HCPC 2016a).

The standards detailed in Box 4.2, along with the *Standards of Proficiency – Paramedics* (HCPC 2014), form the basis on which registered paramedics will be held accountable, should a complaint be made against them. Any such complaint will be considered by

---

Box 4.2 Summary of the standards expected of registered paramedics

Paramedics must:

- promote and protect the interests of service users and carers;
- communicate appropriately and effectively;
- work within the limits of their knowledge and skills;
- delegate appropriately;
- respect confidentiality;
- manage risk;
- report concerns about safety;
- be open when things go wrong;
- be honest and trustworthy;
- keep records of their work.

the Health and Care Professions Tribunal Service (HCPTS), the adjudication service for the HCPC. The HCPTS comprises the Health and Care Professions Tribunal – the Panels which hear and determine cases on behalf of the HCPC's three Practice Committees and the Tribunal Service team which provides operational support to the Tribunal.

The three Practice Committees are:

- First, the *investigating committee* normally looks at every allegation to decide whether there is a case to answer. If a case to answer is apparent, this committee deals with the case or decides to pass it onto one of the other two committees. It is expected that the investigating committee will always deal with cases of fraudulent or incorrect registration.
- Second, the *conduct and competence committee* normally deals with cases of misconduct and/or lack of competence. They will also deal with matters arising from police cautions or criminal convictions.
- The third committee is known as *the health committee* and deals with cases of ill health.

Any fitness to practise hearing is based on current impairment to practise at the time of the hearing. The Council, after dealing with each case, has the power to take action against a health professional if a case is established and current impairment is found. Such action may involve removing the paramedic from the HCPC register. Other action may include suspension from the register or restricting the individual's work or publicly cautioning him or her.

Those prospective paramedics who are trying to join the register will not incur any penalties from the HCPC during education, but will be unable to register if they do not reach the requirements of the HCPC relating to the *Standards of Conduct, Performance and Ethics* that they have to reach in order to apply to be registered with the HCPC. The standards will form part of their educational programme and may be assessed in theory and in the practice environment, depending on the structure and content of the programme approved by the HCPC.

Clinical negligence

Clinical negligence is an area that is often associated with fitness to practise. All paramedics are required by the HCPC to have appropriate professional indemnity insurance, with employees of NHS organisations being covered by their employers' insurance. Those paramedics who undertake private work, or who are self-employed, are required to demonstrate that they have professional indemnity insurance when registering with the HCPC.

Employers are vicariously liable for the actions of their employees, including paramedics. An employer can also be held vicariously liable for an employee's breach of a statutory duty. If the statute imposes a duty on the employee personally, as in the case of the MCA, and makes no reference to the employer, vicarious liability still applies (*Majrowski v. Guy's and St Thomas' NHS Trust* [2006] UKHL 34). If vicarious liability is imposed on an employer, both the employer and employee are held jointly liable, technically enabling the employer to claim a contribution from the employee in respect of any financial loss incurred (Civil Liability (Contribution) Act 1978), however, in practice, this does not happen. The NHS Litigation Authority generally deals with claims of negligence relating to NHS staff or organisations.

For a claim in clinical negligence to be successful, three key elements need to be established by the claimant;

- the existence of a duty of care;
- a breach of that duty of care;
- negative consequences as a direct result of the breach (causation).

The ambulance service itself has a duty of care from the point that it has established the location and identity of a patient, a duty which begins before the paramedic has even got to the scene (*Kent v Griffiths* [2000] 2 All ER 474). A paramedic's duty of care is often straightforward to establish and would begin when the paramedic enters into a patient–carer relationship with the patient by engaging in direct contact with them.

A breach of this duty is when a paramedic has failed to carry out their duties to an expected level of care. In negligence claims, this is an area where expert witnesses may be employed to determine if the paramedic had breached their duty by assessing their actions. It is not expected that paramedics provide best-practice care, rather their actions should be those expected of a 'reasonable' paramedic faced with the same circumstances.

The final element, that of causation, is generally the most difficult to establish and it is on the basis of this that a case may or may not proceed to court. Establishing causation relies on proving a link between the breach and the resultant harm using the 'but for' test (*Barnett v Chelsea and Kensington Hospital Management Committee* [1968] 1 All ER 1068); *but for* the breach, the harm would not have occurred (*Wilshire v Essex AHA* [1988] 1 All ER 871, [1988] AC 1074 (HL)). It is not unusual in clinical negligence cases for duty of care to be established, a clear breach of that duty to be found, but causation not found. An example may be a paramedic who attends a patient and gives the wrong drug during the management of a cardiac arrest, administering a dose of atropine instead of adrenaline. There is a clear duty of care, and the standard of care fell below that reasonably expected in that the paramedic gave the wrong drug. As for causation, in this example, the patient was already in cardiac arrest. Their chances of survival are unlikely to be found to have been reduced as a direct result of the drug error. As such, it is likely that a claim in this case would fail.

The lesson to be learnt from Case study 4.1 is that professionals need to demonstrate that they have reflected on their mishaps and developed themselves appropriately. Engagement in such an approach will very likely lessen the chances of an allegation

Case study 4.1

What happened?

A member of the public complains to the HCPC about the treatment of their relative who died following an acute asthma attack. The attending paramedic failed to identify that the patient was asthmatic, treating instead for a drugs overdose. No bronchodilating drugs were administered and the patient suffered a cardiac arrest. The paramedic failed to maintain the patient's airway and did not attempt intubation.

The employer's perspective

An employer's investigation found that the paramedic had failed to correctly diagnose the patient's condition: a competency issue. This was established through an internal investigation which reviewed the incident, interviewed those present and reviewed all patient report documents. The paramedic reflected on the incident and fully engaged in a period of update training and supervision in practice provided by his employer. He continued to work as a paramedic and self-referred to the HCPC, submitting a full reflective account of the incident and his subsequent update training.

The HCPC perspective

When the case was presented to the HCPTS Investigating Committee Panel, it was considered that there was a reasonable prospect of finding that there had been a lack of competence at the time of the call. When considering the issue of current impairment, however, it was found that the level of insight, remorse and reflection, along with engagement in the remedial plan put in place by the employer meant that the paramedic's current fitness to practise was unlikely to be found to be impaired. No further action was taken and the case did not proceed to a full hearing.

The civil litigation perspective

The patient's relative brought a clinical negligence claim against the ambulance service. Duty of care and breach of duty were clearly established in that the paramedic should reasonably have been able to differentiate between an asthma attack and a drugs overdose. On the basis of expert evidence, causation was also established because, had the paramedic treated the patient with bronchodilators, it is likely that, on the balance of probabilities, the patient would have recovered and survived. The case was settled out of court with damages being paid to the patient's relatives. The paramedic involved in the initial treatment was not involved in the litigation process at any point.

of incompetence going forward to a final hearing. From the litigation aspect, it is worth noting that you may not be aware of a claim made against your employer based on a mistake that you made. Thorough and accurate documentation is essential in the event that such claims are made as the paperwork may be all the evidence that is available.

CAPACITY AND CONSENT

All individuals have fundamental legal and ethical rights in determining what happens to their own bodies – the principle of autonomy. To respect a patient's autonomy, the paramedic has to obtain valid consent in the majority of healthcare encounters. Failure to do so may result in an accusation of assault or battery. A paramedic who does not respect this principle may be liable both to legal action by the patient and to action by their regulatory/professional body (DH 2009).

Capacity

The comprehension required for informed consent is based on the patient's capacity to understand the procedure being explained to him or her. Capacity should not be con-fused with a paramedic's assessment of the reasonableness of the person's decision (DH 2009). The paramedic must have an understanding of the MCA, indeed, paramed-ics are among the professional groups named in the MCA Code of Practice (Department for Constitutional Affairs 2007) who are required to have regard to the Act when car-rying out their duties. The MCA confirms in legislation that it should be assumed that adults (legally classified as aged 16 or over) have full legal capacity to make decisions for themselves (*the right to autonomy*) unless it can be shown that they lack capacity to make a decision for themselves at the time it needs to be made. *Under the MCA, a person is not to be treated as unable to make a decision merely because they make what might be considered an unwise decision.*

1. For the purposes of this Act, a person lacks capacity in relation to a matter if at the material time he is unable to make a decision for himself in relation to the matter because of an impairment of, or a disturbance in the functioning of, the mind or brain.
2. It does not matter whether the impairment or disturbance is permanent or temporary.
3. For the purposes of section 2, a person is unable to make a decision for himself if he is unable—
   (a) to understand the information relevant to the decision,
   (b) to retain that information,
   (c) to use or weigh that information as part of the process of making the decision, or
   (d) to communicate his decision (whether by talking, using sign language or any other means).

(Mental Capacity Act 2005, Part 1, p. 2)

In the circumstances described above, the MCA provides a legal framework for how to act and make decisions on behalf of people who lack capacity to make specific decisions for themselves. In order to assess whether the patient understands the information given, the paramedic should explore the individual's ability to decipher what information is relevant in relation to the nature of the decision, to understand why the information is needed and the likely effects of deciding one way or another or making no decision at all. The Code of Practice advises the practitioner to take time to enable the person to take in the information given to them. It also states that the practitioner must give an appropriate amount of information to the patient and must provide information relating to the risks of any treatment or non-treatment. With respect to taking time with the patient, the Code of Practice provides the following guidance on emergency situations:

> In emergency medical situations, urgent decisions will have to be made and immediate action taken in the person's best interests. In these situations, it may not be practical or appropriate to delay the treatment while trying to help the person make their own decisions. However, even in emergency situations, healthcare staff should try to communicate with the person and keep them informed of what is happening.

The paramedic, in the course of a lifetime career, is likely to come across many difficult and complex situations. Therefore, it is essential the paramedic has an understanding of the above powers and bodies. It is strongly recommended that any student paramedic or registered paramedic in difficult circumstances and who is having problems with the issue of capacity should ask for advice from their employer through the normal emergency channels within their organisation.

In a time-critical situation the paramedic should always take the best interests approach to patient care. As long as the paramedic can justify that their actions were, in their professional opinion, in the best interests of the patient, there can be little comeback.

Adult consent

For consent to be valid, a patient has to have the appropriate information and must be able to comprehend the procedure, treatment, intervention and so forth, being proposed by the paramedic. This means that the patient must be able to understand not only the procedure or treatment to be carried out, but also the consequences of such actions. This will allow the individual to consider the pros and cons of such situations and provide what is termed 'informed consent'. The depth to which the paramedic must discuss these details will be determined by several factors. One may be the severity of the presenting condition and the timescale in which the proposed intervention must take place. The vast majority of invasive interventions are undertaken in circumstances where they are necessary to prevent rapid deterioration of a patient's condition. In such circumstances, it would not be realistic, or expected, for the paramedic to discuss all possible issues surrounding a procedure.

The Department of Health (2001a) advises that consent must be given voluntarily without duress or undue influence from health professionals, relatives or friends. In order for the patient to give consent, it does not have to be written, as this does not exclusively prove the consent is valid. Written evidence is used to record the patient's decision and the events which may have taken place. Consent can only be valid if the patient has capacity.

Chapter 8 to explore the issues of mental ill health in more detail; **Chapter 13** to read about the complexities of safeguarding adults; **Chapter 14** for the variables and complexity associated with establishing consent and capacity when caring for people with dementia and **Chapter 15** for the ethical and legal issues that may arise when caring for people at the end of their lives.

Case study 4.2

What happened?

A paramedic solo responder attends an elderly patient who is resident at a nursing home. The patient is presenting with mild abdominal pain that they have been experiencing for a number of weeks. The paramedic finds that the patient's observations are normal and suggests that an appointment be made for the patient's own GP to attend. The carers at the nursing home insist that the patient is taken to hospital and say that they have spoken to the patient's son who also wants the patient taken to hospital. The patient is able to understand and retain the information given to her and appears content to await a GP visit, but is anxious not to upset the staff at the home.

The ethical perspective

The patient has demonstrated capacity, and therefore is able to give or refuse consent to treatment. Undue influence from the nursing staff and her son may impact on the decision, so that it is not entirely autonomous. Similarly, it is not the paramedic's job to convince the patient either way. The paramedic should ensure that sufficient information is given to the patient to allow her to come to her own decision-enabling autonomy. The principle of justice may be considered by the paramedic; would calling an ambulance to convey this patient remove the resource from others who may need it more or would leaving an unwell patient at the nursing home divert the attentions of the nursing staff away from their other patients? Non-maleficence may also be considered; would conveying this patient to hospital expose them to potential risks from infection or bed sores which would not develop if she were to remain at the nursing home? What course of action would be the most beneficial for the patient? A consideration of beneficence may mean that that the paramedic considers contacting an out-of-hours service rather than waiting for the patient's own GP.

The legal perspective

As the patient has demonstrated capacity, the paramedic cannot remove her to hospital against her will, regardless of the wishes of the patient's family or the nursing staff; to do so would constitute an assault.

Child consent

The Department of Health (DH 2009) explains that before examining, treating or caring for a child, the paramedic must seek consent. Young people aged 16 and 17 are presumed to have the competence to give consent for themselves. Younger children who understand fully what is involved in the proposed procedure can also give consent, although it is better if their parents are involved in the decision at the time it is being made. In other cases, someone with parental responsibility must give consent on the child's behalf, unless they cannot be reached in an emergency. If a 'competent child' consents to treatment, a parent cannot override that consent. Legally, a parent can consent if a child who is deemed competent refuses, but it is likely that taking such a serious step will be rare.

Generally, the complexities surrounding child consent tend to be reserved for debate in the hospital or primary care environment around issues such as immunisation or organ transplantation. It is highly unlikely that paramedics will ever have to deal with a child, or their parent, who refuses a proposed life-saving intervention. If in doubt, adopt the best interests approach.

Patient refusal

In practice, refusal to consent presents a greater challenge for the paramedic. Competent adult patients may refuse treatment (DH 2009); however, any refusal of treatment must be an informed refusal. The only exception to this rule is where treatment is for a mental disorder/illness and the patient is detained under the Mental Health Acts (1983; 2007). If a patient is not competent, then a paramedic may treat the patient if it is in their best interests. This may include the wishes of the patient when they were competent. People close to the patient may be able to give more information and help the paramedic make a balanced, well-informed decision in such circumstances. Patients may make decisions relating to their future care either verbally or in writing. In cases relating to life-sustaining treatment any decisions must be in writing and independently witnessed. The MCA introduced 'advance decisions' which take the place of advanced directives or living wills which may have preceded them. Advance decisions can only refuse consent to certain treatments or interventions in given circumstances, they cannot demand interventions.

Case study 4.3

What happened?

A paramedic ambulance crew are called to a 45-year-old male patient in cardiac arrest. On arrival, the patient's wife presents the crew with a Lasting Power of Attorney (LPA) document that identifies her as the holder of the LPA. The crew initiate basic life support while the document is checked. It is confirmed that the LPA gives the patient's wife decision-making capacity in aspects of healthcare and specifically gives decision-making rights in end of life situations.

The patient's wife indicates to the crew that she wants them to stop CPR as her husband was terminally ill and would not want to be revived.

The ethical perspective

By appointing a lasting power of attorney, the patient has delegated their autonomy to their representative. Although the crew may believe that, considering the principle of beneficence, the best course of action for the patient would be to commence resuscitation, the patient has expressed to his representative that this is not what he would want. Even if the crew do not agree with the decision of the patient, expressed through their attorney, they must still respect it as an autonomous decision. Not carrying out resuscitation may be an uncomfortable decision, but it would be ethically justified.

The legal perspective

If the crew reasonably believe the information given to them is true, then they would be legally obliged to respect the wishes of the patient's representative. If there was any doubt regarding the identity of the attorney or the validity of the documentation, then the crew could commence resuscitation and convey the patient while a definitive answer was sought from the Court of Protection. There can be no legal claim for 'wrongful life', meaning that if the crew did successfully revive the patient and it was later discovered that this was against his wishes, the patient would not be able to sue the crew for taking life-saving action.

CONFIDENTIALITY AND DATA PROTECTION

The NHS Code of Practice, Confidentiality (DH 2003a: 7), clearly defines a duty of confidence as:

> when one person discloses information to another, e.g. patient to clinician in circumstances where it is reasonable to expect that the information will be held in confidence:
>
> a It is a legal obligation that is derived from case law;
> b It is a requirement established within professional codes of conduct;
> c It must be included within NHS employment contracts as a specific requirement linked to disciplinary procedures.

The relationship between healthcare professionals and their patients has always been considered especially significant with regard to disclosure of information. Much of the information given to the paramedic is often of a sensitive nature and there is an expectation that this information will not be passed onto others without the consent

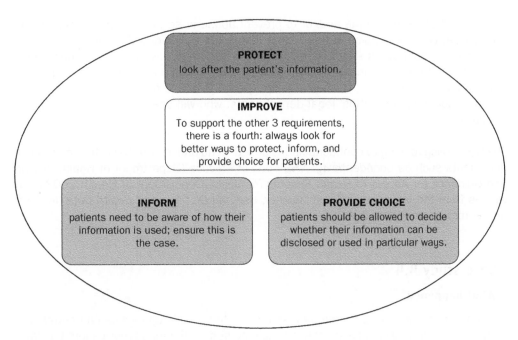

Figure 4.1 The confidentiality model

Source: Adapted from DH (2003a: 10).

of the individual concerned. The confidentiality model (see Figure 4.1) advocated by the Department of Health (2003a: 10) may assist paramedics in their main responsibilities regarding patient confidentiality. This model will naturally involve paramedics in other aspects of quality monitoring, such as clinical audit, in order to establish ways to improve their own and others' professional practice.

It is rare that paramedics are the only healthcare professionals involved in the patient's care; an inter-professional approach is the usual practice. It is necessary to disclose information to health and social care professionals when paramedic practitioners, for example, convey patients to emergency departments (ED) to provide the uninterrupted 'patient care pathway'. In such situations, a copy of the patient record will be left with the relevant ED staff. Patients' consent in such situations should be sought, to enable disclosure of their information wherever possible. When patients are conveyed to hospital, their consent will have been obtained routinely in the vast majority of cases. It is accepted that by agreeing to be taken to hospital, disclosure of information relating to the patient will be shared by the paramedic with those entitled to receive it.

There will be situations where the need for confidentiality has to be balanced against what is termed the 'public interest'. Under common law, practitioners are permitted to disclose personal information in order to support detection, investigation and punishment of serious crime and/or to prevent abuse or serious harm to others where they judge, on a case-by-case basis, that disclosure outweighs the obligation of confidentiality. Practitioners should consider each case on its own merits. On occasions, due to the nature of the incident, it may be difficult to make a decision. In such situations, it may be necessary to seek legal or specialist advice from professional, regulatory or employing authorities' legal departments, who will seek further legal advice as required.

The NHS policy relating to confidentiality is based on guidance from Department of Health documents such as *Confidentiality: NHS Code of Practice* (Department of Health 2003a) and *Guidance for Access to Health Records Requests* (Department of Health 2003b), as well as from the Information Commissioner, *Use and Disclosure of Health Data* (Information Commissions Office 2002).

Case study 4.4

What happened?

You are in the ambulance station mess room with six colleagues when a paramedic arrives back from a call. He proceeds to tell the staff in the mess room about the call that he has just attended. He says that they went to Kipling Rise where he treated a 14-year-old girl called Mary for severe abdominal pain. He diagnosed an ectopic pregnancy and took the girl straight to the emergency department of the hospital where she was transferred to theatre and underwent an emergency operation. The paramedic is very pleased that he correctly diagnosed the presentation.

You notice that one of your other colleagues is very quiet and looks angry. It transpires that this colleague is the uncle of Mary and this is the first he has heard of his niece either being unwell or being sexually active.

Has confidentiality been breached?

Patient confidentiality has definitely been breached in this case. From the information disclosed – name, age and address – the patient could easily be identified.

How could this have been avoided?

Mess room discussions and debriefs are an important element of personal and professional development and should be encouraged, as long as confidentiality is respected. There is no breach if there is no disclosure of identifiable data. This case could just as easily have been discussed as a purely clinical presentation with no reference to the patient's name or address. Identifiable data does not only include names and addresses; if the identity of a patient can be determined by the information disclosed, perhaps due to the unique nature of the presentation within a hospital, then confidentiality can be considered to have been breached.

Reflection: points to consider

Have you observed colleagues try to maintain patient confidentiality in public places during an emergency? Think about the strategies you can use to try and maintain confidentiality in emergency situations. Also think about the possible consequences of ignoring the importance of trying to maintain confidentiality.

The relationship between healthcare professionals and their patients has always been considered especially significant with regard to disclosure of information. Much of the information given to the paramedic is often of a sensitive nature and there is an expectation that this information will not be passed onto others without the consent of the individual concerned.

Data protection

The Data Protection Act 1998 describes the processes for obtaining, recording, holding, using and sharing information. The issue of confidentiality and data protection requires careful management by paramedics. When dealing with the public, healthcare professionals, other professions, emergency services or agencies, there is the potential for information to be leaked about patients and their treatment. It is easy at the scene of an emergency call to declare information about a patient that may be overheard by members of the public. Patient records present another risk to patient confidentiality. Patient records completed by paramedics with respect to patient treatment and details must be recorded as accurately as possible and be protected from viewing by those not entitled to do so. Safe storage and disposal of these are also a requirement of the Data Protection Act 1998 and employing organisations' policies and procedures.

CONCLUSION

It is accepted that the role of a paramedic brings with it a number of important legal areas within their scope of practice. Paramedics need to be aware of the consequences of their actions and be able to maintain a professional, legal and ethical approach at all times. Understanding the law is particularly important as paramedic practice continues to develop and broaden in scope. The HCPC seeks to provide a framework within which paramedics are able to practise to the highest standards and simultaneously maintain their accountability to patients, clients and other professionals. This chapter represents an overview of some of the most common legal and ethical issues facing the paramedic in the twenty-first century. Many of the areas require further investigation and wider reading in order to obtain a more comprehensive understanding of the issues covered in this chapter and the list of suggested reading at the end of this chapter will be useful for this.

Chapter key points:

- Ethical dilemmas are part of everyday practice in the NHS.
- Ethical considerations must underpin the clinical approaches undertaken by the paramedic.
- Paramedic ethical dilemmas occur across the lifespan, due to the nature of the role.
- As registered healthcare professionals, paramedics are accountable for their actions.
- Paramedics therefore require a good understanding of the law in relation to their role.

REFERENCES AND SUGGESTED READING

Beauchamp, T.L. and Childress, J.F. (2013) *Principles of Biomedical Ethics*, 7th edn. New York: Oxford University Press.

Department of Constitutional Affairs (2007) *Mental Capacity Act 2005 Code of Practice*. London: The Stationery Office.

DH (Department of Health) (1983) *Mental Health Act*. London: Department of Health.

DH (Department of Health) (2001a) *Consent: What You Have a Right to Expect. A Guide for Adults*. London: Department of Health.

DH (Department of Health) (2001b) *The Health and Social Work Professions Order*. London: Department of Health.

DH (Department of Health) (2003a) *Confidentiality: National Health Service Code of Practice*. London: Department of Health.

DH (Department of Health) (2003b) *Guidance for Access to Health Records Requests under the Data Protection Act 1998*, Version 2. London: Department of Health.

DH (Department of Health) (2009) *Reference Guide to Consent for Examination on Treatment of Children*, 2nd edn. London: Department of Health.

Health and Care Professions Council (2014) *Standards of Proficiency: Paramedics*. London: HCPC.

Health and Care Professions Council (2016a) *Standards of Conduct, Performance and Ethics*. London: HCPC.

Health and Care Professions Council (2016b) *Guidance on Conduct and Ethics for Students*. London: HCPC.

Her Majesty's Government (1998) *Data Protection Act*. London: The Stationery Office.

Her Majesty's Government (2005) *The Mental Capacity Act*. London: The Stationery Office.

Her Majesty's Government (2007) *Mental Health Act*. London: The Stationery Office.

Information Commissions Office (2002) *Use and Disclosure of Health Data. Guidance on the Application of the Data Protection Act 1998*. London: HMSO.

National Institute for Clinical Excellence (2004) *Self-harm in Over-8s: Short-Term Management and Prevention of Recurrence*. Clinical Guideline 16. London: NICE.

Research and evidence-based practice

Julia Williams, Rachael T. Fothergill and
Joanna Shaw

In this chapter:

- Introduction
- Why is this relevant?
- The role of the paramedic in research
- What is evidence-based practice?
- What is research?
- Involving service users in research
- Using existing evidence
- Types of research
- The importance of the research question
- An overview of quantitative research
- An overview of qualitative research
- Summary of common characteristics of qualitative and quantitative research
- What do we mean by mixed methods research?
- The importance of research ethics and research governance
- Barriers to implementing evidence-based practice
- Conclusion
- Chapter key points
- References and suggested reading
- Useful websites

INTRODUCTION

Research and evidence-based practice are more important in healthcare today than they have ever been in the history of the National Health Service (NHS) in the UK. Research is no longer an 'optional extra' and the message is that research must be embedded as core business for healthcare organisations such as NHS Trusts.

Relevant clinical research is exciting as it has the potential to ensure that we are providing our patients with high quality treatments and optimal patient management grounded in best evidence. Research can be viewed as the 'disruptive technology' which cataly-ses change in clinical practices, if indeed change is required. Clinical research is relevant to paramedics as it can really make a difference to our profession's development, to patients' experiences of pre-hospital and other emergency and unscheduled urgent care, and, ultimately, it can influence and improve patient outcomes. With a renewed emphasis on the value and importance of research in healthcare, there are increasing opportunities for paramedics to be involved in research studies. Such direct involvement enables paramedics to actively influence developments in patient care and the direction of future clinical practices.

However, one chapter can only hope to provide a brief introduction to evidence-based practice and research, and what is offered here is an overview of some of the key compo-nents of these concepts. It focuses specifically on research as a mechanism for inform-ing best practice and evidencing high quality patient care. Further reading will be required in order to fully appreciate and understand the complexities of the processes described.

WHY IS THIS RELEVANT?

Research and evidence-based practice are central to the role of the paramedic, and, in fact, any healthcare professional. Research influences all areas of healthcare provision as well as the development of the paramedic profession as a whole, as it evolves to meet healthcare demand. Research impacts on the currency of clinical guidelines, protocols, development of healthcare systems and policies, and options in treatment and clinical management of our patients. Evidence-based practice has a direct effect on paramedic practice and is something that clinicians are involved with on a daily basis. This is true, no matter where paramedics work. More recently, paramedics are being employed in increasing numbers by a diverse range of organisations other than ambulance services, who have for many years been the largest employer of ambulance clinicians.

As part of professional registration in the UK, all paramedics, irrespective of where they are employed, are expected to meet specific Standards of Proficiency (Health and Care Professions Council 2014) in relation to professional practice, several of which are related to knowledge of research and evidence-based practice. For example, the HCPC (2014) states that registrants must:

- 'be able to use research, reasoning and problem solving skills to determine appropriate actions' (2014: 15);
- 'be aware of a range of research methodologies' (2014: 16);
- 'be able to evaluate research and other evidence to inform their own practice' (2014: 15).

Therefore, a HCPC-registered paramedic must ensure that they are research-aware and have an understanding of what research findings and evidence underpin their profes-sional practice. This is one of several reasons why learning about research and evidence-based care is relevant for paramedics.

THE ROLE OF THE PARAMEDIC IN RESEARCH

Engagement in evidence-based practice is a HCPC registration requirement and every paramedic has a role to play in research, to varying degrees. As a minimum, paramedics need to be research-aware and use current evidence in their professional practice. Some will take their interest in research further, contributing in a number of ways, such as assisting with project design, providing clinical expertise, collecting data or providing recommendations for change. Others will want to follow a full-time clinical research career trajectory as outlined in the College of Paramedics' Career Framework (Figure 5.1), preparing them to become research leaders of the future.

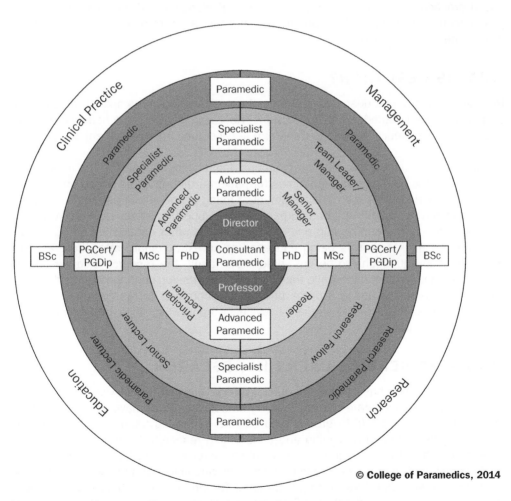

Figure 5.1 College of Paramedics Career Framework (2014)

WHAT IS EVIDENCE-BASED PRACTICE?

Evidence-based practice started its journey as 'evidence-based medicine' and is described by Sackett et al. (1996) as developing its philosophical origins in Paris in the mid-nineteenth century. They define evidence-based medicine as 'the conscientious, explicit, and judicious use of current best evidence in making decisions about the care of individual patients. The practice of evidence-based medicine means integrating individual clinical expertise with the best available external clinical evidence from systematic research' (Sackett et al. 1996: 71).

Over time, evidence-based medicine, originally aimed at doctors, expanded to include other healthcare professionals, moving away from the term 'medicine' towards 'evidence-based practice' or 'evidence-based healthcare'. Evidence-based practice has become synonymous with high quality patient care and has a direct bearing on professional development for paramedics.

WHAT IS RESEARCH?

Research is a term that describes a systematic investigation into a specific area aiming to generate new knowledge and conclusions. Research is vital in the healthcare sector to provide the evidence needed to transform services and improve patient care.

In order to demonstrate that new interventions and developments offer the most effective care and the best possible outcomes for patients, they must be based on research evidence. However, the pace of development of many pre-hospital treatments and practices has been so rapid that it has surpassed the supporting evidence base. While the evidence base is growing rapidly and pre-hospital and other emergency and unscheduled urgent care research is being published at an extraordinary rate, there are still gaps and many questions to be answered. As a result, the research of other professions often needs to be used while the paramedic profession continues to build its own evidence. Paramedics are in a prime position to contribute to research in numerous areas of clinical practice and shape the evidence upon which their profession will be based in the future.

INVOLVING SERVICE USERS IN RESEARCH

In recent years there has been an increase in the involvement of service users and the general public in healthcare research. Many ambulance Trusts have their own Patient and Public Involvement (PPI) groups who can be extremely useful when developing research questions, and designing and undertaking research. Involving service users in research should not be seen just as a token exercise, as having a PPI perspective in all elements of your research can be a valuable and illuminating experience, helping to ensure the study's relevance to patient care. To find out more about how to achieve this, it is worth exploring the INVOLVE programme which was set up in 1996 and is part of the National Institute for Health Research (NIHR). INVOLVE helps 'to support active public involvement in NHS, public health and social care research' (http://www.invo. org.uk/ accessed 8 January 2018) and provides a range of resources to facilitate both researchers and the public to participate in these activities effectively.

Ambulance services' research is demonstrating a high level of engagement with service users in the development of their research and there are published examples of varying levels of public involvement ranging from collaboration in the development of research questions through to participation in data collection and analysis, and on to actual publication of findings (Hirst et al. 2016; Irving et al. 2018).

 Reflection: points to consider

Identify a research study that you know about which is relevant to paramedics. How did they involve service users within this study? Can you think of other ways that this could be done?

USING EXISTING EVIDENCE

The paramedics' regulatory body, the HCPC, expects paramedics to 'be able to draw on appropriate knowledge and skills to inform practice' (HCPC 2014: 14) and, as outlined earlier, there are specific expectations in relation to appraising research and other evidence. To start to meet these requirements, it is, therefore, essential that paramedics possess the skills to find and evaluate relevant published research evidence.

Sourcing research evidence

There are multiple electronic databases available to search for published research evidence. PubMed, CINAHL Plus (Cumulative Index to Nursing and Allied Health Literature), Scopus, Web of Science, and Science Direct are just a few of those that might be relevant to the paramedic profession. It is beneficial to use more than one database as each may cover slightly different publications. To facilitate research and evidence-based practice, all NHS employees have the opportunity to set up an Athens account for easy access to many journals.

To enhance a search, it is possible to look for multiple relevant search terms, or specify terms you do not wish to be included. Box 5.1 outlines the most common BOOLEAN operators which help to connect your search terms to ultimately narrow or broaden your search.

Once articles are found, it is beneficial to search through the reference lists to find further relevant sources. It is also possible to search by author if you know the names of specialists in your area of interest, and hand-search the contents pages of relevant

---

Box 5.1 Common BOOLEAN operators

- AND: Narrows your search to return only articles that include all of your search terms.
- OR: Broadens your search to return articles that include any of your search terms (can be used when there are several terms for a certain aspect).
- NOT: Limits your search to prevent articles that include irrelevant terms.

---

journals. Some electronic databases also allow you to set up citation alerts to send you a message if an article you are interested in is cited elsewhere. Grey literature, such as government reports and guidelines, also provide sources of evidence which may be of interest and can be found on databases such as OpenGrey and NHS Evidence.

Critical appraisal

Not all published articles report on 'good' research, therefore, it is important for a paramedic to be able to critically appraise the evidence to determine its relevance and validity. By studying the research methods used, any potential limitations can be understood and a judgement made as to whether the research is acceptable.

There are many tools available to appraise research articles, some specific to certain research methods while others are more generic checklists. When reading research evidence, it is helpful to consider the general points in Box 5.2.

Box 5.2 Points to consider when reading research evidence

- Was the purpose of the research clearly explained?
- Do you agree with how the research was done? For example, the intervention the patients received? Was the research design appropriate?
- Do the results sound reasonable or is there something odd about them that is not explained?
- Are the conclusions justified? Have the authors provided adequate evidence to support the conclusions?
- What do you think are the positive points about the study in general?
- Are there any negative aspects or limitations? For example, is the research very specific to the country or healthcare system it has been undertaken in?
- Is it a worthwhile piece of work or has it got the 'so what?' factor? Does it provide valuable evidence that contributes to existing literature?
- Would you change what you do based on this research? Do you trust the findings?
- Does the research identify any 'gaps' for future research?
- If you were asked to do the same project, is there anything you would change?

Reflection: points to consider

Self-assess your own skills and abilities in critical appraisal. Do you need to do anything to improve your effectiveness in critical appraisal of published research literature? If so, make a list of what support you think you need and what you can achieve yourself. Then discuss your development needs at your next work appraisal, or with your lecturers if you are on a university programme. In addition you could contact your local Council for Allied Health Professions Research (CAHPR) hub (http://cahpr.csp.org.uk/ accessed 8 January 2018) as there are many CPD events run by these hubs and they have staff who can support you in the development of these skills.

TYPES OF RESEARCH

Research can be broadly categorised as quantitative or qualitative; mixed methods research is increasingly being used within healthcare research to examine phenomena from a variety of perspectives. Research is often confused with other types of projects such as service evaluation and clinical audit as outlined in Box 5.3.

 Clinical audit is discussed in **Chapter 3** where you will find more detail about what it is, its importance and how to undertake this activity.

Box 5.3 Definitions of research, clinical audit and service evaluation

Research

Research generates new knowledge by answering a clearly defined question. It typically requires extra data to be collected to that routinely collected, and may involve interventions not used in standard practice.

Clinical audit

Clinical audit measures the current standard of clinical care against a benchmark standard of care. It is used to inform delivery of best care and may include additional interviews or questionnaires.

Service evaluation

Service evaluation (service development or quality improvement) examines care and interventions already in practice. It generally uses existing data, without reference to a standard, but may include additional interviews or questionnaires.

THE IMPORTANCE OF THE RESEARCH QUESTION

Never underestimate the importance of good research questions or the length of time it might take to refine your research question(s) to get them as clear as possible. As with many areas of research, there is no one way of writing these and it is beyond the scope of this chapter to identify all the conventions used in development of research questions within both qualitative and quantitative research. Many textbooks on research will cover these areas and there are examples of these texts in the suggested reading at the end of this chapter.

Your research question should not fall foul of the 'so what?' factor! So you must ask yourself if your research adds to existing knowledge? Is it relevant? Is there a need? Will it influence clinical practice? Will it improve patient experience/outcomes? If it does not, then your study may have the 'so what?' factor and you should think again before investing further energy and resources in the research.

Hulley et al. (2013) recommend using the FINER framework when developing research questions (see Box 5.4).

It is important to get the research question and any associated aims and objectives as clear as possible, as these will inform the subsequent decisions about choice of research design and methods, as outlined in the following sections.

AN OVERVIEW OF QUANTITATIVE RESEARCH

Quantitative research is largely defined by the collection of numerical data or data that can be enumerated. It is often associated with inductive reasoning where the researcher tests existing theories to prove or disprove them. Quantitative research includes

---

Box 5.4 Characteristics of a good research question

- *Feasible*: Can the study actually be completed? Can it be done in a reasonable time? Do you have the necessary funding? Have you got access to appropriate expertise? Do you have access to an adequate sample size? Is it manageable in scope?
- *Interesting*: Do you and your colleagues think it is interesting? What are the views of patients, funding bodies and other interested parties?
- *Novel*: Will this add to existing knowledge? Does it fill a 'gap' in existing literature?
- *Ethical*: Have you considered all ethical aspects of your study? Would it be approved by a Research Ethics Committee?
- *Relevant*: Has your study got the 'so what?' factor?

Adapted from Hulley et al. (2013).

both experimental studies such as randomised controlled trials and experiments, and non-experimental studies such as surveys, correlational studies and case studies (Cutter 2012). The gold standard of quantitative research is often deemed to be the randomised controlled trial.

An illustration of the general stages involved in quantitative research is provided in Figure 5.2, presenting a framework to show what a quantitative research study might look like in terms of its general overall structure. You should use other research litera-ture (see the references and suggested reading) to learn more about these stages, as it is beyond the remit of this chapter to examine these in further detail here.

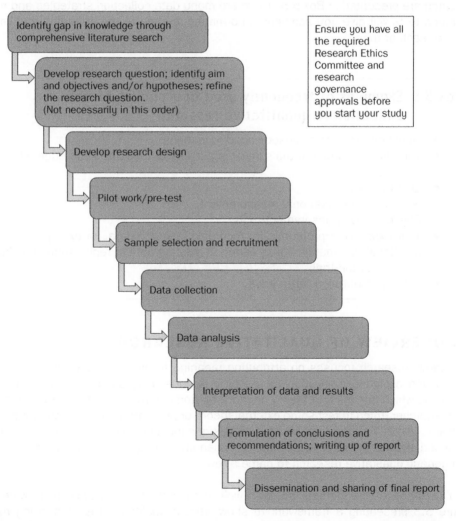

Figure 5.2 Linear process of activities commonly observed in quantitative research

Reflection: points to consider

Find a recent piece of published quantitative research related to the paramedic profession which you find interesting. As you read it, map the key stages identified in this section to your chosen paper and identify the similarities and/or differences between this framework and what the researcher(s) used in your chosen paper.

Some examples of frequently used approaches to data collection in quantitative research are presented in Box 5.5. There are many data collection strategies and most research texts will give you additional information relating to the strengths and limitations of each of these.

Box 5.5 Examples of frequently used approaches to data collection in quantitative research

- Questionnaires with 'closed-ended' questions.
- Various measurement tools including scales to measure knowledge, skills, attitudes, etc.
- Likert scales.
- Structured observational measurement.
- Physiological measurement tools.
- Trial/experiment proformas for recording research data, for example, additional information boxes added to existing patient report forms for the duration of the trial.
- Highly structured interviews.

AN OVERVIEW OF QUALITATIVE RESEARCH

Qualitative research focuses on attributing meaning to human behaviours and experiences, and exploring motivation for people's actions. It is associated with inductive reasoning which 'means that theory or interpretation emerges from the data rather than the researcher trying to *test* some external theory or prior interpretation from the outset' (Williams 2012: 74). Qualitative research designs include various approaches such as grounded theory, interpretive description, phenomenology, ethnography, case study; and generic qualitative research to name a few.

An illustration of the general stages involved in qualitative research is provided in Figure 5.3 presenting a framework to show what a qualitative research study might look like in terms of its general overall structure. As identified in the previous section on

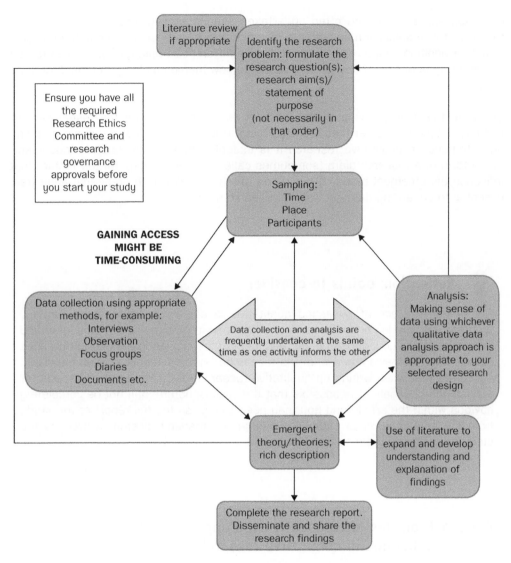

Figure 5.3 Cyclical process of activities commonly observed in qualitative research

Source: Adapted from Williams (2012: 77).

quantitative research, you should use other research methods literature to learn about these stages.

Qualitative research, at first glance at Figure 5.3, might look chaotic and lacking in structure. It contains similar activities to those found in quantitative research (Figure 5.2) but their sequencing may not be the same. Due to its flexible nature, and because data collection and analysis are often undertaken simultaneously, the emerging findings from qualitative analysis may lead the researcher to revisit parts of the research cycle to gather additional data, or perhaps include a different sample group, or even to add in another type of data collection to investigate new themes as they emerge during the study.

Be aware that having this potential flexibility is not a licence for the researchers to just randomly do whatever they feel like doing! Unstructured is not the same as being unsystematic. In qualitative research it is essential that the researchers document, in the form of a research diary (sometimes called a research log), all the factors that influence the emergent research design as this forms part of the research audit trail, essential to enhancing the rigour of the research study.

 Reflection: points to consider

Find a recent piece of published qualitative research related to the paramedic profession which you find interesting. As you read it, map the key stages identified in this section to your chosen paper and identify the similarities and/or differences between this framework and what the researcher(s) used in your chosen paper. Do not forget that when writing up qualitative research, given the word limitations for publishing in journals, it is possible that the cyclical nature may not be completely obvious within the article and you may need to access the full report of the study from the researcher(s) to establish whether the research design evolved as the study progressed, and if so how it changed.

Box 5.6 Examples of frequently used approaches to data collection in qualitative research

- Interviews – usually semi-structured or unstructured
- Focus groups
- Questionnaires using 'open-ended' questions
- Online discussion forums
- Social media including Facebook, texts, etc.
- Observation: participant and/or non-participant
- Diaries
- Photographs
- Videos/films
- Biographies

Table 5.1 Summary of common characteristics of qualitative and quantitative research

Qualitative	Quantitative
Inductive reasoning	Deductive reasoning
Focuses on unknown issues	Focuses on known issues
Purpose is to explore, describe, understand	Purpose is to measure and/or test and/or predict
The study design is cyclical, flexible and emergent	The study design is fully developed before data collection, usually described as a linear process
Gathers non-numerical data	Gathers numerical data or data that can be assigned a numerical value
Methods are frequently semi-structured or unstructured, flexible	Methods are predetermined, highly structured, standardised, inflexible
Researcher frequently interacts with the people being studied, therefore seen as more subjective	Researcher is distanced from subjects, therefore seen as more objective
Criteria used to evaluate methodological rigour usually include credibility, dependability, confirmability and transferability	Criteria used to evaluate methodological rigour usually include reliability and validity.
Findings may be transferable to other settings	Results may be generalisable to other populations
The research process is systematic	The research process is systematic

There are many data collection strategies that are appropriate for qualitative research (examples of which are given in Box 5.6) and most published research methods literature will give you additional information relating to the strengths and limitations of each of these. The common characteristics and differences between qualitative and quantitative research are presented in Table 5.1.

WHAT DO WE MEAN BY MIXED METHODS RESEARCH?

Mixed methods research design is gaining popularity in healthcare research. However, there are complex debates as to how this all fits together philosophically in relation to mixing research methodologies.

For the purpose of this chapter, we just want to highlight that different authors may have different interpretations of the term 'mixed methods' research. Classically (and the more frequent interpretation), 'mixed methods' means using both qualitative and quantitative methods in the same study. However, Creswell (2009: 205) alerts us to the fact that not everyone uses the same terminology to mean the same thing and that sometimes authors use other terms for using both qualitative and quantitative methods in the same study, such as 'multimethod' or 'mixed methodology'. It can be confusing. It would be easier if there were a standardised approach to the use of terminology in general, but do not worry unnecessarily about it. To avoid confusion, just make sure that you are clear what you mean by these terms, and establish what the authors are referring to in each of the papers that you critically appraise.

THE IMPORTANCE OF RESEARCH ETHICS AND RESEARCH GOVERNANCE

During the course of history, there have been some horrific practices undertaken in the name of research, including medical experiments on prisoners in Nazi concentration camps, without the subjects' consent, during World War II (United States Holocaust Memorial Museum 2016). Such ethical atrocities coming to light began a movement which saw the development and implementation of governance frameworks such as the Declaration of Helsinki (WMA 2013), the Nuremberg Code (The Nuremberg Code, undated), Good Clinical Practice Guidance (ICH 2016) and the UK policy framework for health and social care research (NHS HRA 2017). Each framework aims to assure the safety of research participants through the key ethical principles of autonomy, beneficence, non-maleficence and justice. It is a requirement of all NHS Trusts to adhere to ethical and research governance requirements, and for all relevant research to be reviewed by an independent research ethics committee (REC) to protect the rights, interests and safety of participants.

Before any data collection can begin, if your study requires ethical permissions, then this must be achieved before you start your research. You need to be crystal clear as to which governance and ethics committee permissions and approvals you need for your study. If you have any doubts, you should approach the research units within your Trust or organisation where you are going to be undertaking your research. They have staff who will be able to advise you and who are familiar with the frameworks and systems. Additionally, a useful resource is the Health Research Authority's decision tool, called 'Is my study research?', which helps you decide whether your work is actually research and, if it is, whether it will need NHS REC approval (www.hra-decisiontools.org.uk/research/index.html accessed 8 January 2018).

 Chapter 4 for more detail on ethical principles.

BARRIERS TO IMPLEMENTING EVIDENCE-BASED PRACTICE

The process of implementing evidence-based practice requires careful consideration and the decision to use research to change any healthcare practices and/or systems must not be undertaken lightly and would rarely be the sole responsibility of any one individual clinician.

While paramedics have been shown to be receptive to evidence-based practice as a concept (Simpson et al., 2012), as with other healthcare professions, there are many barriers to its implementation (Williams et al. 2015). One of the common challenges is a conflict between guidelines and evidence which is thought to arise from delays in producing new evidence, finite resources for guideline development, and a lack of quality criteria for guidelines (Clark et al. 2006).

Rosser (2012) also identifies time as being a potential barrier and discusses this in relation to clinicians not having or being afforded adequate time to access and review current literature. Additionally she suggests that not having relevant skills and knowledge to effectively critically appraise published literature is an obvious barrier to the implementation of research findings into practice.

Despite these challenges, it is encouraging to see evidence-based practice being successfully implemented in the rapidly developing field of paramedic science with results and findings from research studies being used to make changes in many areas. Some examples are given in Box 5.7.

Box 5.7 Examples of areas being influenced by research related to paramedic practice

- Healthcare service provision
- Policy development
- Clinical skills
- Clinical management and treatments
- Clinical pathways and ambulance response options
- Medical devices and pharmacology
- Interprofessional working
- Paramedic health and well-being
- Educational development
- Expanding roles and scope of practice
- Service users' experiences
- Paramedics' experiences

Reflection: points to consider

How can you become involved in supporting the development and implementation of evidence-based practice in your NHS Trust? Are there any working groups, committees or research projects you might be interested in contributing to?

CONCLUSION

This chapter has highlighted some of the complexities of research and evidence-based practice. It is an exciting area which has direct relevance to paramedic practice and the paramedic profession. Research as a career choice for paramedics is gaining traction and employing Research Paramedics is becoming far more frequent within healthcare organisations. There are many studies now initiated by and led by paramedics in collaboration with other healthcare professionals and discipline experts.

Research is, to coin a phrase, a 'journey' and everyone has to start somewhere. It is a learning process and even after years of working directly within research, we are still learning about research philosophies, methods and approaches within critical inquiry. In part, that is what makes it such a challenging and exciting discipline. We acknowledge that research and evidence-based practice are a vast area and one introductory chapter can only begin to scratch the surface of some of the themes, concepts and challenges. We have identified topics that require further reading and exploration, and signposted you to resources that will hopefully add to your already existing knowledge base on research methods, process and practice. It is hoped that the various sections have raised your awareness of the concepts of evidence-based practice and research, and highlighted the potential for research evidence to inform and improve patient treatment and management.

Chapter key points:
- Research and evidence-based practice are concepts which have direct relevance to the paramedic profession.
- Research is essential to achieve the highest quality evidence-based patient care and management.
- HCPC paramedics must have an awareness of research methodologies and be able to evaluate existing research and other evidence.
- Research is core business for NHS Trusts and is no longer an optional activity.
- There are increasing opportunities for paramedics to engage in research activities at a variety of different levels, from having an awareness of

research findings, through to following a full-time clinical research career pathway.

- It is important to be aware of the characteristics of quantitative and qualitative research and what makes a good research question.
- Service users should be involved in the development of healthcare research to increase its clinical relevance and to avoid the 'so what?' phenomenon.
- These are exciting times as the paramedic profession firmly establishes itself as a serious contender in the discipline of clinical research. In recent years, we have observed a significant increase in published research that has been initiated by and undertaken by paramedics. Paramedics are making a substantive contribution to the health and social care research agenda.

REFERENCES AND SUGGESTED READING

Clark, E., Donovan, E.F. and Schoettker, P. (2006) From outdated to updated, keeping clinical guidelines valid. *International Journal of Qualitative Health Care*, 18(3): 165–6.

College of Paramedics (2014) *Career Framework*. Bridgwater: College of Paramedics.

College of Paramedics/Health Education England (2018) *Paramedics Career Framework*. Interactive web-based version. Available at: https://www.collegeofparamedics.co.uk/downloads/College_of_ParamedicsInteractiveCareer_Framework16.pdf (accessed 8 January 2018).

Creswell, J.W. (2009) *Research Design: Qualitative, Quantitative and Mixed Methods Approaches*, 3rd edn. Los Angeles: SAGE.

Creswell, J.W. and Creswell, J.D. (2018) *Research Design: Qualitative, Quantitative and Mixed Methods Approaches*, 5th edn. Los Angeles: SAGE.

Cutter, J. (2012) Quantitative research in paramedic practice: an overview, in P. Griffiths and G.P. Mooney (eds) *The Paramedic's Guide to Research: An Introduction*. Maidenhead: Open University Press.

Greenhalgh, T. (2014) *How to Read a Paper: The Basics of Evidence-Based Medicine*, 5th edn. Chichester: John Wiley & Sons.

Griffiths, P. and Mooney, G.P. (eds) (2012) *The Paramedic's Guide to Research*. Maidenhead: Open University Press.

Health and Care Professions Council (HCPC) (2014) *Standards of Proficiency: Paramedics*. London: Health and Care Professions Council.

Hirst, E., Irving, A. and Goodacre, S. (2016) Patient and public involvement in emergency care research. *Emergency Medical Journal*, 33(9): 665–70.

Hulley, S.B., Cummings, S.R., Browner, W.S., Grady, D.G. and Newman, T.S. (2013) *Designing Clinical Research*, 5th edn. Philadelphia, PA: Lippincott, Williams and Wilkins.

International Council for Harmonisation of Technical Requirements for Pharmaceuticals for Human Use (ICH) (2016) *ICH Harmonised Tripartite Guideline Integrated Addendum to ICH E6(R1): Guideline for Good Clinical Practice E6(R2)*. Available at: https://www.ich.org/fileadmin/Public_Web_Site/ICH_Products/Guidelines/Efficacy/E6/E6_R1_Guideline.pdf (accessed 8 January 2018).

Irving, A., Turner, J., Marsh, M., Broadway-Parkinson, A., et al. (2018) A coproduced patient and public event: an approach to developing and prioritizing ambulance performance measures. *Health Expectations*, 21(1): 230–8.

NHS Health Research Authority (2017) *UK Policy Framework for Health and Social Care Research,*
v3.2. London: NHS Health Research Authority.

Rosser, M. (2012) Evidence-based practice in paramedic practice, in P. Griffiths and G.P. Mooney
(eds) *The Paramedic's Guide to Research: An Introduction.* Maidenhead: Open University Press.

Sackett, D.L., Rosenburg, W.M.C., Muir Gray, J.A., Haynes, R.B. and Scott Richardson, W. (1996)
Evidence-based medicine: what is it and what it isn't. *BMJ,* 312: 71.

Simpson, P.M., Bendall, J.C., Patterson, J. and Middleton, P.M. (2012) Beliefs and expectations of
paramedics towards evidence-based practice and research. *International Journal of Evidence-*
Based Healthcare, 10(3): 197–203.

The Nuremberg Code (undated) Available at: www.history.nih.gov/research/downloads/
nuremberg.pdf (accessed 8 January 2018).

United States Holocaust Memorial Museum (2016) *Nazi Medical Experiments.* Available at: www.
ushmm.org/wlc/en/article.php?ModuleId=10005168 (accessed 8 January 2018).

Williams, B., Perillo, S. and Brown, T. (2015) What are the factors of organisational culture in
healthcare settings that act as barriers to the implementation of evidence-based practice? A
scoping review. *Nurse Education Today,* 35(2): e34–41.

Williams, J. (2012) Qualitative research in paramedic practice: an overview, in P. Griffiths and
G.P. Mooney (eds) *The Paramedic's Guide to Research: An Introduction.* Maidenhead: Open
University Press.

World Medical Association (2013) World Medical Association Declaration of Helsinki: ethical
principles for medical research involving human subjects. *JAMA,* 310(20): 2191–4.

USEFUL WEBSITES

Athens: www.openathens.net/ (accessed 8 January 2018).

CINAHL Plus (Cumulative Index to Nursing and Allied Health Literature): https://health.ebsco.
com/products/cinahl-plus-with-full-text (accessed 8 January 2018).

Council for Allied Health Professions Research (CAHPR): hub: http://cahpr.csp.org.uk/ (accessed
8 January 2018).

Critical Appraisal Skills Programme (CASP): Making sense of evidence: www.casp-uk.net/
(accessed 8 January 2018).

Defining research: http://www.hra.nhs.uk/documents/2016/06/defining-research.pdf (accessed
8 January 2018).

EQUATOR Enhancing the Quality and Transparency of Health Research: www.equator-network.org/
(accessed 8 January 2018).

INVOLVE: http://www.invo.org.uk/ (accessed 8 January 2018).

Is my study research?: www.hra-decisiontools.org.uk/research/index.html (accessed 8 January
2018).

NICE Evidence Search: www.evidence.nhs.uk/ (accessed 8 January 2018).

OpenGrey: www.opengrey.eu/ (accessed 8 January 2018).

PubMed: www.ncbi.nlm.nih.gov/pubmed/ (accessed 8 January 2018).

Science Direct: www.sciencedirect.com/ (accessed 8 January 2018).

Human factors affecting paramedic practice

Christopher Matthews (written for Isabella)

In this chapter:

- Introduction
- Why is this relevant?
- Communication
- Communication styles
- Situational awareness
- Teamwork
- Escalating concerns
- Leadership
- Conclusion
- Chapter key points
- References and suggested reading

INTRODUCTION

This chapter will provide a brief overview and understanding of human factors (HF) and non-technical skills (NTS). It will include some of the important components that fall under the umbrella of the HF/NTS title (HF and NTS titles will be used interchangeably throughout). Although these specific skills are of increasing importance within the ambulance profession and the wider National Health Service (NHS), they have, historically, rarely been taught on paramedic courses.

WHY IS THIS RELEVANT?

NTS are defined as the cognitive and social skills that enable a clinician to deliver safe and effective care when combined with his/her technical knowledge and skills (Flin et al. 2008). NTS are able to enhance the way one carries out technical (clinical) skills. Health Education England (2015) suggests that human factor principles aim to understand the connection and relationship between a clinician, his/her environment and equipment, including situational awareness, communication, leadership, decision-making and teamwork, to name but a few. The importance of these factors is increasingly being understood, especially within high acuity incidents such as a resuscitation (Resuscitation Council (UK) 2011). The Resuscitation Council (UK) (2011) highlights the growing importance of human factors and leadership in ensuring best patient care and outcome during highly stressful incidents.

Once analysed, many incidents of patient harm across the wider NHS were demonstrated to be attributed to the failure of non-technical skills rather than to actual technical skills (DH 2000; Flin et al. 2008).

The College of Paramedics (CoP) is only too aware that communication, interpersonal skills, leadership and teamwork are fundamental to a paramedic's development, in order to ensure effective team performance and reduce human errors (College of Paramedics 2017).

HF are already an established discipline within many other safety critical industries, such as aviation, which understands the importance of HF and NTS skills in the management of emergencies (Jenkins 2015). Evidence demonstrating these skills is as important within the operating theatre as in an aircraft cockpit and has been around for a number of years (Lingard et al. 2004). Although the NHS has begun to harness HF, it appreciates there is further learning that must be adopted and adapted in order to optimise human performance in healthcare, thereby minimising the risk to patients (National Quality Board 2013).

COMMUNICATION

 Chapter 1 for more on interpersonal communication.

Naturally, communication is an important aspect of paramedic practice. In order to comprehend an incident scene or to assist with a differential diagnosis, one must be able to effectively communicate with patients, relatives, bystanders and other emergency service staff. Patient history taking is an extremely important part of a paramedic's role, and understanding types and ways of communication will be of benefit in obtaining vital information.

It is well known that there are different forms of communication of which the paramedic must be aware. Although verbal communication skills are of immense importance in paramedicine, one must also be mindful of the importance of factors such as non-verbal/body language, listening, emotional awareness and written communication skills.

It is important that a paramedic completes a legible and accurate Patient Report Form (PRF). If the patient is transported to hospital, this documentation will form part of the

Case study 6.1

It is 03:00 and Tim has been working continuously through the night. He has just received a 999 call to attend Charlotte, an elderly lady, who has slipped from her bed and is unable to stand up.

Tim is a professional paramedic who tries to do his utmost for his patients but he is now tired, hungry and cold.

On entering the property, Charlotte is found lying on the floor, unable to stand without assistance. Tim stands over Charlotte looking down at her; he has both hands in his pockets and his facial expression reflects that he is tired, on autopilot and would rather not be there.

Although Tim greets Charlotte using all the correct words and terminology that are associated with professional politeness, she has already witnessed the many non-verbal clues/actions that have betrayed Tim's true feelings. This, in turn, leads Charlotte to feel uncomfortable and may prevent her from calling for an ambulance in the early morning in future. Instead, she may decide to lie on the floor until later in the day so as not to upset anyone, which may lead to further complications in her failing health.

hospital notes. The PRF is often the document that hospital doctors will consult for an accurate, honest and non-biased account of what happened to the patient prior to his/her arrival at hospital and paramedics should be aware of its importance when completing it.

Non-verbal communication plays a significant role in establishing a good rapport between a paramedic and his/her patient (Hart et al. 2016). It may be argued that non-verbal communication is as important as verbal communication: regardless of what sounds and words a clinician may articulate, his/her body language may easily betray the true thoughts and feelings. Case study 6.1 is an example of how body language may affect interaction with a patient.

Obviously Case study 6.1 has been exaggerated, but, nevertheless, demonstrates how it is possible to project negativity through non-verbal communication without the clinician being aware of this.

COMMUNICATION STYLES

Communication may be broken down further into five different 'styles'. This section will focus on the main four, omitting the manipulative style. It is important that a paramedic is aware of the differences, as well as recognising which style he/she most often uses in order to assist with his/her development of communication. We do not always use the same communication as it is dependent on the situation. This section aims to highlight

---

Case study 6.2

Rachel is a newly qualified paramedic working on a single response vehicle, attending an acutely unwell patient suffering a myocardial infarction (MI). She has arranged for an ambulance to transport the patient to hospital and is aware that the patient requires certain medications for the MI but the ambulance arrives before she has administered any medications. Rachel informs the crew that she feels the patient requires these drugs prior to leaving the scene, to ensure best patient care and treatment occurs. The crew is keen to finish the shift and inform Rachel that the patient can be given the medication en route to hospital. Rachel looks at the floor and quietly responds by saying, 'That's okay, I suppose he can wait.'

---

some important differences between communication styles as well as offering some examples for you to consider while following several scenarios.

Passive/submissive communication

Passive or submissive communicators seek to please others and aim to avoid conflict at all costs. They are apologetic in their communication and may speak softly, avoiding eye contact. Passive communicators have developed a pattern of avoiding expressing their opinions or feelings. They will fail to assert themselves and may often feel anxious, depressed and resentful, feeling helpless that their needs are not being met, as can be seen in Case study 6.2.

Can you see from Case study 6.2 how this form of communication has led to the patient not receiving optimal treatment and is not the most appropriate way of ensuring the optimal outcome?

Aggressive communication

Aggressive communicators express their feelings and opinions in a way that projects that any other view is not worth considering or is incorrect (see Case study 6.3). They will stand-up for themselves and express their thoughts in an unhelpful manner – becoming angry or physically aggressive if they do not get their own way. They may use fixed eye

---

Case study 6.3

After the crew inform Rachel that they do not want to medicate the patient at the scene, Rachel adopts an intimidating posture, glaring as she faces the crew 'square on'. She snaps at them and, in a raised and aggressive tone, says, 'I'm fed up of you not bothering to look after your patients. I don't care if you are going to be late finishing your shift, you will administer the medications now. I'm not interested in hearing any other excuses.'

---

contact, increase the volume of their voice and have an overbearing or intimidating posture. Aggressive communicators may use humiliation to control others or seek to force the other party to agree with them.

Not only will this form of communication be detrimental to building a good rapport with colleagues and other healthcare professionals, it will also appear most unprofessional in front of the patient. This is not the most appropriate way of ensuring the best outcome.

Passive-aggressive communication

Passive-aggressive communicators (see Case study 6.4) will appear passive on the surface but are actually displaying anger in a subtle or indirect way. Passive-aggressive communicators tend to mutter to themselves rather than confront an individual or problem directly. Their facial expressions may not match their feelings as they may smile when angry. They often use sarcasm and actually feel powerless, resentful and incapable of dealing directly with the object of their resentment.

Case study 6.4

Rachel turns to the crew with a smile on her face and states in an overtly friendly but sarcastic tone, 'Okay, then, don't worry about giving the medication to the patient now – he can just suffer the consequences instead. Do whatever you want as my ideas are never any good and you obviously know better.' After the incident Rachel will criticise the crew to other clinicians.

Again, this form of communication is not conducive to effective team work or patient care. It will lead to further conflicts when the crew hear about the negative conversations Rachel has had with others about them.

Assertive communication

Assertive communicators clearly, respectfully and appropriately convey their thoughts and feelings, advocating for their rights without showing aggression towards others. These individuals usually have a high self-esteem and listen to the views of others without interrupting; they will feel in control of themselves and make good eye contact. Although they will display confidence in their communication, not allowing others to abuse or manipulate them, they will show respect for others and their points of view, as can be seen in Case study 6.5.

Assertive communication is usually thought to be the most effective style of communication. It allows us to take care of ourselves, aiding our own well-being, as well as ensuring good relationships with colleagues and patients (University College London 2012; University of Kentucky 2014).

Case study 6.5

When the crew do not want to administer medication to the patient suffering from an MI, Rachel turns to face them, displaying confident body language and eye contact. She addresses them in the ideal middle ground between aggressive and passive communication. 'I am sorry that you might be slightly late finishing your shift if we treat the patient on scene and I do understand how tired you must be but, if we administer the medications now, we can be confident that we will have delivered the best possible care. We know that the sooner a patient receives these medications, the better the outcome. If you would like to start sorting out the patient's extrication plans, I am more than happy to administer the drugs.'

Although it is often the best form of communication (helping to boost one's own self-esteem and earning the respect of others), there are times when a paramedic will be required to adapt his/her communication style to be commensurate with the circumstances. It is essential that paramedics are aware of their usual style of communication and have the flexibility to alter this when necessary.

If you consider your own approach to communication, you will be able to determine which style you follow. If you fall within one of the styles other than assertive, do not be disheartened as this is common. What is important is that you are able to recognise this and that you learn the required skills and abilities to step into the assertive communication style when required.

Some tips for assisting with assertive communication from University College London (2012) are:

- What do you want to gain?
- What is the problem?
- Consider and describe your thoughts and feelings.
- Explain what it is you need.
- Be persistent but flexible.
- Recognise there is not always a solution; if required, agree to have a think and discuss it again later.
- Ensure you recognise the difference between what you want and what the other party wants, as they may not always be the same.
- Practise communicating in an assertive manner whenever you can.

SITUATIONAL AWARENESS

Situational awareness is an important skill for a paramedic to learn and develop and many will have already begun their ambulance career with some form of this skill; however, it is important to expand and hone this attribute.

'Bandwidth' is an important concept for all paramedics to be aware of. We all have a finite amount of information that we can absorb at any given time and one's cognitive load is only able to accommodate so much. While long-term memory has unlimited capacity, at any given time, a paramedic's working memory will only be able to process a limited amount of new information (Riem et al. 2012).

A paramedic's 'bandwidth' will only be able to hold and assimilate a certain volume of information. Once capacity is reached, he/she will start to lose situational awareness and will suffer from tunnel vision. In a high-acuity (or any) clinical setting, this 'bandwidth-overload' will present with the paramedic with the possible problems:

- Not hearing anything that is said to him/her.
- Losing peripheral vision.
- Becoming task-focused.
- Losing sight of the 'bigger picture'.
- Increasing stress levels.
- Increasing panic.

As you can imagine, allowing any of the above to develop will lead to the reduced efficiency of the paramedic as well as the wider team. 'Bandwidth overload' can occur almost instantaneously on arrival at an incident or develop later during the incident. 'Bandwidth' can be expanded through education, experiences and exposure to different incidents.

For example, a cardiac arrest incident can be a stressful environment with a high cognitive load due to the number of higher-order cognitive processes that are required such as the challenges of multi-tasking and time constraints. If the paramedic has efficient technical skills – through pre-existing expertise from education, experiences, exposure and practice – he/she may then have a reduced individual cognitive load, freeing up cognitive resources for HF and an expanded 'bandwidth'. It has been evidenced that individuals with high levels of technical skills may demonstrate better NTS performance and vice versa (Riem et al. 2012).

Although all paramedics may eventually reach cognitive overload during certain incidents, having a sound education with a solid underpinning knowledge, coupled with experience and exposure will undoubtedly expand his/her 'bandwidth'.

It is just as important to be aware of the phenomenon of 'bandwidth overload' in order to combat and alleviate the problems associated with it. If a paramedic is aware of his/her own limitations, he/she is able to stay alert and be aware of the warning signs that he/she is approaching his/her cognitive limit (see list above). Being aware can reduce cognitive load, opening up further 'bandwidth'. You may decide to allocate certain technical skills to others, instruct someone else to take an overview enabling you to simply take a step back from the immediate scene in order to 'regroup', re-organise thoughts and look at the bigger picture of the scene. This sharing of cognitive load can be witnessed in many circumstances, with some Helicopter Emergency Medical Services (HEMS) systems being one of these. HEMS clinicians use the above knowledge to their advantage.

For instance, the doctor might be the one undertaking a certain advanced technical skill – taking up most of his/her cognitive load, while the paramedic takes an overview of the scene and directs scene management, focusing on NTS – thereby sharing the load thus freeing up 'bandwidth' and ensuring a high level of care is provided.

TEAMWORK

Although leadership is an important role within paramedicine, the ability to work within a cohesive team is invaluable. Teamwork is essential in ensuring high quality patient care is carried out – especially at larger, more complex incidents. It has been shown that the ability and 'health' of a team has a direct correlation to patient safety (Royal College of Nursing 2017).

It is important to note that each team member will have his/her own strengths and weaknesses. There are different roles that a team member can undertake, but in the fast-moving, dynamic pre-hospital environment there is usually little time to designate certain 'team role behaviours' which have been identified by Belbin (Belbin 1993). Another compounding factor is that pre-hospital teams tend never to be the same mix of people. Due to the nature of paramedicine, crews will change, and different crews will arrive in support of each other, meaning that it is even more important that pre-hospital clinicians have the ability to be flexible and to adapt and overcome the many challenges of teamwork that they may encounter. With this is mind, 'followship' is an important aspect of HF.

'Followship' does not mean that a senior clinician will automatically take the leadership role, with less senior colleagues in the followship roles. Followship is an art in itself, requiring a person to be adept at following direction, allowing a leader to lead while ensuring proactive and appropriate support is available.

An example of good followship might be when an advanced paramedic arrives at an incident scene that is already being competently and appropriately led by a paramedic. If there is no requirement for the lead or clinical skill set of the advanced paramedic, then he/she can easily slot into a followship role and follow the direction of the lead paramedic while offering support and guidance as and when required.

Undoubtedly, there will be times when the team does not form as cohesive a unit as one might prefer. This could, for example, be due to individual conflicts, disagreements regarding the plan/management of the patient/scene or several clinicians may be vying to be the leader of the team. If this occurs, it is down to the individuals within the team, as well as the team leader, to remember and ensure that the patient is at the heart of any conflict and that any issues and disagreements are dealt with at a later time.

The team should work towards the same goal, with the same mental model. This is carried out through skilful communication ensuring that all are aware of the plans and goals. It is good practice for the leader to share information with the team, as well as being beneficial for the leader to use the abilities and knowledge of the team by asking their thoughts and opinions. Team members must have the ability and flexibility not only to work under direction, but to also assist the team leader in decision planning if required. However, given conflicting ideas, one must note that it must be the team leader who should be the person to make the ultimate and final decision. Pre-hospital clinicians will have to be able to interchange between, and embrace several of, the differing team role behaviours: resource investigator, team worker, co-ordinator, plant, monitor evaluator, specialist, shaper, implementer, completer finisher (Belbin 1993).

 Chapter 16 for more on leadership style and **Chapter 17** for theories of decision-making.

ESCALATING CONCERNS

Unfortunately, incidents may not always run smoothly and, regardless of the clinical grade or seniority, every clinician has the right – as well as a professional responsibility – to challenge inappropriate or dangerous practice and behaviours: a daunting prospect in reality. However, all clinicians must feel empowered to voice their concerns and, if required, escalate these concerns until they are addressed and acted upon.

It may simply be a case that the challenging party does not fully understand the plan or treatment being proposed or undertaken. It may simply be due to the challenging person not having been party to pertinent information. If this is the case, the individual being challenged should simply, and without hostility, inform the 'challenger' of his/her plans and reasoning for his/her actions. It is fully justifiable for an individual to seek clarification if there is uncertainty or concern surrounding patient safety and care.

If there *is* a genuine concern and an individual's practice requires challenging, the 'challenger' may be required to escalate this to an appropriate level in order to ensure compliance and, ultimately, patient safety.

There are a number of ways to approach this and differing mnemonics that may be used in order to assist with assertive communication, e.g. P.A.C.E.: **P**robe, **A**lert, **C**hallenge, **E**scalate (Besco 1999). This system uses four escalating levels of graded assertive communication in order to highlight the concern to the individual being challenged. It is important that all clinicians are aware of how to escalate assertive communication as this will ensure that a difficult and potentially dangerous and unsafe situation can be averted, not only as efficiently as possible but in a professional manner which leaves little room for individual uncertainty or confrontation. An example of how to use the P.A.C.E. mnemonic (Besco 1999) can be seen in Case study 6.6.

Case study 6.6

Patrick is attempting to insert a supraglottic airway (SGA) device into a cardiac arrest patient but is struggling to do so appropriately. He is now only focusing on the goal of inserting the SGA.

Sue realises that Patrick is struggling and that, due to his lack of success and tunnel vision, the patient has not been ventilated for an inappropriate amount of time. Sue decides that she needs to raise her concerns and highlight the patient's ventilation need to Patrick, using the appropriate level of assertiveness. Sue states:

> *Are you aware that it has been some time since the last ventilation?*

Sue is 'probing' to see if Patrick is aware of the 'bigger picture' as well as highlighting her concerns in a simple, non-confrontational manner. When Patrick ignores or does not hear Sue, continuing to try to insert the SGA, Sue steps up her assertiveness, with a slight increase in volume:

> *Can we have a look at the airway and ventilation situation now, as it is vital that the patient does not become hypoxic?*

By now, Patrick is displaying signs of cognitive overload and is entirely fixated on the placement of the SGA. As his 'bandwidth' is clearly overloaded, he does not register Sue's 'alert'. Sue realises there is an urgent need to ventilate the patient; she moves next to Patrick and 'challenges' him in a louder, assertive tone. Although Sue has already informed Patrick of the importance of her concerns, she continues this further and informs him of the danger to the patient:

> *Please stop trying to insert the SGA as it is not working. Ventilate the patient with the bag valve mask (BVM), as she is becoming increasingly hypoxic and will be at risk of a hypoxic brain injury soon.*

Although Patrick is not purposefully ignoring Sue, this 'challenge' is not acted upon, with him continuing to fixate on the SGA. Sue now realises that she needs to escalate her assertive level even further, highlighting the 'emergency' need to ventilate the patient. She uses tactile stimulation (if not already undertaken) and places a hand on Patrick's shoulder, addressing him by name (or rank) in a direct, assertive, yet still professional tone:

> *Patrick, STOP trying to insert the SGA and ventilate with the BVM now, as you are causing the patient serious harm.*

Patrick takes note of this, realising his loss of situational awareness and admitting to himself and Sue that he is struggling with the airway. He ventilates the patient with the BVM and allows Sue to assess and manage the airway. Due to the nature of Sue's assertive escalation and communication, Patrick is able to do this without feeling embarrassed or having caused any permanent hypoxic damage to the patient.

LEADERSHIP

Clinical leadership is a key component of paramedic practice and the hope/increasing expectation is that the application and importance of clinical leadership will become established throughout paramedic education programmes and continuing professional development (College of Paramedics 2017). Importantly, this is not simply a paramedic-driven expectation and has arisen from the wider NHS Clinical Leadership Competency Framework (CLCF) (National Health Service Leadership Academy 2011).

By the very nature of the role, all paramedics will, undoubtedly, be put into a leadership position. Many may never have experienced this role prior to being required to step up into this situation in clinical practice. Therefore, it is important that one is aware of many of the HF principles that help when undertaking clinical leadership. Although leadership is, itself, a component of HF, there are many NTS which will aid the paramedic in this role – some of which have been mentioned in this chapter. The clinical lead must be able to draw upon many of these NTS aspects to ensure a competent and expert leadership style is delivered.

Communication plays an important role within leadership. Some incident scenes may be loud and hectic. It is important that any direction or message that you pass as the leader is understood and promptly carried out appropriately. Miscommunication sometimes occurs when the leader thinks the other clinician has heard and understood the command/request but it transpires this was not the case, which may not be beneficial for the patient or colleagues.

Closed loop communication is one way to avoid this and does not have to be carried out in the rigid formality that some always associate with this communication technique. Simply put, the sender verbally gives a message to the receiver. The receiver verbally accepts he/she has heard and understood the message by repeating it back to the sender. Finally, the sender closes the loop by confirming what the receiver has said is correct, see Case study 6.7.

Case study 6.7

Janet (leading paramedic): *Robert, I want you to cannulate this trauma patient and then administer 1g of Tranexamic Acid. Let me know when this has been completed please.*

Robert (2nd paramedic): *Janet, I will cannulate, administer 1g of Tranexamic Acid and inform you when this is complete.*

Janet: *Yes.*

As well as differing communication styles, each of us tend to have a preferred leadership style. Although there are as many as 12 different leadership styles, this section will briefly focus on three styles which one may often witness in clinical practice. These can be interchangeable, and an accomplished leader will be able to alter his/her leadership style, if required, in order to achieve his/her goals.

Autocratic leadership

This is an extreme form of transactional leadership. Members of the team will have little to no input into decisions or the ability to make suggestions, even if these are in the best interest of the patient. Although autocratic leadership may alienate the team, leading to feelings of resentment or lack of appreciation, one might choose to use this sometimes efficient leadership style during a high acuity, stressful incident, when decisions must be made quickly and without dissent (Leadership Foundation for Higher Education 2016).

Democratic leadership

Democratic leadership usually adopts a more approachable and inclusive style than that of autocratic leadership. The democratic leader may well be much more open to team members offering up their ideas and being more engaged in the decision process. However, democratic leaders still make the final decisions. Although this style seems to motivate and empower team members during incidents, it may hinder a hectic, time-critical scene where speed or efficiency is essential.

Laissez-faire leadership

'Leave it be' leaders appear more easy-going, allowing their team to work independently. Although the *laissez-faire* leader will offer support with resources and advice, he/she will not otherwise become involved at the incident scene and will leave all the decisions to the team members. There is a place for this leadership within an experienced, skilled team and it has been shown to lead to high job satisfaction and increased productivity. However, it can be counter-productive and possibly dangerous to patients if the team members do not manage their skills, time or themselves appropriately – especially if they do not possess the correct level of knowledge, skills and motivation to do their work effectively (Leadership Foundation for Higher Education 2016).

As you can see, each of the styles has its own positive and negative aspects and it will be up to the skilled leader to ensure he/she utilises the best style is adopted when required.

CONCLUSION

It is evident that NTS are an important aspect of paramedicine. In order to be an effective and safe clinician, it is important that you develop a good understanding of the different aspects of HF. Self-reflection on your adopted communication and leadership styles is important and challenge yourself to use other styles when appropriate.

Consider how you would interact and feel if you were one of the individuals discussed in the case studies provided throughout this chapter.

Chapter 2 for more on reflection. See Chapter 16 for more on leadership styles.

It is important to note that you will not always achieve the desired result or achieve the objective in the most appropriate way. When this is the case, it is important that you have the ability for self-reflection in order to develop your NTS, to ensure you do not repeat the same mistakes during the next situation.

Chapter key points:

- Human factors are an increasingly important factor in paramedicine.
- There are many aspects that form human factors.
- Failures in human factors can be attributed to many patient harm incidents.
- Ensuring you have an awareness of the different communication and leadership styles is important, as well as the adaptability to interchange between the different styles.
- Be aware of the importance of non-verbal communication.
- Develop your ability as an assertive communicator.
- Be aware of your situational awareness and understand that your 'bandwidth' is finite. However, with experience, expertise and continued education, this can be expanded and honed.
- Teamwork is essential in ensuring high quality patient care.
- Be aware of the different roles that form a cohesive team and develop the ability to interchange between these roles.
- Competent 'followship' can be as essential as strong leadership in ensuring the effectiveness of the team.
- The ability to calmly, professionally and assertively challenge colleagues and escalate concerns is important to patient safety.
- Find an approach to escalating concerns that suits you, then practise and develop it.
- Leadership is a key component of paramedic practice.
- Competent and strong leadership can be developed and honed with practice and experience.

REFERENCES AND SUGGESTED READING

Belbin, R.M. (1993) *Team Roles at Work*. Oxford: Butterworth-Heinemann.

Besco, R. (1999) PACE: Probe, Alert, Challenge, and Emergency Action. *Business and Commercial Aviation*, 84(6): 72–4.

College of Paramedics (2017) *Paramedic Curriculum Guidance*, 4th edn. Bridgwater: College of Paramedics.

DH (Department of Health) (2000) An organisation with a memory. Available at: https://www.aagbi.org/sites/default/files/An%20organisation%20with%20a%20memory.pdf (accessed 11 December 2017).

Flin, R., O'Connor, P. and Crichton, M. (2008) *Safety at the Sharp End: A Guide to Non-Technical Skills.* Farnham: Ashgate.

Hart, Y., Czerniak, E., Karnieli-Miller, O., et al. (2016) Automated video analysis of non-verbal communication in a medical setting. *Frontiers in Psychology Journal.* 7: 1130. Available at: https://www.ncbi.nlm.nih.gov/pmc/article/PMC4993763/ (accessed 12 December 2017).

Health Education England (2015) *Human Factors.* Available at: https://hee.nhs.uk/printpdf/our-work/hospitals-primary-community-care/learning-be-safer/human-factors (accessed 11 December 2017).

Jenkins, B. (2015) Training and assessment of non-technical skills in the operating theatre: Where next? *Journal of the Association of Anaesthetists of Great Britain and Ireland,* 70(8): 897–902. Available at: http://onlinelibrary.wiley.com/doi/10.1111/anae.13182/full (accessed 10 December 2017).

Leadership Foundation for Higher Education (2016) 10 x Leadership Styles. Available at: https://www.lfhe.ac.uk/en/general/lf10/ten-times-tables/10-leadership-styles.cfm (accessed 17 December 2017).

Lingard, L., Epsin, S., Whyte, S., et al. (2004) Communication failures in the operating room: an observational classification of recurrent types and effects. *Quality and Safety in Health Care,* 13(5): 330–4. Available at: http://www.ncbi.nlm.nih.gov/pubmed/15465935 (accessed 15 December 2017).

National Health Service Leadership Academy (2011) *Clinical Leadership Competency Framework.* Coventry: NHS Institute for Innovation and Improvement.

National Quality Board (2013) *Human Factors in Healthcare: A Concordat from the National Quality Board.* Available at: https://www.england.nhs.uk/wp-content/uploads/2013/11/nqb-hum-fact-concord.pdf (accessed 15 December 2017).

Resuscitation Council (UK) (2011) *Advanced Life Support,* 6th edn. London: Resuscitation Council (UK).

Riem, N., Boet, S., Bould, M., Tavares, W. and Naik, V. (2012) Do technical skills correlate with non-technical skills in crisis resource management? A simulation study. *British Journal of Anaesthesia,* 109(5): 723–8. Available at: https://www.ncbi.nlm.nih.gov/pmc/articles/PMC3470444/ (accessed 10 December 2017).

Royal College of Nursing (2017) *Teamwork.* Available at: https://www.rcn.org.uk/clinical-topics/patient-safety-and-human-factors/professional-resources/teamwork (accessed 9 December 2017).

University College London (2012) *Session 5: Communication Styles.* Division of Psychiatry. Available at: https://www.ucl.ac.uk/psychiatry/start/startmanual/accordion/CARER_Session_5_FINAL_14.11.12.pdf (accessed 9 December 2017).

University of Kentucky Violence Intervention and Prevention Center (2014) The four basic styles of communication. Paper presented at Wellness Conference. Available at: https://www.uky.edu/hr/sites/www.uky.edu.hr/files/wellness/image/Conf14_FourCommStyles.pdf (accessed 10 December 2017).

Introduction to psychology and child development

Jackie Whitnell and Chris Preston

In this chapter:

- Introduction
- Why is this relevant?
- Psychology: what is it?
- Different approaches to psychology
- Child development
- Why is this relevant?
- Theories of development
- Psychological approaches linked to practice
- Atypical development
- Conclusion
- Chapter key points
- References and suggested reading

PSYCHOLOGY: AN INTRODUCTION

Psychology is the study of behaviour and mental processes. A person's actions, why they do or say what they do or say is psychology. There are a number of different approaches that psychologists adopt in their attempt to gain a greater understanding of human behaviour. Some approaches appear similar, such as cognitivism and learning theory (or behaviourism) and some approaches are very different. This chapter will endeavour to provide the reader with an introduction to the understanding of psychology in order to enhance the care and compassion offered to clients.

WHY IS THIS RELEVANT?

Psychology is a core subject for the paramedic as it serves to underpin their knowledge of health and health behaviours. Brady (2012) found that the majority of 999 calls were psycho-social in origin, leaving 10 per cent only as life-threatening emergencies, thus, evidencing the importance of knowledge and understanding of psycho-social health behaviours. In order that paramedics and healthcare professionals can help patients/ clients who are ill or disabled, it is important that they understand how humans function when they are healthy. To work successfully in the paramedic profession, you will need a thorough grasp not only of how the individual person functions but also how they interact with each other and in groups. It is especially useful to understand those who are potentially vulnerable, including babies, children, the mentally ill and elderly, plus those who have a disability or learning needs, among many others. As a healthcare professional you will spend many working days caring for those who experience socio-economic disadvantage and those who cannot cope with life. You will also be aware that in today's society, people are living longer and you will care for those with chronic illness and life-limiting conditions. Consequently, an understanding of psychology can help in the care of such people. Psychology also informs us of individual patterns of behaviour and of the difficulties with behaviour change (Gerrig et al. 2012).

PSYCHOLOGY: WHAT IS IT?

There are many factors that determine our behaviour, for example:

- the genes we are born with;
- our physiological system (brain, nervous system, endocrine system);
- our cognitive system (thoughts, perception, memory);
- the social and cultural environments in which we develop over time;
- our life experiences including those from childhood;
- our personal and individual differences including our IQ, personality and mental health (Whitnell 2012a).

 Reflection: points to consider

You are called to a nightclub following a collapse of a man from an altercation outside the establishment. Could it be one of the following?

- the attacker has inherited his genes from his parents, plus his father is known for his short temper (genetics and physiology);
- the attacker experienced violence in his childhood in his family home (learned behaviour);
- the patient has a history of personality disorder and is experiencing mental health problems (social/cultural experiences);
- the attacker was frustrated with the other person and this gave him thoughts of anger and aggression (cognitivism);
- the attacker thought the other person was insulting his family and in his culture it is acceptable to defend his family in that way (social/cultural).

Having read the above, one could be excused for thinking 'that's just common sense', but it is more than that. The study of psychology can be usefully applied in many different situations and life experiences. For the purposes of this chapter, psychology will be considered in brief to provide the reader with a thirst for further exploration of this subject. Psychology is not a single subject; rather it is a coalition of different special-isms (Gerrig et al. 2012).

The different schools of thought are many, as the example in the previous 'reflection: points to consider' box shows, and include biological, cognitive, developmental, social, health and clinical psychology, to name but a few. This chapter will provide an overview of psychology and child development, which will include discussion on atypical development. Chapter 8 will further discuss abnormal psychology and child and adolescent mental health, as well as adult mental health. These areas have been chosen not because they are essentially more important than others but because paramedics and allied health professionals in their day-to-day working life will benefit from an understanding of the theoretical underpinning around these topics, thus linking theory to practice.

Psychology is an academic discipline and characterised by many different theoretical approaches to behaviour and mental functioning of individuals. Psychology emerged as a distinct discipline approximately 150 years ago. It has its roots in physiology, physics and philosophy and is a discipline which relies on theories to understand how people behave and think, and attempts to make predictions about how processes, such as memory, will occur. In order to do this, psychologists design and undertake carefully planned experiments and observations and use specific scientific methods to collect data, which after careful analysis enables them to make such predictions. However, theories are ever evolving, and psychologists may modify them over time when they continue to investigate their chosen approach/es (Gerrig et al. 2012). Theorists investigate from many different viewpoints. Some viewpoints or approaches that are important in current psychology are biological, psychodynamic, learning theory, cognitivism and humanism.

Psychology is concerned with human beings, but the nature of 'the human' is subject to much debate. Questions have been asked as to whether a person is a product of pre-wiring (according to laws of nature) or develops from a person's nurturing environment (laws of behaviour), in that they are a product of creativity, free-willed and responsible for their own actions. This question has, over decades, been transposed into what is commonly called the 'nature/nurture' debate. This is the long-standing debate among philosophers, psychologists and educators concerning the importance of heredity and learning.

Theoretical perspectives also vary in terms of the time span that psychologists consider, for example, psychologists, including Freud, consider past experiences to explain present behaviour, including experiences in childhood, and effects of abuse and family break-up. However, the focus could be on the present, observing behaviour here and now and how the behaviour is shaped by reward and reinforcement (operant conditioning) (Whitnell 2012a). This chapter continues with a brief introduction to some of the approaches in psychology.

DIFFERENT APPROACHES TO PSYCHOLOGY

Biological theory

This approach seeks to explain human functioning in terms of underlying physical structures and biochemical processes; it seeks to explain behaviour in terms of its physiology, its development, its evolution and its function (Kalat 2014). Psycho-biologists argue that the causes of behaviour come from within the nervous system and are pre-wired, affected by hormones and biochemical brain structures. The trigger for action comes from chemical and electrical activities taking place within and between nerve cells. Biological theory is often considered reductionist, whereby individual components are examined in order to understand behaviour instead of understanding behaviour as an embodied whole (Barker 2016).

Psychodynamic approach

Sigmund Freud (1856–1939) is a name that often springs to mind when people think of psychology. Freud was credited for making the unconscious worthy of serious inquiry. His techniques (used to investigate people who had mental health problems), termed psychoanalysis, were that of free association and dream analysis. Freud, in essence, believed that these techniques led him to an understanding of the patient's problems and by bringing that source out in dialogue, into conscious awareness, the emotional release (or catharsis) would assist in helping the patient towards a solution to the problem. However, he has been criticised for his theory being that of mythology, drama and legend as opposed to sound empirical theory. Freud's ideas and evidence are open to many differing interpretations and cannot be tested or verified in the way that modern psychology believes to be essential. Freud's views of the human mind and behaviour have highly influenced psychological thinking over time, although they are not central to it and have been adapted and developed by other theorists in this field, including Erikson, Jung and Klein (Barker 2016).

Learning theory (behaviourism)

Learning theory argues that the process of learning can be defined as that which has occurred when a relatively permanent change in behaviour or behaviour potential has been produced by experience. Watson, Pavlov and Skinner from 1912 onwards were influential theorists who dedicated their studies to observable behaviour. They argued that our capacity for learning depends on both genetic heritage and the nature of our environment. The study of learning has been dominated by the behaviourist approach, as represented in their work. Two main areas of study are those of classical conditioning and operant conditioning (Whitnell 2012a).

Social cultural theory

This theory was brought about by contemporary social scientists in the analysis of the social origins of mental processes. In this view, mental functioning in the individual can be understood only by examining the social and cultural processes, for example, the family, environment, culture, and so on, from which the individual derives. Humans are nurtured in a social world and within differing cultural diversities. Consequently, this must have an impact on the behaviour of the individual. Development commences with a human being totally dependent and supported in learning a new skill ('scaffolding'), then being facilitated and guided (guided participation) to becoming independent in a new skill (Banyard et al. 2010).

Cognitivism

Cognitivism had its origins in learning theory with emphasis on controlled observation of behaviour but with different considerations, such as how people think, make decisions, and so on. Since the inception of computers, researchers have examined the ways in which people mentally process information. The term cognitivism usually refers to mental representation of events, to the process of interpretation, prediction and evaluation of the environment, as well as to beliefs, thoughts and expectations (Gerrig et al. 2012). The so-called 'cognitive revolution' has emerged over the past few decades as a direct challenge to learning theory, and cognitivism is unconcerned with intra-psychic dynamics as in psycho-dynamic theory.

There has been much critique of this perspective and it is argued by cognitive theorists that a person's life can be planned like a computer; however, it can be counter-argued that emotions get in the way and all too often can ruin the life plan! For instance, people are not usually emotionally moved by things they see or experience literally, but more by the view, or interpretation, they take of what they see or experience.

Humanism

Known as the 'third force' in psychology developed in the United States in the 1950s, the humanistic approach is an alternative to psychodynamic and learning theory. Humanistic psychologists neither hold the Freudian view that people are driven by forces, or the behaviourists' view that they are manipulated by the environment. Humanism argues that people learn from individual experiences, their personal view of events and from life histories of other people, and conclude that this provides more understanding about the meaning of life experience. Humanistic psychologists argue that people are active creatures, essentially good, and capable of choice. There were two main contributors: Carl Rogers and Abraham Maslow; both argued that human health, growth and positive self-concept come from individual natural tendencies. Maslow developed a humanistic psychology of motivation; he argued that the individual has a need for self-actualisation, is personally responsible, free-willed and will strive towards personal growth and fulfilment (Gerrig et al. 2012). In Maslow's hierarchy, basic needs must first be granted, then the individual can move on through other needs to reach a peak in performance (see Figure 7.1).

Social constructionism

Social constructionism is a non-scientific approach to psychology along with humanism. This approach is based on the assumption that our knowledge of ourselves and of others is socially constructed. In other words, social construction is about understanding the behaviour of human beings based on what the current thinking is, so what are called

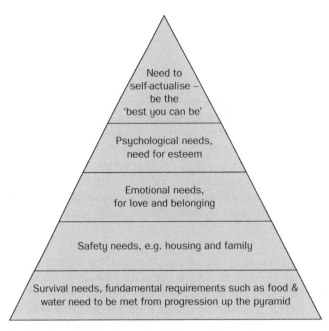

Figure 7.1   Hierarchy of needs

Source: Based on Maslow (1970).

facts are simply versions of events, which in modern-day society are acceptable. Social constructionism argues that human beings are always a product of their cultural and personal history and of their immediate social contexts. This approach directs study away from individual behaviour, towards a study of relationships examining human practices and discourses (experiences and language). Social constructionism informs us of how to behave in a given group.

Summary

The approaches discussed briefly above are not exhaustive; they have been chosen to provide readers with an awareness of the topic of psychology, and hopefully encourage them towards pursuing further reading. Theories often contradict, but sometimes complement, each other. However, they all pursue the accumulation of knowledge. In psychology there are many theories based on several schools of thought or approaches. In order to relate the perspectives discussed above to the practice of the paramedic, this chapter will follow with a case study that considers a situation from some of these perspectives. Hopefully this will aid the reader in terms of the application of psychology to practice.

While reading Case study 7.1, you may well have come to the conclusion that David suffers from anxiety; you would be correct.

Case study 7.1

David is a 21-year-old first-year student at university. He is doing well in his studies and enjoying his programme so far. However, he finds it extremely difficult to participate in seminars and workshops and experiences extreme stress prior to these sessions and suffers physiological symptoms of nausea, sweating, stammering, dry mouth and cough. In these situations, David feels faint and gets angry with himself, as he has no control over these experiences.

 Reflection: points to consider

What would the differing approaches to psychology above make of David's experience?

Psychodynamic approach

From a psychoanalytic view, David's anxiety may well be a symptom of problems dating back to his childhood. He may have had difficulty in speaking out in the family home; it may be that one of his parents was very dominant and David found it easier to remain silent. It could be that David experienced conflict at the stage of development in which he was trying to find his own identity when he was trying to establish sexual, political and career identities or was confused about what roles to play. Identity crises can create storm and stress. A psychotherapist could help David to find out and come to terms with his anxiety or repressed issue and help him to alter his responses to the situational factors that make him anxious (Turner-Cobb 2014).

Learning theory (behaviourist approach)

David could have experienced in his early life a situation in which he felt extreme anxiety in a classroom: that could be enough to generate anxiety in similar future situations. This is known as a conditioned emotional response or learned behaviour, and arises, according to learning theory, from classical conditioning. Classical conditioning (in essence) occurs when a stimulus (event or situation) triggers anxiety because it has previously been associated with another threatening stimulus and negative response.

Behaviourists would be most concerned with the circumstance in which the anxiety occurs Antecedent (A), the behaviour itself (B) and the consequence (C) and not concerned with the thoughts and feelings being suffered. This is termed functional analysis of behaviour. It may also be that David has previously experienced, for argument's sake, a situation in which he gave a presentation and forgot his note cards and felt very embarrassed, which produced anxiety. This situation would have negative consequences for further presentations in this situation. This behaviour is brought about by operant conditioning based on the law of effect (Mukherji and Dryden 2014).

Cognitivist approach

The cognitivist would consider David's situation in terms of his previous experience, like the behaviourist, but would want to know how David interprets the problem and how he has processed the information that causes the anxiety (Gerrig et al. 2012). A cognitivist would consider the interpretation as the basis for changing the way David thinks about the problem that causes the anxiety. If the anxiety was such that it became debilitating, David might be offered cognitive behaviour therapy (CBT).

Humanist approach

The humanist would be interested in David's self-esteem (Banyard et al. 2010). How does he perceive his abilities? Does David have a perception of himself as a failure when having to 'speak out' in public? The humanist may consider that David would benefit from client-centred therapy and maybe refer him to the student counselling service. This would provide David with the opportunity to talk through his fears and to gain insight into what worries him and why. The intended outcome would be that David gains confidence and feels better about himself and would experience far less anxiety when participating in seminars or workshops and speaking out in class.

Psychology can be considered a difficult subject to understand and the study of it can be divided in two: one that deals in the absolute scientific reality, learned through experimentation, and the other that appears to be common sense, logical and easily understood, which is socially constructed and can change over time and in different situations and circumstances. The study of human behaviour has over many years enabled psychologists to understand how certain psychological problems may arise and how they can be managed. In terms of providing healthcare, the understanding of how people think and why they behave as they do can support paramedics in their care practice and be a valuable resource.

Hopefully, this introductory section of the chapter has provided you with a taste of the exciting subject of psychology and a thirst for more. Psychology is a core subject for the paramedic, along with sociology and physiology. However, it can be a difficult subject to follow in terms of its relevance to healthcare. Psychologists like to debate differing ideas; if you have an interest in psychology you will join this interesting debate (Banyard et al. 2010; Gerrig et al. 2012; Barker 2016).

 Reflection: points to consider

Consider the differing approaches. Which do you think makes most sense? Which aligns to your practice more readily? Challenge the basic assumptions and ask your own questions.

CHILD DEVELOPMENT

The lifespan approach is commonly used in developmental psychology – from conception onwards. This introductory section will consider child development from birth to young adulthood, however, I would advise the paramedic to take time to read about the important development that occurs at conception and throughout pregnancy. Development through pregnancy will also have an effect on an infant's post-natal development.

Research can be conducted over different time spans, from a few seconds or minutes of observation to months, years or even an entire lifetime, as with longitudinal research. This is seen in developmental psychology and is vital in terms of understanding what can occur at periods in a child's development. This section of the chapter will first look at the importance of the paramedic having an understanding of child development (developmental psychology). Having previously taught this subject to student paramedics, I am often greeted in the first instance with a query as to why they need this knowledge, therefore I am taking this opportunity of providing the answer to this question, with the intention that this part of the chapter will not be skipped! This chapter will also consider, albeit briefly, atypical development (learning disabilities), to provide the reader with an overview of the diversity of children's development.

WHY IS THIS RELEVANT?

After considering some of the approaches of psychology earlier in this chapter, you could ask 'How will the theory link to my practice?' The answer is that, you will maybe for a short, yet extremely valuable period of time, be caring for children and their family members. In that time, your knowledge of how a child develops and what constitutes atypical development could be essential.

 Reflection: points to consider

Before reading further, why not note down why you think it is important for you to have an understanding of child development?

Below we outline why knowledge of child development is of paramount importance. If you have an awareness of normal child development, you will be in a better position to do the following:

- understand why children and families behave the way that they do;
- have an awareness of what to expect in terms of the child's language, in an appropriate manner, in accordance with a range of expected development, which will aid communication in order to obtain accurate information regarding the child's health needs;

- make a more accurate assessment regarding learning needs, special needs, disability, pain, and so on. Only the child can tell you how he feels (if able to express it, aiding accuracy of assessment);
- help the mother/father describe what she/he has seen or heard;
- observe the child's behaviour and social interaction with her carer. This can be extremely valuable information, especially for situations where non-accidental injury is a possible concern;
- identify inappropriate behaviour for the expected range of development of the child and be able to inform the professional of your worries when handing over the child's care (Mukherji and Dryden 2014);
- use evidence-based knowledge from differing perspectives of child development including psycho-social influences when caring for the child;
- have an awareness of children's rights (Jones and Welch 2010);
- inform Emergency Department staff and other healthcare professionals of concerns, in order that the child can be followed up appropriately, safeguarding the child at all times (Whitnell 2012b);
- be able to complete appropriately, and with child development knowledge, the patient report form and, if necessary, the safeguarding children report form.

 Reflection: points to consider

Review your last call to a child of any age.

- Were you confident communicating with the child?
- Was your knowledge of the range of development expected for their age clear to you?
- How well did you do with assessment?
- Could it have been improved, if so, how?

THEORIES OF DEVELOPMENT

Attachment theory

Most infants' early learning is in social development. There are two main aspects of this early learning that are very important: sociability and attachment. As a paramedic you will observe relationships between child and carer and you may well try to administer care to the infant/child. You may experience a crying child, clinging to its carer and trying to get away from you; this could be due to what is termed 'stranger awareness'. This usually occurs around the age of 4–6 months when the child develops object permanence (Bradford 2012).

Piaget's sensori-motor stage of development is discussed later in this chapter.

At this stage the child knows the difference between a familiar face and that of a stranger; this highlights that the child's cognitive development and social development is taking place. At approximately 6–10 months most children will try to cling on to their carer. When you try to remove them for a short while, they will cry out, but will stop crying and smile almost as soon as you pass them back to their familiar carer. There has been much research on attachment theory and you might like to read Mary Ainsworth on infant-mother attachment, who discussed what she termed 'strange situations'.

John Bowlby (1907–1990) was a child psychiatrist and psychoanalyst, and one of the first theorists to describe the importance of attachment in human development. His interest in the study of animal behaviour led to his theory that human children, like young animals, have a need for a figure that provides a source of safety, comfort and protection.

Bowlby (1979) identified the 'critical period' and argued that although the main attachment of an infant is usually to its mother, strong bonds occur to significant others with whom the infant has regular contact. If as a paramedic it is essential you administer treatment to a child, it would always be better (if possible) for you to have the person to whom the child is attached to help you; this may make your administering care a lot easier. Look up the work of Bowlby for greater knowledge on attachment theory.

Reflection: points to consider

Consider the relationships between parent and child that you have cared for. Have they always been warm and caring? As a paramedic you are in a prime position to notice the interaction between the child and carer and it is important that you report anything that is untoward or inappropriate when you hand over the care of the child. You will note that not all attachment is positive (Whitnell 2012b).

According to Bowlby, in the first three years of life, bonding must occur. In contrast, Ainsworth (1979) found that the relationship between the mother and baby develops over time, rather than being fixed shortly after birth. In reality, not all infants and children are parented sensitively or responsively. As a paramedic you will observe many different/diverse parenting skills. Deprivation can lead to long-term difficulties when it occurs due to problems with social relationships, more than from ill health. Bowlby (1979)

Case study 7.2

You are tasked to attend a 999 call for a 2-year-old girl who has been hot and unwell for three days and has a rash. On first assessment the child is alert, appears to be breathing normally, is well perfused and has a wide spread blotchy rash on the visible areas of her arms and legs. However, she is very clingy to her mum and making it quite clear that she wants nobody to examine her. Consider:

- What are the necessary assessments and investigations you must undertake?
- How can you balance distressing the child against your professional duty of care?
- How does the child's development stage influence your plan of care?
- To what extent is observing the behaviour and interactions between the carer and child important for your assessment and why?

argued that adverse effects of maternal deprivation are normally irreversible. Cultural differences in parenting practices reflect differences in terms of adults' cultural expectations and values. Parental acceptance and rejection can vary in different cultures but, in the main, rejection is generally associated with poor outcome in the children, for example, low self-esteem, delinquency and poor educational attainment. However, it is incumbent upon me to say that most infants in most cultures have a secure attachment and as a paramedic you will most often see positive attachment between child and carer throughout your daily practice (Whitnell 2012b).

Psychoanalytical and learning theory

Grand theories are comprehensive theories that have inspired and directed thinking about development over decades, but no longer seem as adequate as they once did. However, they remain influential.

During the first half of the twentieth century, two opposing grand theories dominated the child development 'scene':

1. psychoanalytic theory in two strands: psycho-sexual = Freud and psycho-social = Erikson.
2. learning theory (behaviourism) – Thorndike/Watson/Skinner/Pavlov.

These began as psychological theories and later were applied to human developmental psychology theories more broadly. A fundamental assumption of psychoanalytic theory is that development over the lifespan is determined during early childhood.

Psycho-sexual theory

Freud was interested in the role of unconscious mental processes and inner forces (id, ego, and superego) that he considered influenced people's behaviour. Freud argued

Table 7.1 Freud's stages of psycho-sexual development

Stage	Average age	Development
Oral	0–18 mths	Eating and sucking provides satisfaction
Anal	18–36 mths	Anal area is interesting and satisfying
Phallic	3–5 yrs	Satisfaction from the genitals
Latency	6 yrs–puberty	Boys and girls spend little time together
Genital	Onset of puberty	Main pleasure from genitals

that urges are gratified by three parts of personality, through stages of development which reflect erogenous zones (see Table 7.1). These underlying forces (id, ego and superego) and urges influence people's thinking and behaviour in the smallest decisions and in crucial life changes.

Drives and motive provide foundations for universal stages of development in human experience. A critique of this theory of development is that it is one-sided, the emphasis being on sexuality as the dynamic factor in development. Theorists from other approaches acknowledge Freud's thinking even though it is considered empirically weak (Gerrig et al. 2012), as mentioned earlier in the chapter. An important example of radical reformulation of psycho-sexual development theory is Erikson's psycho-social theory.

Psycho-social theory

Erik Erikson (1902–1994) was a Jewish German developmental psychologist who coined the phrase 'identity crisis'. He was one of Freud's followers who accepted some of Freud's theory and expanded it to take into account people's lifestyle and culture.

Erikson acknowledged the importance of the unconscious; he agreed that unresolved childhood conflicts at certain stages affect adulthood, but expanded and modified Freud's ideas. Erikson proposed eight developmental stages, each characterised by a particular challenge or developmental crisis, which is central to that stage of life. He placed the emphasis on a person's relationship to his family and culture, not just sexual urges.

Erikson's stages are as follows:

1 Trust vs mistrust (birth to 1 year): Babies learn either to trust that others will care for their basic needs, including nourishment, warmth, cleanliness and physical contact, or will lack confidence in the care given by others.
2 Autonomy vs shame and doubt (1 year to 3 years): Children learn either to be self-sufficient in many activities, including toileting, feeding, walking, exploring and talking, or they may doubt their own abilities.

3   Initiative vs guilt (3 years to 6 years): Children want to undertake many adult-like activities, sometimes overstepping the limits set by parents. That can lead to the child feeling guilty, thus resulting in poor self-esteem.

Reflection: points to consider

As a paramedic you will identify Stages 2 and 3 in terms of children who have attempted something that may well have been out of their range of development, which results in an accident.

4   Industry vs inferiority (6 years to 11 years): Children busily learn to be competent and productive in mastering new skills or they may feel inferior and unable to do anything well, thus leading to the potential for child and adolescent mental health issues, e.g. depression.
5   Identity vs role confusion (adolescence): Adolescents try to figure out 'Who am I?' They establish sexual, political and career identities or may be confused about what roles to play. Identity crises can create storm and stress for the young person. Sociological theory suggests that changes within social roles cause conflicts, e.g. girlfriend and daughter, schoolgirl and work experience. In addition, the mass media and peers can cause conflicting values for this age. It can be a very difficult time for the young person going through this stage of development.
6   Intimacy vs isolation – (young adult): Young people are working on establishing intimate ties to others. However, if they have experienced earlier attachment problems, some young adults cannot form close relationships and remain isolated (Gerrig et al. 2012).
7   Generativity vs stagnation – (middle adulthood): This stage involves giving to and guiding the next generation through child rearing, caring for others or reproduction. If a person cannot achieve this, they may feel an absence of meaningful accomplishment.
8   Ego integrity vs despair (the elderly person): This is the final stage where people reflect on the kind of person they have been and become. Integrity comes from feeling that life is worth living. However, older people who are not happy with their life fear death (Berger 2011).

Learning theory (behaviourism)
Learning theory holds the view that all development involves a change in an individual. It avoids references to the unconscious which cannot be observed. Behaviourism and the law of learning theory are based on the premise that learning can be explained by the forming of associations. Learning involves a *stimulus* (action which elicits a response) and *response* (instinct or learned action taken upon the stimulus) through *conditioning*.

There are two types of conditioning associated with behaviourism: classical conditioning and operant conditioning.

- *Classical conditioning*: John Watson (1876–1958) was opposed to Freud and Erikson's ideas on development and offered a new type of psychology. He argued that psychologists should study only what they could see and measure, not the unconscious. According to Watson, anything could be learned; in the right environment, he could train anyone to be anything regardless of talents, tendencies, abilities, vocations and cultures. He argued that the study of actual behaviour is objective and far less difficult than the study of unconscious motives and drives. Watson extended Pavlov's research with dogs and showed that classical conditioning occurred also in humans (Whitnell 2012a; 2012b).
- *Operant conditioning*: This conditioning occurs when behaviour produces a consequence. The principle is that the consequence (effect) of behaviour will determine how likely it is to reoccur; for example, if the consequence of behaviour is useful/pleasure/relieving (a positive reinforcement, such as medication), a child will take the medication again, when instructed, to achieve that same consequence (effect). Conditioning is used quite widely in behaviour management of children and in managing people who suffer with phobias (Gerrig et al. 2012).

 Reflection: points to consider

If a child experiences an asthmatic attack and is given a nebuliser, which makes the child feel much better and less scared, the child will be happy to use it again. Reinforcement and reward are very useful when managing a child who is scared; learning theory used in practice can be very useful. The child using the nebuliser has learned that the response to her difficult breathing comes from the positive reward = operant conditioning.

Social learning theory

Conditioning does not adequately explain where new behaviour comes from; social learning theory may help to explain this. This approach argues that not all learning has occurred from the child's experience of direct classical or operant conditioning (behaviourism). Children learn to behave in ways that are rewarding and avoid ways that are punished by others. Social learning theory, a more recent approach, accepts that children learn from reinforcement and punishment but also suggests that they learn by observing, imitating and modelling others. Modelling occurs when the observer is uncertain or inexperienced and models on a more senior, admired, or powerful role model (Bandura 1977).

Reflection: points to consider

If a child needs medication or a plaster, for example, you could consider this theory to aid administration. You could use modelling in terms of pretending to give the medication to the child's doll or teddy or put the plaster/bandage on the doll or teddy. Upon seeing this situation and with the intention of modelling the behaviour, the child may have more confidence in your care.

Cognitive theory

Jean Piaget (1896–1980) was a biologist and zoologist from Switzerland. Piaget's basic idea argued that it is more useful to understand how a child stores and uses information than how much knowledge and intellect a child has.

He made a study of three areas:

- how the senses take in information about things around us;
- how the brain processes and stores information;
- how the subsequent behaviour changes as a result of stored information = cognitive theory of development.

Piaget was a very influential and extraordinary intellectual leader/researcher who fashioned the framework of cognitive theory. Piaget argued that development does not occur through what has been forgotten (Freud and Erikson's ideas) or what has been learned (Pavlov and Skinner's ideas), but from what and how children think.

Piaget argued that children develop in stages. There are four age-related stages of development in which changes take place, the first, sensori-motor stage being the most dynamic in a child's life.

Let us look at these stages in turn:

1 Sensori-motor
2 Pre-operational
3 Concrete operational
4 Formal operational

Sensori-motor stage, 0–2 years

Most changes take place in this stage, from simple physical reflexes through to beginning to symbolise. Initially an infant's interactions are basic and reflexive but after a very short time the baby will learn to use some muscles and limbs for movement, and will begin to understand some information received through her senses (Sharma and Cockerill 2014).

Reflection: points to consider

What are the senses? Jot them down and consider why they are important.

The first ideas babies develop are around how to deal with their world; these are called 'action schemas' (construct representations of events, people and relationships from the real physical world). Babies are totally egocentric; they are unable to take anyone else's needs or interests into account. They start to develop fine and gross motor skills, become social beings and develop language (see Sharma and Cockerill 2014 for detail on the development of these skills over weeks, months and early years). Infants learn about objects and what they can be made to do. Some intellectual behaviour is occurring, for example they will hold a rattle and shake it, then throw it and watch what happens to it. Objects start to have meaning and babies/infants begin to do more with them. This is the time when object permanence occurs (Whitnell 2012b).

Pre-operational stage, 2–7 years

Operations at this stage will require combining schemas in an orderly, sensible, logical way, although at this stage they will be somewhat limited. The child's vocabulary and imagination are expanding at 2 years, seen in the use of words in play such as house, mummy, car, bird, dog, cat, and so on, and they may not be heard clearly. At the beginning of this stage, the child understands much of what is being said to him but can find it difficult to express himself; this brings about frustration. There is again a great deal of difference in development from 2 years to 7 years (Sharma and Cockerill 2014).

Within this stage the child is beginning to use:

- Symbolism – children's thought processes are developing; they are starting to make sense of their world and make use of symbolisation – for instance, a thumbs-up symbol for agreement/happy.
- Egocentrism – children generally see things from their own point of view.

Reflection: points to consider

You could use a doll or teddy to aid assistance when caring for a child at age 2–7 years. Not all children at this stage are egotistical; if the task is simple, the child may be able to see it from others' perspectives depending on where the child is in the stage of development.

- Animism – the child holds with the belief that everything that exists has some kind of consciousness. For example, if the car won't start, the car is tired; if the child is hurt in a collision with a chair, she will blame the 'naughty chair'.

- Moral realism (towards the later stage) – the child thinks that her way of thinking about what is right and wrong will be shared by everyone else. She will have respect for rules. The use of moral realism may well help you to administer treatment, if you explain that the treatment is essential.

Case study 7.3

You are called to a 5-year-old boy who has developed paraphimosis (a painful and retractile foreskin which constitutes a medical emergency). Considering different theories and stages of the boy's development, what conclusions could you reach on the nature of this condition being idiopathic, self-inflicted or symptomatic of abuse? What would be your plan of care?

Concrete operational stage, 7–11 years
At this stage you will experience a child with more rational and adult-like thinking. There is more logical reasoning and grasp of the idea that illness and death have biological causes. At this stage the child recognises her own mortality. This is an easier stage in the child's life, where you can explain what has happened and what you are going to do about it.

Children can think logically, if they can manipulate the actual object that they are thinking about. At this stage the child learns that objects are not always what they appear, for example, conservation, number, volume, length, mass (Whitnell 2012b).

Formal operational stage, 11–16 years
At this stage children can manipulate their own thoughts, and do not need the real object at hand. Around puberty, the ways in which children think change again. They

Table 7.2 Domains of development

Biological	Cognitive	Psycho-social
Genes	Perception	Temperament
Hormones	Memory	Family
Information processing	Imagination	Culture
Motor skills	Learning	Value
Fine motor skills	Thinking	Beliefs
	Decision-making	School
	Hearing and speech	Socialization and play
		Significant others

work things out in their heads, without seeing the object; they think more abstractly, consider a range of societal issues and can take others' reasons for behaviour into account. However, not all young people, nor indeed some adults, can do this, as they may not have developed to this stage cognitively.

Contemporary thinking on child development tends to lean towards ranges of development as opposed to stages (Berger 2011). Children develop different skills at differing times. All children are unique! (Whitnell 2012b).

Table 7.2 highlights the areas of development according to the main domains: biosocial, cognitive and psycho-social.

 Reflection: points to consider

Can you jot down from memory what is expected in terms of physical gross and fine motor skills according to ages and stages of child development, from birth to 5 years? It would be valuable for the paramedic and other health professionals who come into contact with children to have an understanding of the range of 'normal' development milestones to aid assessment of children. See a useful text entitled *Mary Sheridan's from Birth to Five Years: Children's Developmental Progress* (Sharma and Cockerill 2014). This text breaks down detailed ranges of development.

Piaget was criticised by social constructivists for his underestimation of the role of social and cultural factors in knowledge development, hence the emergence of the socio-cultural theory of development (Vygotsky 1962).

Socio-cultural theory

Lev Vygotsky (1896–1934) was one of the most important Russian psychologists of the twentieth century. He is famous for research into the development and structure of human consciousness, and the theory of signs, which explains the way children internalise language in the course of their social and cultural development.

The socio-cultural theory is relatively new when compared with the grand theories of development. Vygotsky argued that development results in a dynamic interaction between child or learner and people, surroundings and culture (normally parents, teachers, peers) that provides instruction and support to the child in order that she can acquire knowledge and capabilities. This theory considers the importance of social factors; children are apprentices in thinking. The concepts of 'scaffolding' and 'guided participation' in acts of everyday life are important for children to draw on. This is acquired through the child learning from experienced members of a social group. Vygotsky developed the concept of the Zone of Proximal Development (ZPD), shown in Figure 7.2.

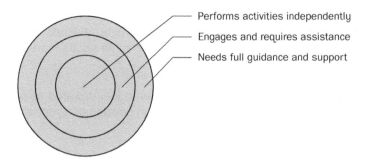

Performs activities independently

Engages and requires assistance

Needs full guidance and support

Figure 7.2   Process of proximal development

Source: Based on Vygotsky's Zone of Proximal Development.

Figure 7.2 highlights the process a child goes through, in terms of learning. The child moves through the learning process from the outer zone (being totally dependent and supported) through the middle zone (being facilitated) to the inner zone where the child becomes fully independent.

Vygotsky (1962) also emphasised the importance of language as a learning tool for children and language being valuable in terms of communicating feelings. He argued that inner speech is a form of language spoken to oneself, for instance, in an examination a student could use inner speech to talk through the answer to a question before writing.

This chapter has provided the reader with an understanding of children's development. It will be apparent that there are not only different theoretical approaches to child development but also different stages/ranges at which the child develops. Below are examples of two situations that can be related to children of different ages, in terms of practical care.

PSYCHOLOGICAL APPROACHES LINKED TO PRACTICE

When caring for children at different ages and stages/ranges of development, there will be differing ways to approach the child in order that you can care appropriately. The ages and stages examples below provide a guide to the range of development, bearing in mind all children are unique.

Below highlights the different ways in which you may care for a child with breathing difficulties who is requiring an oxygen mask and makes the link to the developmental theory behind the management:

- At 6–9 months of age, you may show the child what the mask looks like on a teddy or doll before attempting to use it on the child in order that he allows you to care for him. A child will copy/mimic behaviour if it appears to be 'OK'. This aligns to modelling behaviour within social learning theory.

- At 5 years of age, the child grasps and understands that illness has a biological cause and she needs help, but may be assertive and refuse. It is necessary to explain to a child of this age the importance of the mask and the reasoning behind its use in quite simple terms. The child may want to take control of the mask. This situation in terms of development aligns with cognitive theory; this child is likely to be at the pre-operational stage of development. This child's efforts to act independently can lead to pride or failure. This age child is at the initiative vs guilt stage within psychosocial theory.
- At 12 years of age, this child would be within the formal operational stage of cognitive development. His thinking is more refined and he can comprehend more immediate risks and will accept help and try to understand why he requires the oxygen via a mask to make his breathing easier.

Below highlights the different ways in which you may care for a child who is experiencing pain at different ages and considers theories of development:

- At 2 years of age the child may cry out, 'it hurts' or 'sore' and possibly hold the painful area while crying. This age child is unlikely to communicate clearly verbally. You will need this child's comforter to help settle her if possible. This child will be 'stranger aware' and cling to the carer; you may need to administer the treatment to the child in the carer's arms. This child is at the end of the sensori-motor stage according to Piaget, and has made attachment to the carer.
- At 5 years of age, the child will show you where the pain is on her body by pointing at the area that hurts. She will be able to point at a pain chart of images/faces to gauge the amount of pain she is experiencing. She may also be able to show you on the teddy or doll where the pain is. According to the cognitive pre-operational stage of development, this child may have a cognitive understanding of moral realism.
- At 11 years, the child will be able to tell you on a scale of 1–10 how bad it is. Pain experience can be mediated by socio-cultural factors (e.g. verbal/non-verbal cues given off by the carer). However, it is imperative that as a paramedic you always believe what the child says until the child is investigated. If the child has been rewarded for his behaviour, previously he may have learned to behave in this way. The theory behind this idea comes from positive reinforcement/operant conditioning. This child may have experienced pain in the past and had a positive outcome from medication in which case the child may be happy to accept pain relief; this situation links with the theory on classical conditioning.

ATYPICAL DEVELOPMENT

As a paramedic, you are likely to care for and transport children with special needs or a learning disability. As this is an introductory text this chapter includes limited discussion of emotional, behavioural and social problems and learning disabilities that children can experience. Therefore, this section will include an example of disorders that will lead to atypical development such as attention deficit hyperactive disorder (ADHD), autistic spectrum disorder and children who have Down's syndrome. It is important that you have an understanding of the diversity of children's development in order that you care for them appropriately. In the first instance, it is incumbent upon me to say that children with learning disabilities should be considered as children in the first instance, with needs and rights similar to those of any other child. Their disability and care needs are secondary. They will have other special needs but the understanding and management of those needs (albeit in some instances challenging) will affect the outcome. There are many difficulties that all children can face and it is important that paramedics are aware of the potential additional risk of harm for children with learning disabilities and the need to protect them and consider their rights along with all other children (Jones and Welch 2010). I hope that this section will offer 'food for thought' and that you will be interested enough to search for further information on children with atypical development by way of self-directed learning.

The study of developmental psychopathology is thought of as a relationship between psychology and the study of childhood disorders. A range of functions will be taken into account when assessing a child's development, for example, biological, genetic, socio-cultural and cognitive. Psychologists generally assume a continuum of behaviour, with the child's behaviour showing somewhere along it (Comer 2017). There are a number of factors that may contribute to, or result in, learning disabilities. The preconceptual, prenatal, perinatal and postnatal periods are distinct and differing times, before and during pregnancy and after birth, when learning disabilities can occur, as these are the times when possible causative factors operate. These factors are:

- Heredity: the gene is a discrete segment of the chromosome and the basic unit for the transition of heredity instructions, e.g. hair and eye colour traits. The chromosome is the carrier of genes. An example of chromosomal abnormality is Down's syndrome; see the section on Down's syndrome in this chapter for further details.
- Environment during and after pregnancy: toxic agents, birth trauma, oxygen starvation, nutrition (Gates 2011).

How do professionals diagnose children with atypical development? How do they know when normal behaviour ends and developmental psychopathology begins? Children differ considerably in their rate of development, and it makes sense to continue to think in terms of the stages of development that most children go through at around the same ages. However, these stages are less relevant to those children who, for a number of reasons, are not developing as per the 'normal' age and stage/range.

There are many ways of determining whether someone has a learning disability; however, no one criterion will provide a definitive answer. Over time, psychiatrists and researchers have highlighted the confusion of diagnosis and the use of different tools (Morton 2004). Defining learning disability is difficult as it means different things to different people. Generally, it is agreed that learning disability comprises sub-average intellectual functioning that coexists with below-average social functioning that manifests before the age of 18 years (Gates 2011).

Children with learning disability fall into three main areas and can be assessed using differing diagnostic tools:

1   Intellectual ability (Intelligent Quotient = IQ) (APA, 2013); Child Behaviour Checklist (Achenbach 2013);
2   Legislative definitions: Mental Health Act (1983/2007);
3   Social competence criterion.

Children who have a learning disability will have an IQ which is below the average IQ of 100. IQ is useful only up to the age of 18 years. IQ within the population is evenly distributed, therefore it is possible to measure how far an individual is from what is considered 'normal'. Using this system, a child who has an IQ of less than 70 is said to have a learning disability (scores more than two standard deviations (SD) from the average of 100; score of 15 = 1 SD).

- 70–84 = borderline of intellectual functioning;
- 50–69 = mild learning disability (25–30 people in UK per 1000 population);
- 35–49 = moderate learning disability;
- 20–34 = severe mental retardation (3–4 people in UK per 1000 population);
- <20 = profound mental retardation (people with complex additional disabilities, e.g. sensory, physical or behavioural).

                    Adapted from NICE Guideline (May 2015) and www.bild.org.uk

In legislative terms, children who have physical and sensory impairment, for example, who are blind or deaf or suffer from cerebral palsy, are considered to have a learning disability (DH 2007).

Children with emotional and behavioural problems, such as autistic spectrum disorders (including Asperger's disorder) and Attention Deficit Hyperactivity Disorder (ADHD), are likely to have impaired social functioning and may be assessed using the social competence criterion (Wilmshurst 2017).

An example of a diagnostic tool is shown in Box 7.1.

Box 7.1 *Diagnostic Statistical Manual of Mental Disorders* (DSM-V)

DSM-V uses categories to classify behaviour, signs and symptoms logged to enable diagnosis. DSM-V is not concerned with classification, more with the behaviour expressed; suggesting this helps to remove the negative stigma of labelling which only leads to derogation and uninformed understanding.

Critique: DSM-V considers developmental issues but does not consider changes in children over time. Disorders can occur as a function of age and change at different ages, e.g. Attention Deficit Hyperactive Disorder = in young child; more hyperactivity than in older child (American Psychiatric Association 2013).

Diagnostic tools

Another useful diagnostic tool is shown in Box 7.2.

Box 7.2 Child Behaviour Checklist (CBCL)

CBCL is dimensional and provides information about the way and how much the individual shows disturbance. Deviation is viewed as continuous from normal (continuum). It allows for changing behaviour. CBCL looks at internal and external scales. Internal disorders include anxiety and depression; external are outward (ADHD) 'acting out' a form of distress, including aggression and delinquency. Children can show both, e.g. be sulky and aggressive at the same time.

Critique: CBCL does not include some major disorders, e.g. autism, eating disorders, which DSM-V includes (Achenbach 2013).

It can often be difficult to confirm a diagnosis of behaviour, because co-morbidity (where two different conditions are present in one child) can occur. For some children with learning disabilities, a precise diagnosis is not possible and a more comprehensive, multiagency assessment of the child's needs is required. This is obtained using the *Framework for the Assessment of Children in Need and Their Families* (DH 2011). This assessment includes the parents' needs for support with caring for the child.

This section will consider a small sample of some significant childhood disorders that children experience which will bring into being learning disabilities of one form or another; during your working practice, it is very likely you will care for children with a developmental disorder.

Attention Deficit Hyperactivity Disorder (ADHD)

Signs and symptoms:

- unable to sit still for any length of time (pattern of restlessness/overactivity);
- loses things;
- cannot concentrate on tasks, even fun tasks;
- easily distracted;
- doesn't appear to listen (inattentive);
- much energy, fidgets, runs, climbs, talks incessantly;
- shows anti-social behaviour (impulsive);
- interrupts conversation.

Adapted from APA (2013)

ADHD is an externalising form of maladjustment. The name of this disorder highlights the issues that arise. It involves the ongoing presence of inattention and hyperactivity

Case study 7.4

You are called to a 14-year-old boy who has punched a brick wall and has suspected fractures to the fingers and hand. The child is both aggressive and uncooperative and finds it difficult to articulate his situation. A carer introduces himself and explains that the child has ADHD. Consider how you would assess and treat this young boy.

with impulsiveness, all of which are beyond the norm and are more frequent and severe. In true ADHD, symptoms are evident in children younger than 7 years of age and the behaviour occurs at school and at home.

It is difficult to diagnose this in toddlers, as at this age you would expect inattention, but it can be detected if extreme, frequent and chronic. It is easier to detect in middle childhood, as one would expect a child to have more control in their activities, be socially competent and be able to concentrate for a period of time. These children can show anti-social behaviour in adolescence and young adulthood, consequently, this disorder may go hand in hand with conduct disorder (co-morbidity). Conduct disorder is defined as 'a repetitive and persistent pattern of behaviour in which the basic rights of others or major age-appropriate societal norms or rules are violated' (APA 2013). Indeed, co-occurrence of conduct disorder and ADHD and their symptoms is so strong that researchers have questioned whether they are separate disorders (Morton 2004).

Autism

Autism lies at the extreme end of the autistic spectrum and is characterised by a triad of social communication difficulties. Vygotsky (1962) stated that language, thoughts and social interaction are inextricably linked around the age of 2 years. Consequently, this disorder may not be noticed in infancy. These children have impairment in communication and socialisation, and restricted and repetitive interests, movements and activities. The factors suggested for this disorder are prenatal (genetics/uterine environment, brain structure and function), perinatal (birth trauma) and postnatal (vaccination = MMR, food intolerance) (Boucher 2009; Gates 2011).

Signs and symptoms:

- deficits in sociability and empathy;
- deficits in communicative language;
- deficits in cognitive flexibility;
- delay with speech development;
- restricted, repetitive and stereotyped patterns of behaviour, interests and activities;
- detectable before the age of 3 years;
- 70 per cent of children have IQ < 70.

Asperger's syndrome

Signs and symptoms:

- poor social skills, lack of insight;
- behavioural inflexibility, narrow range of interests;
- IQ > 70. Note: these children have an IQ that is greater than the criteria for learning disability and indeed can have strengths in verbal areas (Wilmshurst 2017).
- no delay with speech; often well-developed vocabulary basis but deficit in communication at a social level;
- visual motor clumsiness with typical stiff gait and posture.

The word 'autism' was first used by a Boston physician called Leo Kanner in 1943. There are three main characteristics forming the triad of social communication of this disorder:

1. Social interaction – poor eye contact and use of gestures and facial expressions. These children have no interest in others or joining in. They cannot understand the effect of their behaviour on others and have no insight into their own or others' behaviour.
2. Communication – there is delay in speech. These children misinterpret sarcasm, jokes and non-verbal cues. They also take things literally.
3. These children have restrictive, repetitive patterns of behaviour, interests and activities. They are excessive in rituals and routines and have unusual interests. These children can be prone to self-injury, e.g. head banging or biting.

There is another form called Pervasive Developmental Disorder (PDD) that is not otherwise specified. PDD applies to less severely affected children who do not meet the criteria for either autism or Asperger's syndrome (APA 2013).

Autism can be co-morbid with:

- learning disability;
- epilepsy;
- speech and language difficulties;
- ADHD;
- dyspraxia (motor coordination problem);
- tics and Tourette's syndrome;
- feeding and eating difficulties (refusal, hoarding, overeating) (www.nas.org.uk).

Parents are usually the first to note that their child's development is unusual and may feel relief to know there is a reason/diagnosis. However, it should not be underestimated that having a child with autistic spectrum disorder (like other disorders) can cause considerable stress in raising a child. There are three main factors that are particularly stressful: (1) societal lack of understanding (stigma and challenging behaviour); (2) poor service provision (pre-school and school provision); and (3) the permanency of the condition (relationships and work). However, there is an emerging political movement of autistic people which is gaining media attention in the hope that society will alter its attitudes towards autistic spectrum disorder (Gates 2011).

Prior to the inclusion of Asperger's disorder in the DSM, there was considerable controversy regarding differential diagnoses among disorders and syndromes that share common features, such as autism, Asperger's syndrome, and semantic pragmatic disorder. Even though these disorders now sit within a spectrum of pervasive developmental disorders, it remains difficult to distinguish between Asperger's disorder and 'high-functioning autism' (Wilmshurst 2017).

Down's syndrome

British physician John Langdon Down (1828–1896) first described the abnormality of the twenty-first chromosome in 1866, hence the name Down's syndrome. The most common chromosomal disorder leading to a learning disability is Down's syndrome (Gates 2011). Definitive diagnosis is available by obtaining a small sample of cells from the tissue of the placenta from the pregnant woman, called chorionic villous sampling by amniocentesis.

There are three types of chromosomal abnormality resulting in Down's syndrome:

* Trisomy 21 accounts for 94 per cent of people with Down's syndrome. The individual has three instead of two twenty-first chromosomes.
* Translocation – the individual has two normal twenty-first chromosomes and a third twenty-first chromosome fused with another chromosome (15th or 13th).
* Mosaicism – this is extremely rare and involves cells with two twenty-first chromosomes and cells with three twenty-first chromosomes found in the same person.

Signs and symptoms (Gates 2011; Comer 2017):

* IQ between 35 and 49 (level of intellectual impairment differs in individuals);
* may have difficulty with pronunciation due to protruding tongue and intellectual disability;
* may develop slower than expected range of development;
* this child will age quickly so may look older than his biological age;
* may develop dementia in older age (40–50) due to genes of dementia being located close to each other on chromosome 21 (ongoing research);
* facial features = small head, flattened facial appearance, high cheekbones, hair is dry and sparse;
* congenital heart disease affects around 40 per cent;
* thyroid disease occurs in about 20 per cent.

A useful website is: www.downs-syndrome.org.uk. Many different characteristics are associated with Down's syndrome, but it should be noted that not all children and adults with this condition will exhibit them all.

Reflection: points to consider

As a paramedic, you are in a prime position to notice differences and atypical behaviour in terms of a child's development. Some things to think about:

- A child may not be developing according to the age and expected range of development; this is where your knowledge of the well child and stages/ranges of development will be very useful.
- You need to pick up cues from the carer and from the response that you get from the child when communicating with her. (For ideas on communication, see Chapter 1.)
- Make sure you collect whatever enables the child to maximise his ability to understand, if possible, and most certainly allow the child to take her comfort, e.g. toy, doll, blanket. Remember that this child may have an 'unusual' interest in an object, for example, the batteries in a toy, as opposed to the toy.

How to relate to a child/adult with learning disability

Children and adults with learning disability, as with the rest of the population, will display a range of behaviour. As a paramedic you will need to use your acute assessment and communication skills in order to establish a rapport and maximise communication with the child/adult/family/carer as soon as possible. This is so that you get the best from them and they trust your professional care. As a paramedic you will use the clues around you, in terms of their living situation and how their carer communicates with them, to determine how you should communicate with them, in either a child-like or adult-like manner. Children can show challenging behaviour towards you; indeed, this can be a characteristic of a child with learning disability, such as ADHD or autism. You would be wise to gain the assistance of the carer who will know how best to manage the child. In contrast, one of the most endearing (or possibly awkward, depending on your personal experience) characteristics of children with Down's syndrome, for example, is their loving nature and very often public demonstration of the same (Whitnell 2012b).

Reflection: points to consider

While children with Down's syndrome are generally happy and loving and are often keen to express their love (even to strangers), this can be a disadvantage as they can be vulnerable.

You may be called to a person with learning disability who lives alone, in a supported community, with carers or with family as back-up support. Observing the environment in which the person lives may provide you with clues about how independent she may be.

If a person with learning disability lives in a supported community, it is likely that she may have been encouraged with and taught some social and practical skills to enable her to live relatively independently. If, however, a person with learning disability lives with his family, it may be that he is unable to live independently or has not been given the opportunity to do so.

People with learning disability who have been socialised to be more independent may have been taught to curb their affections with strangers. However, in general terms, if a person, especially a child, with learning disability takes a liking to your personable nature, she will generally cooperate with you in your assessment and possibly even treatment. In contrast, if a child or adult with learning disability does not want to cooperate, she can be extremely stubborn and possibly obstructive.

CONCLUSION

This chapter has provided a taste of the exciting subjects of psychology and child development. In order for the paramedic to assess and treat patients accurately and effectively. it is of paramount importance to have knowledge and understanding of why children and families behave in the way that they do. This chapter has provided the paramedic with information on the many approaches to psychology and child development theory.

This chapter also considered atypical development to provide you with an overview of the diversity of children and young adults and their needs. There are many positive changes that have occurred in the care of children and adults with learning disabilities. However, changes need to continue if this group is to be included, valued and afforded an equal status in society.

Chapter key points:

- Paramedics require an understanding of psychology in order to care holistically for patients/clients and their families.
- An understanding of the work of the key child development theorists will help the paramedic understand more about the development and behaviour of clients requiring their care and treatment.
- In addition to 'normal' development, the paramedic also requires an understanding of atypical development and disability, in order to provide holistic care to the patient.

REFERENCES AND SUGGESTED READING

Achenbach, T. (2013) *Assess Adaptive and Maladaptive Functioning: Achenbach System of Empirically Based Assessment (ASEBA)*. London: Harcourt Press.
Ainsworth, M.D.S. (1979) Infant–mother attachment. *American Psychologist*, 34: 932–7.

APA (American Psychiatric Association) (2013) *Diagnostic and Statistical Manual of Mental Disorders, DSM-V*. Philadelphia, PA: American Psychiatric Association.

Bandura, A. (1977) *Social Learning Theory*. London: Prentice-Hall.

Banyard, P., Davies, M.N.O., Norman, C. and Winder, B. (2010) *Essential Psychology: A Concise Introduction*. London: Sage.

Barker, S. (2016) *Psychology for Nursing and Health Care Professionals: Developing Compassionate Care*. London: Sage.

Berger, K.S. (2011) *The Developing Person Through the Lifespan*, 8th edn. New York: Worth Publishers.

Boucher, J. (2009) *The Autistic Spectrum: Characteristics, Causes and Practical Issues*. London: Sage.

Bowlby, J. (1979) *Attachment and Loss*. Vol. 1: *Attachment*. Harmondsworth: Penguin.

Bradford, H. (2012) *The Wellbeing of Children Under Three*. London: Routledge.

Brady, M. (2012) Pre-hospital psycho-social care: changing attitudes. *Journal of Paramedic Practice*, 4(9): 516–25.

British Institute of Learning Disabilities (BILD) (2018) *Statistics*. Available at: www.bild.org.uk. (accessed 1 January 2018).

Comer, R.J. (2017) *Abnormal Psychology*, 9th edn. New York: Worth.

DH (Department of Health) (2007) *Mental Health Act*. London: HMSO.

DH (Department of Health) (2011) *Framework for the Assessment of Children in Need and Their Families*. London: TSO.

Dogra, N., Parkin, A., Gale, F. and Frake, C. (2009) *A Multidisciplinary Handbook of Child and Adolescent Mental Health for Front-Line Professionals*, 2nd edn. London: Jessica Kingsley.

Gates, B. (2011) *Learning Disabilities: Towards Inclusion*, 6th edn. London: Churchill Livingstone.

Gerrig., R.J., Zimbardo, P.G., Svartdal, F., Brennen, T., Donaldson, R. and Archer, T. (2012) *Psychology and Life*. Harlow: Pearson Education.

Jones, P. and Welch, S. (2010) *Rethinking Children's Rights. Attitudes in Contemporary Society*. London: Continuum.

Kalat, J.H. (2014) *Biological Psychology*, 11th edn. Pacific Grove, CA: Brooks/Cole Publishing.

Maslow, A.H. (1970) *Toward a Psychology of Being*, 3rd edn. New York: Van Nostrand.

Morton, J. (2004) *Understanding Developmental Disorders: A Causal Modelling Approach*. Oxford: Blackwell Publishing.

Mukherji, P. and Dryden, L. (2014) *Foundations of Early Childhood: Principles and Practice*. London: Sage.

NICE (2015) *Challenging Behavior and Learning Disabilities: Prevention and Interventions for People with Learning Disabilities Whose Behaviour Challenges*. London: DH.

Sharma, A. and Cockerill, H. (2014) *Mary Sheridan's From Birth to Five Years: Children's Developmental Progress*. London: Routledge.

Turner-Cobb, J. (2014) *Child Health Psychology: A Biopsychosocial Perspective*. London: Sage.

Vygotsky, L. (1962) *Thought and Language*. Boston, MA: MIT Press.

Wilmshurst, L. (2017) *Child and Adolescent Psychopathology: A Case Book*, 4th edn. London: Sage.

Whitnell, J. (2012a) Psychology: an introduction. In A.Y. Blaber (ed.) *Foundations of Paramedic Practice: A Theoretical Perspective*. Maidenhead: Open University Press.

Whitnell, J. (2012b) Developmental psychology: an introduction. In A.Y. Blaber (ed.) *Foundations of Paramedic Practice: A Theoretical Perspective*. Maidenhead: Open University Press.

8 Mental health
Children, young people and adults
Jackie Whitnell

In this chapter:

- Introduction
- Why is this relevant?
- Child and adolescent mental health (CAMH)
- An overview of abnormal psychology
- Legislative powers and mental health
- Conclusion
- Chapter key points
- References and suggested reading

INTRODUCTION

'Defining mental health and illness is difficult. In our society the word "mental" has negative connotations and, over time, has been used as a term of abuse' (Whitnell 2012c: 38). The field of mental health and abnormal psychology is the area of psychological investigation directly concerned with understanding mental health and the nature of individual pathologies of mind, mood and behaviour (Gerrig et al. 2012). Abnormal psychology focuses on the causes and treatment of psychological disorders and adjustment problems, including mood, personality and dissociative disorders, colloquially referred to as 'mental health problems/disorders' or 'mental ill health'. Estimates of the prevalence of mental ill health in Britain vary. The Mental Health Foundation (2018b) and Mental Health Network (2016) put the figure at one in six adults at any one time. The one in six figure represents those people defined as having 'significant' mental health problems. Mental health problems are common at all ages, affecting one in four people at some point in their life, consequently there is a burden of cost to the National Health Service (NHS). Indeed, McManus et al. (2016) put the burden in the NHS budget for mental ill health at 28 per cent compared with heart conditions and cancer, both being 16 per cent. Mental health problems can be recurrent, remitting and enduring (Whitnell 2012c).

Box 8.1 Guidance for assessment of abnormal behaviour

1 *Distress or disability*: an individual experiences disabled functioning or personal distress which puts the client at risk of psychological deterioration.
2 *Maladaptiveness*: an individual acts in ways that hinder the client's or others' goals and thus hinders the personal well-being of self or others.
3 *Irrationality*: an individual talks or acts in ways that are incomprehensible or irrational to others.
4 *Unpredictability*: an individual behaves erratically or unpredictably, experiencing loss of control.
5 *Unconventionality and statistical rarity*: an individual behaves in a way that is rare; that violates social norms.
6 *Observer discomfort*: an individual creates discomfort in others, making them feel distressed or threatened.
7 *Violation of moral and ideal standards*: an individual violates expectations for how they ought to behave in the normal social world.

Adapted from Gerrig et al. (2012) and DSM-V (APA 2013)

How do health professionals decide what is abnormal behaviour? The distinction between normal and abnormal is not a difference between types of behaviour; it is more a matter of the extent to which a person's actions resemble a set of agreed criteria of abnormality (DSM-V, APA 2013). Mental disorder is best thought of as a continuum, as normal and abnormal are relative and not absolute. One end of the continuum defines optimum mental health, at the other end are behaviours that define minimal mental health and in between are gradual rises in maladaptive behaviours (Gerrig et al. 2012). For guidance on assessment of abnormal behaviour, see Box 8.1.

Professionals are more confident in labelling behaviour as 'abnormal' when more than one criterion is present and valid (Gerrig et al. 2012). The frequency of mental health problems is well documented statistically. However, these figures need to be considered with some caution. Often widely differing figures will be given for the same mental health problem, making it difficult to determine exactly how common the problem is. This is partly because these figures are not always measuring the same thing. There are often controversial challenges to the DSMV (Field and Cartright-Hatton 2015). For example, in order to reflect the fact that mental health is not fixed but likely to change over time, a variety of different figures are used. The most common are:

- *Prevalence*: this measures the number of people with a particular diagnosis at a given time.
- *Lifetime prevalence*: this measures the number of people who have experienced a particular mental health problem at any time in their lives.
- *Incidence*: this measures the number of new cases of a particular mental health problem that appear in a given time period (Comer, cited in Whitnell 2012c).

Often these figures are compared in order to provide further information about a mental health problem. For example, comparing the number of new cases (the incidence) with the number who are ill at any one time (the prevalence) can give us a rough idea of the average amount of time a mental health problem is likely to last. Another important factor is the kind of sample used to arrive at a particular figure. Often the number of people treated by health professionals is used to determine how common a mental health problem is. However, this is likely to ignore all those who have not come into contact with services. Furthermore, psychiatric diagnosis is often far from straightforward – a person's diagnosis may be changed several times in the course of their treatment.

Mental health problems may be associated with, provoked by and maintained by alcohol or other substances, possibly making the care of these individuals difficult. Indeed, while some patients will volunteer to accept your help, others will not and may need to be compelled to receive an assessment and treatment, possibly against their will, using the powers of legislation (DH 2005; 2007).

Due to the introductory nature of this text, this chapter will provide the reader with only a brief overview of mental ill health. The chapter will commence with an overview on child and adolescent mental health and will continue with discussion on mental health disorders that people can suffer.

Children can experience most of the disorders that adults experience. This chapter cannot cover all of them, therefore we will consider: deliberate self-harm, depression, eating disorders and anxiety. I must mention here that when assessing and caring for children, the age and stage of development should be taken into account (Field and Cartright-Hatton 2015; Wilmshurst 2017).

WHY IS THIS RELEVANT?

It is extremely important that paramedics have at least an understanding of some of the most common mental illnesses which children, young people and adults may have, and an idea of some of the signs and symptoms that the client/patient may exhibit. Paramedics will be in the position of caring for clients with mental ill health and will make assessments during their working practice. It is the aim that this overview will at least provide some information and excite an interest and thirst for further exploration of this area of ill health.

CHILD AND ADOLESCENT MENTAL HEALTH (CAMH)

It is now recognised that many mental health problems can manifest in childhood. One in three mental health conditions relates directly to adverse childhood experiences (APA 2013). There are a wide range of mental health problems that can affect children and adolescents. Children who experience three or more stressful life events, such as serious illness, family bereavement or divorce, are significantly more likely to develop emotional and behavioural disorders (Whitnell 2012c). Many studies have been conducted to identify the number of individuals experiencing specific problems. These studies generally use one of two classification and diagnostic criteria (DSM-V in APA 2013 or ICD10 in WHO 1992). Studies will give different results depending on the measures used and the cultural context in which they are used. Results will also differ, depending on many variables, for example, different populations and environments. Consequently, it can be very difficult to understand why there are still such variable rates of recorded prevalence of mental health problems in young people today. One in 10 children (roughly 3 in every classroom) aged 5–16 years has a mental disorder which is clinically recognisable based on the International Classification of Disease Related Health Problems (WHO 1992; 2018a), which is a classification of mental and behavioural disorders with strict impairment criteria. Half of all mental health problems manifest by the age of 14 years; 75 per cent by age 24 (Field and Cartright-Hatton 2015). Some 2 per cent of children suffer from more than one type of disorder (co-morbidity); this poses a greater challenge in terms of diagnosis and also in the care of the child.

To **Chapter 7**. Read the section on atypical development for more information on child-related conditions (Whitnell 2012a; 2012c).

Deliberate self-harm (DSH)

Children as young as 7 have been found to self-harm, however, the average age for children commencing self-harm is 13 years old. DSH is common in the 10–14-year age group. One other important factor is that DSH is four times more common among girls. However, until the age of 12 years, DSH is more common in boys than girls (Gerrig et al. 2012).

DSH is considered an intentional act of self-injury with a non-fatal outcome in which an individual acted in one of the following ways:

- ingested a substance in excess of the prescribed dose or generally recognised therapeutic dose;
- initiated behaviour (for example, self-cutting, jumping from a height) which they intended to cause self-harm;
- ingested a recreational drug or illicit substance that was an act that the person regarded as self-harm;
- ingested a non-ingestible substance or object.

Reflection: points to consider

Before continuing, jot down some of the risk factors for mental health problems in children and young people.

Field and Cartright-Hatton (2015) identified a number of environmental, family and individual factors that can lead to a higher level of risk of mental health problems in children and young people. These include living in families where the main 'breadwinner' is unemployed, having a parent with a mental illness, and having some form of learning disability. Other possible causes are genetic predisposition, stress at home or school, over-protective parents and an over-controlling environment.

It is estimated that 80 per cent of children and adolescents with mental health problems are also likely to experience family life and relationship difficulties. Thankfully, suicide is rare in childhood and early adolescence, but it becomes more frequent with increasing age. Suicide is the most common cause of death for boys aged 5–19 and the second cause of death for girls of the same age. The relationship between psychiatric disorders and adolescent suicide is now well established. Previous suicide attempts, mood disorders and substance misuse are strongly related (Dogra et al. 2009; Gerrig et al. 2012).

Depression in childhood

The criteria for depressive disorders are the same or similar for children and adults (depression in adults will be discussed later in this chapter). However, there are differences in how this disorder shows itself for different ages. Depression is thought to occur in 1 per cent of children and young people, with children as young as 5 suffering signs and symptoms of depression (see Box 8.2) (Achenbach 2013; RCPSYCH 2017). However, depression is not very common before adolescence (Field and Cartright-Hatton 2015).

In terms of gender and depression in childhood, prior to age 12, males report greater rates of depression, following which there is a reversal in the gender ratio (Dogra et al. 2009). In puberty, more girls than boys suffer with depression and the same into adulthood. By mid-adolescence, approximately 2–3 per cent of children will experience a diagnosis of depressive disorder. Girls internalise their feelings and depression tends to show in mood state, whereas boys externalise their feelings and act out (Dogra et al. 2009) (Box 8.3). Consequently, one could argue that as girls express this disorder more outwardly in their mood, it is more noticeable and easier to detect. One approach used to explain the occurrence of depression in childhood derives from attachment theory

---

Box 8.2 Depression in childhood; signs and symptoms for differing stages

- *Infant/toddler* – loss of developmentally appropriate behaviour, e.g. toilet training and intellectual function.
- *Pre-school* – sad appearance or irritable, regression to earlier development, e.g. separation anxiety and sleep problems.
- *School age* – eating and sleep disturbances, being self-critical, and having low motivation. They may act out their distress.

(Whitnell 2012a: 98)

> ## Box 8.3 Depression in childhood
>
> Signs and symptoms
> - sadness or irritability
> - tiredness
> - self-pity
> - loss of appetite
> - disturbed sleep pattern
> - thoughts of death.
>
> (Whitnell 2012a: 99)

(Field and Cartright-Hatton 2015). This suggests that insecure attachment can lead to depression in infants, children and adolescents. Feeling insecure leads to unworthiness and the feeling of being unloved can predispose children to being vulnerable, fearing disapproval and abandonment. A further consideration from the social-cultural theory suggests the cause could derive from problems in the home, in school or with peers (Berger 2011; Whitnell 2012c, Field and Cartright-Hatton 2015).

 Chapter 7 for discussion of David in Case study 7.1.

There are different types of anxiety, for example:

- specific phobias;
- obsessive-compulsive disorder (boys > girls);
- separation anxiety disorder;
- social phobia;
- panic disorder (girls > boys).

Anxiety will be discussed in more detail later in this chapter.

 Reflection: points to consider

You may attend to and transport a child/adult who suffers from anxiety. What would your approach be? How would you try to calm the child/adult in order to care for them and transport them safely?

When children and young people present with mental health problems, the solution to their difficulties is rarely straightforward. Munir (2016) argues that children often present with more than one problem. The most frequent number of problems is four or five, while half of children referred to CAMH services have at least two severe problems (co-morbidity)

(Whitnell 2012c; Field and Cartright-Hatton 2015). As a paramedic you will attend and possibly transport children and adolescents with mental health problems. It is important that you have a good understanding of the types of issues and difficulties facing these children as well as report your findings of the interactions you observe between the child/ young person and significant others, noting anything that you find unusual, inappropriate or unsafe (Brown et al. 2016).

AN OVERVIEW OF ABNORMAL PSYCHOLOGY

Self-harm and suicide

The incidence of self-harm, which has always been high, does not seem to be abating. Attempted suicide and self-harm are considered both the same entity: called 'suicide-related behaviour'. The term 'suicide-related behaviour' is used to describe all behaviours where the person intended to kill or harm himself. Deliberate self-harm is frequently encountered by paramedics and healthcare professions alike; it is a hidden health prob-lem worldwide (Rees et al. 2015). Self-harm is one of the leading five causes of acute medical admission for women and men. The myth around self-harm is that it is a cry for attention; this is not totally accurate. While deliberate self-harm can communicate to others the person's suffering, it can also express that the individual needs help and is in crisis. Self-harm is commonly completed in private. It is true to say that family, friends and therapists may be unaware of the episodes of self-harm a person is experiencing (Whitnell 2012a; Mental Health Foundation 2018b).

Without doubt, there is no greater problem facing mental health practitioners than suicide-related behaviour. Since the mid-1970s, the data gathered has consistently indicated that suicide is a leading cause of death in young people. The possible contrib-uting factors could include:

- decriminalisation of the Suicide Act in 1961;
- drug-prescribing increase since the 1960s;
- the rise in unemployment at the end of the 1970s and early 1990s.

There is one death from suicide every 90 minutes across the UK and Ireland (ONS 2017). Almost three-quarters of these suicides are among men.

Suicide rates for men are higher than for women in all age groups, and currently men are almost three times more likely than women to commit suicide. However, suicide rates in the UK decreased in 2016 by 3.6 per cent (ONS 2017). From 2015–2016 the suicide rate fell for males and females in England and Wales.

The likelihood of a person committing suicide depends on many factors: social problems – especially those related to family stress, separation, divorce, social isolation, death of a loved one and unemployment (an unemployed man is two to three times more at risk of suicide than the general population); mental and physical illness; and access to the means of suicide. Certain occupational groups such as healthcare professionals, vets and farmers are at higher risk of suicide (ONS 2017). Alcohol and drug use are also factors which can influence suicide risk. Men are known to have far higher drug and alcohol consumption rates than women, and the figures are particularly high for younger men (ONS 2017). Suicide by self-poisoning is an important cause of death worldwide. A substantial proportion of those with a fatal outcome may come into contact with a paramedic and/or emergency department before they die.

Box 8.4 highlights some risk factors for suicide.

There are a variety of tools available often used by specialist paramedics and approved mental health professionals (AMHP), and the paramedic has a professional responsibility and should be encouraged to expand and update their knowledge of mental health assessment to improve their competence and confidence. Such knowledge may aid their skill of appropriate referral and subsequently the care of their patient. An example assessment tool used by paramedics in practice can be found in JRCALC (Brown et al. 2016) – the IPAP suicide risk levels (Brown et al. 2016: 10, Tables 3.16 and 3.17).

Box 8.4 Suicide: a serious mental health and public health problem

Facts about suicide

- Suicide rates vary by culture.
- Suicide is the most common cause of death among men aged between 15 and 44 years (ONS 2017).
- In all cultures, men are more likely than women to complete suicide.
- Rates of suicide in children and adolescents are on the increase (Gerrig et al. 2012).
- People with mental disorders, especially depression, schizophrenia and borderline personality disorder, are at high risk for suicide.

Risk factors

- Past history of attempted suicide.
- Talking about committing suicide.
- A clear plan to commit suicide.
- Available means (e.g. access to a gun, drugs).
- Depression.
- Substance abuse.
- Hopelessness.
- Impulsivity.
- Stressful life events.
- Lack of social support.
- Saying goodbye to people.
- Giving away personal items.

Adapted from Whitnell (2012a: 102)

Chapter 18 for your continuing professional development responsibilities.

Anxiety disorders

Anxiety is an illness that becomes problematic enough to interfere with a person's ability to function effectively or enjoy everyday life. Anxiety produces an intense, often unrealistic and excessive state of apprehension and fear. This may or may not occur during, or in anticipation of, a specific situation, and may be accompanied by a rise in blood pressure, increased heart rate, rapid breathing, nausea and other signs of agitation or discomfort. MIND (2017) estimates that 6 per cent of adults experience generalised anxiety disorders (GAD) (not including depression) at any one time. GAD is an anxiety disorder in which the individual feels anxious or worried most of the time for at least six months when no threat is apparent (Field and Cartright-Hatton 2015). A further 7.8 per cent of the population has mixed anxiety and depression. Mood, stress-related and anxiety disorders are the most common groups of problems and often represent the extremes of normal emotion. They are recognised by a set of symptoms:

- depressed mood (to be discussed further on in this chapter);
- emotional – fear, worry;
- physical – shortness of breath, sweating, upset stomach, heart pounding;
- cognitive – fear of dying, losing control, 'going crazy'.

Adapted from APA (2013).

Anxiety is a usual part of our everyday lives, however, how do we differentiate between 'normal' or manageable fear from anxiety, and impairment due to unmanageable anxiety? A disorder can be classified when there is fear and anxiety in response to something that is not inherently frightening or dangerous (see Box 8.5). This may be termed the 'target of fear'.

Box 8.5 Anxiety disorder

Anxiety disorders have four things in common:

- Each is defined by a specific target of fear, this is the situation/item the person is afraid of.
- Encountering the target of fear may induce anxiety or panic attacks.
- The sufferer avoids the target of fear.
- Anxiety disorders tend to be persistent – so are chronic in nature, rather than being episodic.

Adapted from Whitnell (2012a: 104)

Types of anxiety disorder

1   *Specific phobias* – fear and avoidance of a particular object or situation (e.g. dogs, heights, flying). People can live a 'normal' life, by avoiding their phobia, unless they are asked to confront their fear. Phobias are present in 18 per cent of adults and 1 per cent of children and more in females than males (Field and Cartright-Hatton 2015).

2   *Social phobia* – tends to be more impairing as it involves significant social isolation. People with this type of phobia are afraid of rejection and negative evaluation, so they avoid it at all costs. These phobias can be mild (fearing public speaking – see Case study 7.1 of David in Chapter 7) or severe (fearing all social interaction). Some 1.9 per cent of adults in Britain experience phobias and women are twice as likely as men to suffer (Mental Health Foundation 2018b).

3   *Panic disorder* – can be debilitating, especially when accompanied by agoraphobia. Panic disorders are related to anxiety. An anxiety disorder in which sufferers experience unexpected, severe panic attacks that begin with a feeling of intense apprehension, fear or terror. The anxiety begins with panic attacks that occur *out of the blue*. The disorder gets worse when people worry about having another panic attack and begin to avoid places and situations associated with the panic attack. Panic disorder accounts for 2–3 per cent of the population with an onset in childhood or adolescence and often are co-morbid (RCPSYCH 2017).

4   *Obsessive-compulsive disorder* (OCD) – can be quite specific but can also cause obsessive domination and impairment of someone's life. Symptoms are unwanted, persistent, intrusive, repetitive thoughts, also typical ritualistic repetitive behaviours that a person feels compelled to engage in, including hand washing, checking, counting and hoarding. It is traditionally regarded as a neurotic disorder, like phobias and anxiety states and 7–9 per cent of the population can suffer this disorder (Field and Cartright-Hatton 2015).

5   *Post-traumatic stress disorder* – see specific section below.

6   *Generalised anxiety disorder* – is characterised by a period of over six months of chronic, uncontrollable worry about numerous things. Sufferers are worried and tense at all times, easily irritated and have trouble sleeping and concentrating (Gerrig et al. 2012).

Post-traumatic stress disorder (PTSD)

PTSD is characterised by the persistent re-experience of traumatic events through recollections, dreams, hallucinations or flashbacks (Gerrig et al. 2012). It is one of the anxiety disorders but is worthy of specific attention due to the nature of the role of a paramedic.

 Reflection: point to consider

Consider the local and global situations that people have found themselves in over recent years that may predispose to a person suffering from PTSD.

Box 8.6 Post-traumatic stress disorder

Signs and symptoms/presentation:

- Fear of the trauma itself creates anxiety so the person will avoid anything associated with the trauma (avoidance).
- The person may lose their memory for the event, or be plagued with intrusive and unwanted thoughts, such as flashbacks and nightmares (re-experience).
- People tend to be psychologically numb, emotionally 'shut down', find no pleasure in things and cannot look to the future (emotional numbing).
- Conversely the person may have symptoms of 'hyper-arousal' – startle easily, cannot sleep or concentrate, be irritable and easily angered.

Specific recognition for children and young people:

- Do not rely wholly on an adult's assessment; if possible, ask the child or young person to explain how they feel and what they are experiencing.
- Ask the adult/child about sleep patterns or significant changes to it.

(RSPSYCH 2017) and (NICE 2015)

PTSD was first noted among war veterans. It can be equally seen in victims of trauma and in observers who witness or are involved in the event. Stress is the cause of PTSD (Box 8.6). Up to 80 per cent of adults experience a traumatic event in their life which may develop into PTSD. PTSD sufferers have a high suicide rate (Dogra et al. 2009). It can present in children following a traumatic event such as experiencing the divorce of their parents, seeking asylum, child abuse and/or living with domestic abuse. Emotionally the responses to PTSD can occur in an acute form immediately after the trauma and may not subside until after a period of several months. Globally people are migrating and seeking asylum: hence refugees are a vulnerable group.

Depression in adults

Depression is considered to be the 'common cold' of psychopathology, it aligns to learned helplessness. It occurs frequently and almost everyone has elements of this disorder at some time in their life. Depression with anxiety is experienced by 1 in 6 adults living in Great Britain. All neurotic disorders are more common in women than men, except panic disorder, which is equal for both. Women have a higher prevalence of mood disorders, however, studies suggest depression occurs as often in men, although women are twice as likely to be diagnosed and treated. It is argued that men tend to express their symptoms differently, for example, through the use of alcohol and drugs, and are unwilling to admit to the symptoms of depression. It is therefore interesting to note that the figures for men are rising faster than the figures for women. This may indicate that men now are more likely to admit to feeling depressed (Gerrig et al. 2012).

Box 8.7 Unipolar depression/major depressive disorder

The primary symptom is sad or depressed mood, but it is much more than this. Other symptoms include:

- lack of interest or pleasure in things that are usually enjoyed;
- changes in appetite;
- changes in sleep habits;
- low energy level, poor concentration and extreme fatigue;
- feeling bad about themselves, low self-esteem, negative self-concept; self-reproach and blaming themselves for what has 'gone wrong' in their life, 'paralysis of will' (Gerrig et al 2012);
- hopelessness about the future;
- preoccupation with ailments and death – suicidal ideation.

(Whitnell 2012a: 106–7)

Mood disorders may have some common symptoms but they have very different causes and prevalence to other disorders. Unipolar depression or major depressive disorder is one of the most common (see Box 8.7). Less prevalent are the bipolar disorders (otherwise known as manic depression). Depression is a disorder that affects people of all age groups, including children (Dogra et al. 2009; Wilmshurst 2017). The age of onset of major depressive disorder is reducing; early onset predicts a worse course of depression over time. Depression follows a recurrent course. Most people have multiple episodes that become worse with time, while some may have isolated episodes. Mild depression with a few symptoms may indicate the person will suffer with more serious depression later on. The feelings of major depressive disorder should not be negated. Some 15 per cent of depressed people commit suicide, due to the feelings of hopelessness and long-term suffering (Mental Health Foundation 2018b).

Bipolar affective disorder: commonly known as manic depression

Bipolar disorder is a mood disorder characterised by alternating periods of depression and mania (Gerrig et al. 2012). Most studies give a lifetime prevalence of 1 per cent for bipolar disorder and equal prevalence rates for men and women. Bipolar is a common health problem affecting between 1 and 2 per cent of the population and it affects people of all ages (see Box 8.8). However, hospital admission rates are much higher owing to the recurrent nature of the illness. It is a serious mental illness, but if it is well managed with help from family, friends, support groups and health professionals, then a person with bipolar can lead a productive and satisfying life. Manic depression has no known cure; a person may require psychiatric treatment for the rest of their life, although it is estimated that 20 per cent of people who have a first episode of manic depression do not get another (MIND 2017). It is considered that sufferers of bipolar depression have a predisposition genetically, but the manic state can be triggered by

---

> ## Box 8.8 Bipolar affective disorder
>
> Signs and symptoms/presentation
>
> - Highs and lows are increasingly disconnected from everyday events and out of control.
> - People feel excessively self-important, expansive and over-confident with inflated self-esteem or grandiose ideas.
> - There is an increase in goal-directed activity.
> - The person may become sexually promiscuous, excessively religious, financially irresponsible, intolerant, verbally aggressive, irritable, over-communicative and incapable of listening to or empathising with other people.
> - They may suffer from hallucinations, delusions and paranoia in extreme depression.
> - The person may suffer from sleeplessness and over-active behaviour.
> - Bipolar disorder occurs in 1 per cent of the population in contrast to unipolar disorder which occurs in 17 per cent of the population.
>
> (Whitnell 2012a: 107)

the stresses and strains of everyday life, or a traumatic event. Sufferers experience sudden onset lasting anything from one or two days to weeks or months. The average age of people with bipolar affective disorder used to be 32 years, but in the last decade it has dropped to under 19 years of age.

The symptoms of this disorder may only be spotted with the onset of a severe crisis in a person's life and may require compulsory treatment under the Mental Health Act (DH 2007). It may only be then that the person is referred to a psychiatric unit and diagnosed for treatment.

Postnatal depression

Another form of depression seen less frequently is that of postnatal depression. The most common form of postnatal disturbance is the 'baby blues', which is said to be experienced by at least half of all Western mothers. This usually lasts between 12 and 24 hours, generally occurring between the third and sixth day after the birth. This is perfectly normal and the mother and family may just need reassurance. An incidence figure of 10 per cent of all new mothers is most often quoted, with other studies showing a figure between 3 per cent and 22 per cent. It is likely that around 50 per cent of these cases will never come to medical attention. However, puerperal psychosis is a severe and relatively rare form of postnatal depression affecting between 0.1 and 0.2 per cent of all new mothers and as a paramedic you may be called to a patient suffering from this, where the husband/partner/carer is very concerned about the mother's behaviour (Comer 2017).

> ## Box 8.9 Personality disorder
>
> All personality disorders have some things in common:
>
> - long-standing – begin at a relatively early age;
> - chronic – continue over time;
> - pervasive – occur in most contexts.
>
> The behaviour, thoughts and feelings seen in personality disorder are:
>
> - inflexible – resistant to change and are applied in a rigid manner;
> - maladaptive – they do not enable the person to get what they expect/want.
>
> (Whitnell 2012a: 108)

Personality disorder

Another disorder that you may identify in a patient/client is personality disorder (see Box 8.9). Personality disorder is defined by instability and intensity in personal relationships as well as turbulent and impulsive behaviour (Gerrig et al. 2012). In Britain, the prevalence of personality disorder ranges from 2–6 per cent, according to different studies.

Sufferers of personality disorder will generally consider their behaviour perfectly normal and will blame the other person for the behaviour shown. Consequently, this may lead to treatment issues. It is always wise to consider your own safety as well as that of your patient in difficult situations (Comer 2017).

The DSM-V (APA 2013) describes the main disorders and their traits. There are 10 personality disorders that form three clusters:

Cluster A – the odd and eccentric cluster

- paranoid – suspicious, distrustful, makes hostile attributions;
- schizoid – interpersonally and emotionally cut off, unresponsive to others, a 'loner';
- schizotypal – odd thoughts, behaviours, experiences, poor interpersonal functioning.

Cluster B – the dramatic and erratic cluster

- histrionic – dramatic, wants attention, emotionally shallow;
- narcissistic – inflated sense of self-importance, will feel entitled, low empathy, hidden vulnerability;
- anti-social – behaviours that disregard laws, norms, rights of others; lacking in empathy – commonly men;
- borderline – instability in thoughts, feelings, behaviour and sense of self – commonly women.

Cluster C – the fearful and avoidant cluster

- obsessive-compulsive – rigid, controlled, perfectionist;
- avoidant – fears negative evaluation, rejection and abandonment;
- dependent – submissive, dependent on others for self-esteem.

Personality disorders are long-term patterns of emotional functioning. Each of the 10 disorders has a low prevalence in the general population. Most people with personality disorders do not seek, want or comply with treatment, consequently, treatment is not always effective (Field and Cartright-Hatton 2015; Comer 2017).

 Reflection: points to consider

Consider the three clusters and think about how you would manage a person expressing these symptoms towards you, who may require immediate treatment and who may be resistant.

Psychoses

Psychosis is a collection of signs that constitute a current mental state and may indicate the presence of a physical cause or a 'functional' disorder, such as schizophrenia or bipolar affective disorder. It is not a diagnosis in itself. Psychoses and functional psychoses are disorders that produce disturbances in thinking and perception that are severe enough to distort the person's perception of the world and the relationship of events in it. Psychoses are normally divided into two groups:

1 *Organic psychoses*, such as dementia and Alzheimer's.
2 *Functional psychoses*, which mainly cover schizophrenia and bipolar depression (although 'functional psychosis' does not necessarily have to belong to either one of these two diagnoses and can exist as a diagnosis in itself).

 Chapter 14 for more detail on caring for people with dementia.

Schizophrenia

The diagnostic label in ICD10 and DSMV sits schizophrenia alongside a group of psychotic disorders whereby personality seems to disintegrate, there is withdrawal from reality, thought and perception are distorted and emotions are blunted. When considering schizophrenia people often think of 'madness' or 'insanity'. Schizophrenia (see Box 8.10) is a complex and puzzling illness; experts in the field are not exactly sure what causes it.

Box 8.10 Schizophrenia

Presentation of positive, negative and disorganised symptoms:

- perceiving things that are not there – auditory hallucinations, may also be visual and tactile;
- paranoid delusions – believing things that are not true, delusions of grandeur, delusions of persecution;
- using bizarre language, 'word salad' (jumbled words);
- their behaviour may be reported by others as seriously disordered or irrational;
- lack of demonstrating emotions facially, inappropriate laughing, crying and anger.

Behaviour disturbances can be grouped into four areas:

- repetitive movements and mannerisms;
- significant lack of motivation – this can be termed 'avolition';
- struggle to take care of themselves with 'basic' care such as washing or dressing;
- social withdrawal, poor social skills and strained relationships with others.

(Whitnell 2012a: 110)

This is a common and often severe mental illness. It may present acutely with severe change in behaviour or insidiously as a slow but progressive change over a period of time. Some physicians think that the brain may not be able to process information correctly. Genetic factors appear to play a role, as people who have family members with schizophrenia may be more likely to inherit the disease themselves (Field and Cartright-Hatton 2015). While prevalence rates are the same for men and women, age and gender together form an important factor: one study shows incidence for men aged 15–24 years is twice that for women, whereas for those aged 24–35 years, it is higher among females. This reflects a common late onset of the illness for females (Comer 2017).

Positive symptoms describe unusual occurrences, such as hallucinations, delusions and odd speech. Negative symptoms describe the lack of behaviour that is normal for the rest of society, for example, good social skills, motivation, expression of emotion and being able to look after oneself (see Box 8.10).

Paramedics should be aware that some of the features of schizophrenia can occur alongside the presence of physical disease, intoxication with licitly or illicitly obtained substances or being under the influence of psychotropic drugs. It is important that the paramedic attempts to ascertain what the person may have taken in the form of drugs or substances in order that you can report it and at the same time identify risk factors to the patient/client and to yourself (Hawley et al. 2011a).

LEGISLATIVE POWERS AND MENTAL HEALTH

This chapter has provided the reader with a brief overview of mental ill health with consideration for the relatively common mental health problems/disorders that paramedics are likely to encounter during their working practice.

Mental Health Act 1983 (DH 2007)/Mental Capacity Act 2005 (DH 2005)

The Mental Health Act of 2007 was passed through Parliament in July 2007; it serves to update the previous Mental Health Act of 1983. There are seven major amendments to the 1983 Act and a further eighth amendment, updating the Mental Capacity Act of 2005 (Amblum 2014). See JRCALC (Brown et al. 2016), Tables 3.15, 3.16, for detailed information on the Mental Capacity Act (DH 2005: 108, 109). The amendments provide better safeguards for mental health service users, the new rights to advocacy, a say in who their nearest relative is, and the right to refuse electroconvulsive therapy and other treatments (Jones et al. 2014).

Criteria for application for admission under the Mental Health Act 2007

A person suffering from a mental illness, who is either a danger to themselves or to the public, may be removed from a public place or their home to a place of safety (usually a police station or hospital) by a police officer.

As a paramedic, you would usually be empowered by the appropriate Approved Mental Health Professional (AMHP) or family member to convey the patient compulsorily under a Section Order to hospital or a mental health facility. You may have to call on the services of a police officer to aid with the escort of the patient, especially in the presence or threat of violence. It is vitally important that a bed has been secured for the patient, if required. However, in reality, it may be some time before a bed is available and the hospital may enlist the help of a psychiatric nurse while the patient remains in the emergency department, until the patient has been fully assessed and decisions made. Where there is an AMHP on scene, the services of the police may not be required, as the AMHP may have the powers to issue the Section (DH 2007).

Reflection: points to consider

- In your practice area, do AMPHs work alongside paramedics regularly?
- Do you know their jurisdiction?
- Consider the value of their expertise and write down some points that highlight the importance of the AMPH role alongside that of the paramedic.

The Mental Health Act (DH 2007) was designed to protect the individual from potential abuses to their freedom, while protecting the public and the patient from any consequences of the mental illness. AMHPs, GPs and specialist approved doctors (psychiatrists) are usually involved in assessing the patient for a Section Order. This multidisciplinary approach to invoking the Section Order is designed to protect the patient from unnecessary admission and removal of human rights.

There are a variety of Sections within the Act that may be used to secure a patient's admission; see Box 8.11.

Box 8.II Sections of the Mental Health Act (DH 2007) relevant to the paramedic

- *Section 2 (Admission for assessment)*: Admission for up to a period of 28 days. Two doctors make recommendation for admission, one of whom must be approved. Assessment from both doctors within a period of five days of each other.
- *Section 3 (Admission for treatment)*: Admission for up to a period of six months, renewable for periods of up to one year at a time for severe mental illness/impairment/disorder, which requires treatment in hospital.
- *Section 4 (Admission for assessment in an emergency)*: Admission for a period of up to 72 hours (the patient can be placed under Section 2 or 3 after examination) for urgent assessment.
- *Section 131 (Informal admission)*: The patient voluntarily agrees to be admitted, but can change his/her mind and refuse. There is no time limit.
- *Section 135 (Place of safety order – private)*: Admission for a period of up to 72 hours. A person suffering from mental illness can be removed from a private dwelling to a place of safety for assessment. The patient should not be removed directly to hospital under Section 135 unless an AMHP/Approved Social Worker or GP has attended.
- *Section 136 (Place of safety order – public)*: Admission for a period of up to 72 hours. A person suffering from a mental illness can be removed from a public place to a place of safety (usually a police station or possibly a hospital) by a police office or an AMHP/Approved Social Worker.

Under the 2007 Mental Health Act, both Sections 135 and 136 have been amended to allow transfers between places of safety, within the 72-hour detention period. Transfer during the 72-hour detention period was not allowed under the 1983 Mental Health Act. Paramedics may be asked to provide safe transfer of patients under either of these two sections.

For further reading, see JRCALC (Brown et al. 2016; DH, 2007).

CONCLUSION

This chapter has attempted to provide the reader with an understanding of some of the psychological problems that a child, young person and adult can face. We may agree to define psychological abnormalities as patterns of functioning that are:

- dysfunctional (interfering with the person's ability to conduct daily activities in a constructive way);
- deviant (different, extreme, unusual, perhaps even bizarre);
- distressful (unpleasant and upsetting for the sufferer and significant others);
- dangerous (to themselves or to others, hostile and careless).

However, we should be clear that these criteria are often vague and subjective and not all sufferers will show all behaviours. It is also important to mention that, despite popular misconceptions, most sufferers with anxiety, depression and even 'bizarre' thinking and behaviour pose no immediate danger to themselves or to others. However, as a paramedic, you should at all times make an assessment of your personal safety when approaching an upset, disorientated, agitated or threatening patient. If you think you are at considerable risk, you may need to call the police who are suitably trained for these situations (Brown et al. 2016). It may be wise to regularly refresh your knowledge of conflict resolution training/education to aid your care of a patient.

As a paramedic, you will encounter sufferers of psychological problems in your working life. It is essential that you have an awareness of the theoretical underpinnings of your practice in order that you can assess and care for these sufferers holistically and competently (Hawley et al. 2011a; 2011b). It is important that your approach to these patients should be calm and you should take your time to communicate during assessment

 Reflection: points to consider

Here is a useful mnemonic (GASPIPES), in terms of thinking through the assessment of a patient/client's mental state. Ask yourself and the patient whether the patient is experiencing any of the following:

Guilt and self-reproach
Appetite is disturbed
Sleep disturbance, suffering insomnia
Paying attention to your questions or not, orientation to time, place and person
Interest in things is lacking, such as football, music, etc.
Psychomotor disturbance – slow, agitated, pacing, mood, hallucinations and belief expressed
Energy – loss, tired, slow
Suicidal – expressed thoughts

(Whitnell 2012a: 114)

(Palmer 2011). Do not rush, because a distressed or agitated person may react negatively to being hurried, and always be honest about what is going to happen in order to help gain their compliance and trust.

Chapter key points:

- The paramedic requires knowledge and understanding of mental ill health for children, young people and adults.
- The paramedic requires an awareness of the signs and symptom and the guidelines given by the Mental Health Act (DH 2007), the Mental Capacity Act (DH ,2005), JRCALC (Brown et al. 2016) national guidelines and local Trust policy, in order to assess a patient's condition correctly and instigate appropriate treatment or obtain specialist assistance.
- Paramedics should be aware of the personal safety of the patient and themselves at all times.

REFERENCES AND SUGGESTED READING

Achenbach, T. (2013) *Assess Adaptive and Maladaptive Functioning: Achenbach System of Empirically Based Assessment (ASEBA)*. London: Harcourt Press.

Amblum, J. (2014) A critical appraisal of the impact of Section 3 of the Mental Capacity Act 2005. *Journal of Paramedic Practice*, 6(8): 422–8.

APA (American Psychiatric Association) (2013) *Diagnostic and Statistical Manual of Mental Disorders (DSM-V)*. Philadelphia, PA: American Psychiatric Association.

Berger, K.S. (2011) *The Developing Person Through the Lifespan*, 8th edn. New York: Worth Publishers.

Brown, S.N., Kumar, D. and Millins, M. (eds for JRCALC and AACE) (2016) *UK Ambulance Service Clinical Practice Guidelines*. Bridgwater. Class Professional Publishing.

Comer, R.J. (2017) *Abnormal Psychology*, 9th edn. New York: Worth.

Culbert, K.M., Racine, S.E. and Klump, K. (2015) Research review: what we have learned about the causes of eating disorders: a synthesis of sociocultural, psychological, and biological research. *Journal of Child Psychology and Psychiatry*, 56(11): 1141–64.

DH (Department of Health) (2005) *Mental Capacity Act*. London: HMSO.

DH (Department of Health) (2007) *Mental Health Act*. London: HMSO.

Dogra, N., Parkin, A., Gale, F. and Frake, C. (2009) *A Multidisciplinary Handbook of Child and Adolescent Mental Health for Front-Line Professionals*. London: Jessica Kingsley.

Field, M. and Cartright-Hatton, S. (2015) *Essential Abnormal and Clinical Psychology*. London: Sage.

Gerrig, R.J., Zimbardo, P.G., Svartdal, F., Brennen, T., Donaldson, R. and Archer, T. (2012) *Psychology and Life*. Harlow: Pearson Education Limited.

Hawley, C., Singhal, A., Roberts, A.G., Atkinson, H. and Whelan, C. (2011a) Mental health in the care of paramedics: part 1. *Journal of Paramedic Practice*, 3(5): 230–6.

Hawley, C., Singhal, A., Roberts, A.G., Atkinson, H. and Whelan, C. (2011b) Mental health in the care of paramedics: part 2. *Journal of Paramedic Practice*, 3(6): 304–12.

Jones, S., Williams, B. and Monteith, P. (2014) Decision making for refusals of treatment: a framework to consider. *Journal of Paramedic Practice*, 6(4): 180–6.

Kalat, J.W. (2009) *Biological Psychology*, 10th edn. New York: Brookes Cole.

Kerrig, P.K., Ludlow, A. and Wenar, C. (2012) *Developmental Psychopathology: From Infancy Through Adolescence*, 6th edn. Maidenhead: Open University Press/McGraw-Hill.

McManus, S., Bebbington, P., Jenkins, R. and Brugha, T. (eds) (2016) *Mental Health and Wellbeing in England: Adult Psychiatric Morbidity Survey 2014*. Leeds: NHS Digital.

Mental Health Foundation (2018a) *Eating Disorders*. Available at: https://www.mentalhealth.org.uk/a-to-z/e/eating-disorders (accessed 2 January 2018).

Mental Health Foundation (2018b) *Statistics*. Available at: www.mental health.org.uk/statistics. (accessed 2 January 2018).

Mental Health Network NHS Confederation (2016) *Key Facts and Trends in Mental Health*. Available at: http://www.nhsconfed.org/resources/2016/03/key-facts-and-trends-in-mental-health-2016-update (accessed 2 January 2018).

MIND (2017) *Mental Health Facts and Statistics: Types of Mental Health Problems*. Available at: https://www.mind.org.uk/information-support/types-of-mental-health-problems/statistics-and-facts-about-mental-health/how-common-are-mental-health-problems/#.Wk3aBpfLjcs (accessed 4 January 2018).

Morton, J. (2004) *Understanding Developmental Disorders: A Causal Modelling Approach*. Oxford: Blackwell Publishing.

Munir, K.M. (2016) The co-occurrence of mental disorders in children and adolescents with intellectual disability/intellectual developmental disorder. *Current Opinion in Psychiatry*. Available at: https://www.ncbi.nlm.nih.gov/pmc/articles/PMC4814928/ (accessed 2 January 2018).

NHS Confederation (2016) *Mental Health Network Factsheet: Key Facts and Trends in Mental Health*. Available at: http://www.nhsconfed.org/resources/2016/03/key-facts-and-trends-in-mental-health-2016-update (accessed 2 January 2018).

NICE (National Institute for Health and Care Excellence) (2015) *Post Traumatic Stress Disorder: Management*. Available at: https://www.nice.org.uk/guidance/cg26 (accessed 4 January 2018).

ONS (Office for National Statistics) (2017) *Suicide by Occupation: England: 2011–2015*. London: Office for National Statistics. Available at: https://www.ons.gov.uk/peoplepopulationand community/birthsdeathsandmarriages/deaths/articles/suicidebyoccupation/england 2011to2015 (accessed 2 January 2018).

Palmer, A. (2011) Improving the assessment and referral of mental health patients. *Journal of Paramedic Practice*, 3: 496–503.

Rees, N., Rapport, F. and Snooks, H. (2015) Perceptions of paramedic and emergency staff about the care they provide to people who self-harm: constructivist metasynthesis of the qualitative literature. *Journal of Psychosomatic Research*, 78(6): 529–35.

RCPSYCH (Royal College of Psychiatrists (2017) *Mental Health Factsheet* Available at: www.rcpsych.ac.uk/healthadvice/problemsdisorders.aspx (accessed 2 January 2018).

Whitnell, J. (2012a) Abnormal psychology: an introduction. In A.Y. Blaber (ed.) *Foundations of Paramedic Practice: A Theoretical Perspective*. Maidenhead: Open University Press/McGraw-Hill Education.

Whitnell, J. (2012b) Developmental psychology. In A.Y. Blaber (ed.) *Foundations of Paramedic Practice: A Theoretical Perspective*. Maidenhead: Open University Press/McGraw-Hill Education.

Whitnell, J. (2012c) Child and adolescent mental health. *Early Years Educator*, 13(11): 38–44.

WHO (1992) *The ICD-10 Classification of Mental and Behavioural Disorders: Clinical Descriptions and Diagnostic Guidelines*. Geneva: World Health Organisation.

WHO (2018a) *The 11th Revision of the International Classification of Diseases (ICD-11)*. Geneva: World Health Organisation. Available at: www.who.int/classifications/icd/revision/en (accessed 2 January 2018).

WHO (2018b) *ICD-11 Version for Morbidity and Mortality Statistics (ICD-11 MMS)*. Geneva: World Health Organisation.

Wilmshurst, L. (2017) *Child and Adolescent Psychopathology: A Casebook*, 4th edn. London: Sage.

An introduction to sociology, social factors and social policy

Amanda Y. Blaber and Chris Storey

In this chapter:

- Introduction
- Why is this relevant?
- Introduction to sociology
- Review of classical sociology theorists
- Socialisation
- Social stratification
- Case studies and associated theory
- Introduction to social policy
- Conclusion
- Chapter key points
- References and suggested reading
- Useful websites

INTRODUCTION

This chapter will briefly summarise the classical sociologists and their theories. More reading of 'pure' sociological texts is essential to aid further understanding, particularly if this is not a subject you have studied before. There are, however, other areas of our lives where contemporary sociologists have focused their work, such as social aspects of health and illness and the changing role of families. Whatever is happening within our society is of interest to sociologists and their subsequent research and theories reflect the dynamic nature of the society we live in now.

This chapter will use a case study approach to explore a few of the main factors that affect all of our lives and how we function within society. All the factors discussed will seem familiar and probably are areas you may not have thought much about previously, taking things for granted, such as age and culture. The second edition of the *Foundations* text contains more theoretical information on these and other areas, as will sociology textbooks. Finally, the chapter closes with an introduction to the importance of social policy and its relevance to paramedic practice.

WHY IS THIS RELEVANT?

All professionals working in the NHS have contact with members of Britain's society. So why do paramedics require an understanding of sociology and its key concepts? Paramedics and other healthcare community workers are unique in the sense that they see people in their own social world, i.e. their homes, with families, friends and in their part of society (location). Hospital-based workers do not see people functioning in their own environments because the fact of being hospitalised brings them into the hospital organisation, with its own culture. If paramedics have a wider understanding of why people talk and act, respond to illness and operate within society in the way that they do, clinicians may be able to adjust their own behaviour accordingly, when dealing with patients. This would obviously improve the experience for both clinician and patient and may enhance the overall quality of care provided.

As well as introducing some new concepts/theories, the chapter is intended to invite you to question areas of your life that you may take for granted and have grown up with. Although brief (in comparison with sociology texts), the chapter hopes to raise the student's awareness of sociology and how it can assist us in understanding ourselves and others. Readers are invited to explore their thoughts on certain areas of social life. Many areas will require further reading in order to avoid 'skimming the surface' of a subject: suggested reading has been included.

INTRODUCTION TO SOCIOLOGY

Many people find the study of sociology frustrating because it does not have concrete answers and is the cause of disagreement between clinicians and academics. The study of anatomy and physiology is very different: you know it or you don't and there is little ambiguity about the facts. Successful sociology requires students to open their minds and eyes, be curious, ask questions about the world around them, and to think about and discuss their own ideas and beliefs.

There are many key theorists who have done just that, have become eminent in their field and have created concepts that can still be applied to our social world today. This is perhaps a good starting point for students who have not studied sociology before, as it provides concepts to explore and discuss in relation to the twenty-first century.

Every one of your actions results in a reaction from the person you are caring for, their families, your colleagues and other social and healthcare practitioners; sociology may assist you in experiencing positive rather than negative reactions on a daily basis (Blaber 2012a). This chapter is asking you to challenge the obvious, think about things you take for granted and be curious to try and understand (a little more) about people and the society in which we all live. Students may also learn something about themselves.

REVIEW OF CLASSICAL SOCIOLOGY THEORISTS

Table 9.1 summarises the main classical sociologists and their main theories that have relevance to society today. Although at first glance this may not be immediately obvious, many of the contemporary theories draw upon the seminal works of these sociological 'masters'. If you are not familiar with the work of the classical sociologists, then please delve further into 'pure' sociology textbooks for more detail.

These three classical sociologists whose work originates in the eighteenth century still have relevance today. Durkheim developed the concept of 'social solidarity' to explain the various ways in which societies can be integrated. Durkheim also explained other types of solidarity, such as mechanical solidarity, where individuals identify with each other, usually because they have similar lives. Durkheim applied this to pre-modern societies, with respect to clans and tribes. Regarding modern societies, Durkheim identified that no individual or section of society could function without engaging in interaction with others; he termed this organic solidarity. Durkheim states that a complete society is reliant on the close interrelationship between individuals and sections of society. Where individuals act independently (or outside) of commonly recognised norms of behaviour or social standards, Durkheim used the term 'anomie' to explain their behaviour. He believed societies were at greater risk of social disintegration because of the growth of individualism and self-importance. With this comes the increase of divergence of experience and values for members of society.

Functionalism assumes that society works as a social system and is not just made up of social facts. The ways we think and live are established in a culture and can be called institutionalised behaviour and beliefs, in sociological terms. The integration, solidarity and balance of a society are maintained by institutions such as the family, the political system, the education system and the legal system, each performing their functions properly and interdependently. For students who prefer human biology, think of our society as a human body: there are organs that perform necessary functions to keep a human healthy. This is, in essence, the basis of a functionalist principle.

Suicide was a subject that Durkheim studied in terms of social causes, rather than explaining it in terms of individual or psychological factors. Durkheim believed suicide was due to social factors more than anything else.

Reflection: points to consider

In your experience of suicide, was this the case? Have you seen an increase in people committing suicide? What were their ages? Could there have been a social cause, such as bullying, unemployment, debt, substance misuse?

Table 9.1 Summary of classical sociologists and their key theories

Name	Date of birth-death and country of origin	Key points that may have influenced their work	Key theories
Emile Durkheim	1858–1917, France	1860–71 Franco-Prussian War – France defeated by Prussia 1914–18 First World War Brought up as Orthodox Jew Father was a Rabbi Converted to Catholicism in adulthood	Explores the nature of societies Develops the concept of 'social solidarity' Mechanical solidarity Organic solidarity Anomie Functionalism Suicide
Karl Marx	1818–1883, Germany	Political ideas became more radical at university Lived in Paris Worked as a journalist Visited Germany during 1848 revolution Exiled in London in 1849	Examined dynamics of society and changes over time Evolution of capitalism Conflict in society 'Mode of production' Power relations
Max Weber	1864–1920, Germany	Huge changes in Germany's industrial status during his lifetime Worked as an academic in economics and political economy Suffered with depression: nervous breakdown after his father's death	Explored becoming a modern society 'Rational-legal' authority 'Social action' Protestant work ethic

Sources: Collated and adapted from Giddens and Sutton (2017), Punch *et al.* (2013) and Denny *et al.* (2016).

Karl Marx, like Durkheim, was interested by and examined the dynamics of societies and the changes that take place in societies over time. Marx wanted to explain the evolution of capitalism and how this, he believed, would eventually lead to a communist system. Marx is concerned with exploring conflict in society. One of Marx's concepts, the mode of production, describes ways in which the production of goods, needed for individuals to survive and prosper, was organised in society. Marx argued that in a capitalist society the motivation for the production of goods is for profit. Workers generate more wealth for their employers but only keep a small percentage of the profit, a case of the rich getting richer at the expense of the poor. This can be seen in modern twenty-first-century societies to this day.

After visiting Germany during the 1848 revolution, Marx was exiled in London in 1849 until his death. During this time Marx tried to build a workers' party while analysing capitalism, as he believed political power is closely linked to economic power. Marx used class analysis as one of his central themes. Marx saw power as being unequally distributed across societies and believed that economic power is the basis for other forms of power. Two distinct forms of Marxism have developed since Marx's death: (1) structural Marxism, concerned with class exploitation and the importance of economics; and (2) humanist Marxism, focused upon the alienation of the human spirit due to capitalism.

Max Weber's work expresses his own fears and anxieties about modernity (becoming a modern society), which he believed was irreversible. Weber believed that an individual's needs would not be fulfilled by the material gain, increased power and economic dependence that modernity brings. One of Weber's central themes was that rules, regulations and laws naturally accompany capitalist modernity and that society would become dependent on this organised structure. Weber believed 'rational-legal' authority characterised modern society. He believed this is based upon impersonal rules that have been rationally formalised and organised without emotion or intuition and have created bureaucracy. Weber introduced the concept of 'social action' and called on sociologists to examine the consequences of individuals (or as he termed them 'social actors'); these may not always be intended or anticipated (Punch et al. 2013; Giddens and Sutton 2017).

 Reflection: points to consider

How many rules and regulations are there in your university and clinical placement provider? We accept these and take these for granted, but are they all required? Are they impersonal? Is there too much bureaucracy? These are the points Weber was trying to make.

The classical theorists' work still has resonance in the twenty-first century. Other sociologists have developed their thinking and theories based upon the classical sociologists' concepts. There are key areas of our lives that have an influence on 'who we are': our social class, our family, our education and our work are examples. Some of these areas will be examined in terms of sociological theory, in order that students can link theory to their own lives and the lives of patients.

SOCIALISATION

Socialisation is an important sociological term and is perhaps an appropriate starting point for students to begin to question why they are who they are. This process commences at birth. Denny et al. (2016: 9) define socialisation as 'processes by which individuals acquire the roles, norms and cultures of society'.

The initial stages of a child's development are primarily with parents and members of the family and are face-to-face. As a child grows up, other influences, such as school and friends, are involved in a child's development; this is when formal social rules are predominantly learnt. Charles Cooley (1864–1929) was a US sociologist who developed his theory of symbolic interactionism in the 1920s and 1930s. Another writer in this area is George Mead, who linked social behaviour with social psychology. Cooley (1909, cited in Ritzer 1996) describes the initial face-to-face socialisation as being undertaken by a primary group and the latter stages as secondary group socialisation. It is when children enter other social institutions, such as school, that they realise they form part of a 'larger picture' and are, perhaps for the first time, judged by society's rules and standards. This is described as Cooley's 'primary group' theory. Another of Cooley's concepts (1902, cited in Kornblum 1997) was the 'looking-glass self', where we judge ourselves as we imagine others see us. This concept has three steps:

1   We imagine how we present ourselves to others; for example, are we smart, caring, tall, funny?
2   Then we interpret how people react to us; for instance, do they see us as we see ourselves, or do they see something else?
3   We then use interpretations of others' reactions to us, to develop our sense of self. If we sense that people disagree with our perception of our self, then our 'self-concept' will diminish; we may change our behaviour. If we think we agree with others, our self-concept will become stronger.

Cooley's approach is described as symbolic interaction.

 Reflection: points to consider

Think about yourself. Who would you say constituted your primary group during your socialisation? Who constituted your secondary group? Does this process ever stop? Has your paramedic education socialised you in a different way?

During socialisation with both primary and secondary groups, an individual forms an identity. Sociologists suggest that identity formation is a combination of the physical, the personal and the social. During the process of growing up the individual does not take on all influences, but reflects, negotiates and incorporates (or rejects) them.

Erving Goffman (1922–1982), another important US sociologist, considered all individuals to 'act' for their audiences in everyday life. His approach is interactionist. Goffman argued that our behaviour follows patterns and that individuals follow a set of instructions that influence and determine behaviour.

Our interactions between ourselves and the world we live in help establish our identity. Sociologists, such as Cooley (1902, cited in Kornblum 1997; and 1909, cited in Ritzer 1996), Mead ([1934] 1967) and Goffman (1963) believe our identities are subject to change and not assigned at birth. Most of us have a variety of identities that we adopt according to our varying roles in society, for example, parent, colleague, paramedic, student (Goffman 1963; Cohen 1994).

Punch et al. (2013) suggest that as our socialisation with the secondary group increases, we will influence others' views of us by using dress and language. For example, consider the influence (either positively or negatively) of your uniform (see Case study 9.4). In order to challenge your own first impressions, you should take time to discover as much as possible about the person you are treating. Obviously in out-of-hospital care, this is unrealistic; as paramedics you make guesses or predictions about others, based on your own socialisation and your own experiences. Being aware of how we are socialised into society should enable you as paramedics to appreciate the influences on development of identity and challenge your first impressions of members of society (see Case studies 9.1 and 9.2).

 Reflection: points to consider

What factors influence the first impressions you have when you arrive on scene when at work?

SOCIAL STRATIFICATION

Having briefly explored how we develop our own identities it is logical to explore our position in society and introduce some sociological concepts/approaches.

Inequality

The effects of not being able to escape poverty are sometimes clearly seen in our varying environments, but the effect poverty can have on children's educational attainment may not be so obvious. Even before they reach school age, some children from poorer backgrounds are already at a substantial disadvantage. Children from financially poorer backgrounds have significantly lower language skills than those children from financially richer homes, by the time they commence school. There is a link between annual income and the time spent reading to children in the home, during the pre-school years. There is a link between reading at home, language development and the finances of the family (Punch et al. 2013; Denny et al. 2016; Giddens and Sutton 2017).

The paramedic is faced with consequences of such financial inequalities on a daily basis, manifesting in the wide variety of homes that are visited. Inequalities are also demonstrable in the types of illness people succumb to, some of which are indicative of the person's living conditions, for example, childhood asthma worsens in damp living conditions.

Crompton (2008) suggests that inequality leads to social stratification – members of society being ranked in a hierarchical manner. This ranking system depends on factors such as income, wealth, age, power, status and gender. The importance of inequality must not be underestimated; it has been the subject of much research and profoundly affects a person's quality of life and can specifically affect the length of life (Giddens and Sutton 2017).

A term that students may be more familiar with is that of social class. Prior to industrialisation, societies were relatively closed. This refers to people not really moving far from where they were born and not having any other prospects, other than those associated with the social group they were born into. With industrialisation a more open system developed, due to competition and more opportunity for social mobility (Punch et al. 2013; Giddens and Sutton 2017). It is commonly accepted by sociologists that modern societies are stratified on the basis of social class (Crompton 2008).

 Reflection: points to consider

Would you classify yourself as being from the same social class as your ancestors?

With a stratified approach to society, it is important that we can all explore where we are in the hierarchy. The Office for National Statistics (ONS) classification has not been updated since 2010 and remains the current recognised system of occupational class hierarchy (see Box 9.1).

Classification systems are rarely perfect and Punch et al. (2013) highlight some criticisms of this eight-class scale. Marxist writer Coser (1977) believes a scale does not reflect the relationship between each class and therefore negates the importance

---

Box 9.1 The ONS socio-economic classification analytic classes (2010)

1   Higher managerial and professional occupations:

    1.1 Large employers and higher managerial occupations
    1.2 Higher professional occupations

2   Lower managerial and professional occupations
3   Intermediate occupations (e.g. clerks, secretaries, computer operators)
4   Small employers and own account workers
5   Lower supervisory and technical occupations
6   Semi-routine occupations (e.g. cooks, bus drivers, hairdressers, shop assistants)
7   Routine occupations (e.g. waitresses, cleaners, couriers)
8   Never worked and long-term unemployed.

https://www.ons.gov.uk/methodology/
classificationsandstandards/
otherclassifications/thenationalstatisticssocio
economicclassificationnssecrebasedonsoc2010

---

of division, conflict and dynamics of class struggle. Other criticisms of a class scale are that variations between occupations are not taken into account. Despite being in the same category, for example, a consultant doctor and a junior doctor do very different jobs and have different standards of living. The scale is based on the working population, so how are retired people and housewives represented? Crompton (2008) criticises the scale, as the occupation of the male head of household dictates the category. The terms upper, middle and working classes are still commonly used within society, but are they valid sociological concepts in twenty-first-century Britain?

There is no argument that social class affects opportunities and lifestyle for all of us. It is a common perception that we are all able to move up the social class 'ladder', if we have the right conditions to do so (education and employment opportunities, for example). This is commonly referred to as social mobility. One would assume that in twenty-first-century Britain, people have the opportunities to change and shape their lives; however, inequalities still exist.

There are many inextricably linked aspects of our lives that sociologists have been researching, observing and commenting on for many years. Within the scope of this text it is not possible to explore all of them, but the following have been chosen as being most relevant for paramedics to have a sociological appreciation of and will be accompanied by a case study and questions.

Age

Our social world is structured and ordered by age. At times we may not be able to do something because of our age, for example, enter a pub alone under the age of 18 years; or it is more acceptable to behave in a certain way because of our age – a child having a tantrum, for example. We can be both enabled and constrained by our age. Age can be classified into three areas: chronological age, biological age and social age. Our chronological or numerical age results in us being able to access certain privileges and may be linked to laws, for example, being able to drink alcohol legally in pubs. Biological age and chronological age are linked. Biological age is linked to physical appearance. One of the reasons why we are so concerned with our biological age and appearance is centred on society's response to biological age. It is about how you look and the way people respond to the way you look. How a person feels in relation to his age group and life experiences is termed social age. Here, a 70-year-old may biologically look older, but may feel socially 'young' and no different to when he was 40 years of age. Society expects people to act and look their age – hence comments like 'mutton dressed as lamb' when an individual acts outside the social norm.

Age stratification as a sociological concept refers to the 'unequal distribution of social resources, including wealth, power and status, which are accorded to people on the basis of their age' (Punch et al. 2013: 301). Childhood, youth, young adulthood, mid-life and old age are key groupings. Some sociologists also refer to the 'old old' as an additional stratified group. Care must be taken not to apply groupings to people without considering people as individuals. People's life chances, education, family upbringing, and employment will all have an impact on how they experience older age. Talking about age 'groupings' is only useful to describe people's chronological age, e.g. 'the retired'. Paramedics will also be interested in the physiological changes that happen over the lifespan. But it is also important to take time to understand an individual's experience of the life course. This will be dependent upon where the individual is located at a particular point in time when they require your assistance (Denny et al. 2016). Old age and childhood are prime examples in British society where we ascribe less status and value to some age groups, compared with others. Just the titles of some organisations indicate this to be true. Why is there a *National* Society for Prevention of Cruelty to Children (NSPCC) and a *Royal* Society for the Protection of Cruelty to Animals (RSPCA)?

In addition to having fun and socialising during our older years, communication technology has a major part to play in many older people's lives and can be an enriching experience. We must be mindful that this also has the potential to isolate and exclude older people who do not have access to the internet, especially if we take its use for granted. Healthcare professionals need to think about their communications with older people and suggest appropriate advice for the 'age' and circumstance (people/families in poverty may not have internet access) in respect of technology and using it to support healthcare, such as re-ordering prescriptions, checking symptoms via the NHS website before making an appointment with your GP, and so on.

Reflection: points to consider

When was the last time you heard a paramedic give advice that required the individual to access information or appointments online? Was their advice 'age and circumstance appropriate'?

CASE STUDIES AND ASSOCIATED THEORY

Case study 9.1

Norman is a 90-year-old man who lives alone in a small bungalow. Due to his frailty, he struggles to clean his home or do any repairs needed. As a result, he lives in very unkempt conditions. Norman also struggles with personal care. He washes his face and hands every day (he cannot get in or out of a bath or shower) and he always wears a shirt and tie (though his clothes are rarely washed). He has several medical conditions including chronic obstructive pulmonary disease (though he gave up smoking 30 years ago), atrial fibrillation and Type 2 diabetes for which he is on medications (including a blood thinner). Norman has frequent falls due to decreasing mobility. After a spate of falls he was seen by the falls service team who fitted his home with 'grab' rails, boosters for his chair and toilet, and gave him a walking frame to aid his mobility. Norman now also has carers twice a day who come in the morning to get him up and give him breakfast and medications and then again in the evening to put him to bed. Norman has two grown-up children who live several miles away and he does not see them very often.

Consider the following questions and reflect upon your answers:

- How does society view Norman?
- What is Norman's place in society now that he no longer works or contributes through his taxes or through raising his children?
- Is Norman a 'problem' for society/for the NHS?
- How has Norman's role within the family changed over the years?
- How do employment, age and family role affect our view of each other within our society?
- How might the paramedics who attend Norman reinforce a negative social view of him or challenge it, presenting a more positive one?
- Though Norman has carers, he is just one of the clients they have to see each day. How might this impact upon Norman's life? (The time he wants to go to bed or get up, for example.)

Common perceptions of what constitutes 'old age' are being challenged by older people themselves, and paramedics should be questioning their own beliefs and stereotypes of the older generation.

In addition to being a biological process, age is also socially constructed and our experiences of age depend on our society. As with gender, ethnicity and class, age is a social variable. There can also be social divisions associated with age; for example, the experience of ageing for a working-class woman will be very different from the experience of an older middle-class man (Giddens and Sutton 2017).

Prior to 1990 the sociology of childhood was mainly concerned with the child's future worth as an adult. This changed in the 1990s to focus on the children's present-day lives, not their future as adults. Now sociology takes children's views seriously and considers them to be able to shape their own lives, within certain constraints. There is a dichotomy in society about how children are viewed. On the one hand, they are seen as vulnerable and innocent, in need of protection from the adult world. On the other, they are vulnerable and corruptible and in need of control. Children are subject to many age-based institutions, which clearly show the different status given to children and adults, where they learn about power and authority, for example, playgroups, nurseries, Cubs/Brownies and youth clubs. These experiences and membership of age-related groups enable children to understand the way society is structured through age. Our perceptions of the very young and very old are shaped by our society. The influences on our perceptions are also interrelated factors: social, political and historical context, language, ideologies and media (Punch et al. 2013; Giddens and Sutton 2017). The policies and politics associated with a particular age group also influence our thinking; this may change over time. For example, the concept of retirement is generally thought to be positive and associated with enjoyment but many older people find retirement frustrating and boring.

Case study 9.2

During concurrent 12-hour shifts where the youngest patient I had cared for was in their early eighties and where every patient had a number of age-related conditions, I had cause to reflect.

The frailty of age along with the cruelty of chronic illness started to make me think negatively about the ageing process and my view of elderly people. I started to look at some patients I went to and thought 'I don't ever want to end up like that.' This soon became, 'I don't want to live beyond 80 years old . . .'

I was then called to an elderly lady (over 80 years old) who had 'difficulty breathing'. It transpired this was a diagnosed chest infection and was being treated with antibiotics.

Her reason for calling had been more to do with anxiety, which my crewmate and I were able to address by reassuring her.

As part of our assessment, I took her blood pressure which was 120/80. 'Wow, that's Olympic standard blood pressure!' I told her. Then she giggled, lent forward and whispered in my ear . . . 'I went to three Olympic Games.' In that moment I suddenly stopped seeing her as some 'generic old lady' whose 'presenting complaint' I needed to address before moving on to the next 'elderly patient'. I saw her with a value I had not considered her to have before, due to the negative opinion of ageing I had allowed myself to adopt. She then showed me photos of herself at each of the Olympics she had attended along with her GB Team Olympic blazer and other Commonwealth Games medals she had won. Attending her as a patient transformed her from being a pressure into a privilege.

During that visit I had reassured an elderly lady over her anxiety, but she had changed my view of every elderly person I have met ever since. Now I love meeting the old fighter pilots, Bletchley Park code breakers, athletes who ran a hundred marathons who now need my arm to lean on as they walk to their chair. Now I feel that we all have an enduring value which outlasts our 'finest hour' when we might have done something society would count as productive. We do not stop being 'productive' but we sometimes need a change of perspective to see it.

The paramedic experience of elderly people is not a normal one. The vast majority of elderly people we see are not well at all. We do not spend time with the 80-year-olds who are improving their handicap on the golf course or heading off for their weekly Pilates class, they are not the ones who call for an ambulance. This can cloud our judgement about ageing if we're not careful, which in turn could affect our attitude towards patients.

I'd like to live to be over 80 now . . . though I'll probably never make the Olympics.

Answer the following questions and reflect on your answers:

- What is your view of the ageing process: is it fatalistic or hopeful?
- Have you found yourself viewing different sections of society negatively due to your exposure to them in emergency situations? In what way is this realistic or representative of these groups as a whole?
- How could you as a paramedic ensure you do not let 'the job' cloud your opinion of people?
- How could you as a paramedic act to change any negative opinion of diverse social groups you encounter in your role?

People can be 'stereotyped' within social groups and this can prevent paramedics from exploring the wide diversity of experiences or knowledge the person may have. All retired people had a 'life' before retirement, in addition to their retired 'life', as can be seen by Case study 9.2. Do you ever ask what they did prior to retirement? It may provide valuable insight into their decision-making and illness behaviour. Lives, in any age grouping, will vary according to other variables – class, gender, ethnicity, disability. This stereotyping is reflected in the terminology and language used in society today. Older people are sometimes referred to as 'little old ladies', 'the old boy', 'old biddy', as a few examples (Blaber 2012b).

In relation to the other variables, women are more likely to live in poverty (as their pensions tend to be less than those of men). Women also tend to live longer than men, meaning they are more likely to end up living alone in later life (Denny et al. 2016). Exploring the social construction of age and ageing may assist clinicians to question their own practice, language and general approach to people.

Culture

The term 'race' is often used to describe a person's heritage, ancestry or biological differences, whereas 'culture' tends to link people to particular religious beliefs, social customs and social norms (Giddens and Sutton 2017).

Society and culture are so closely linked that one could not exist in any 'meaningful' way without the other. Punch et al. (2013) remind us that what is regarded as normal and acceptable behaviour by one society or cultural group may be punished as a crime in another part of the world. We all have a set of values and beliefs which shape the way we view the world; the opinions we hold and judgements we make about others. Often our world view has its foundations in our upbringing (via the people who shaped our early development, parents, extended family and teachers) but also it develops through our own experiences, both positive and negative. Socialisation alone in a child's early years is not sufficient for physical, intellectual, emotional and social development. The quality of a child's cultural experience is crucial for her development, as exhibited by cases of physical child abuse and neglect. Sociologists believe cultural deprivation can help explain differences in patterns of criminal behaviour and educational achievement between varying social groups (Giddens and Sutton 2017).

Historical events like the acquisition and relinquishing of empire, combined with globalisation, world wars and the resulting mass movement of peoples have meant that people from across the world holding different world views now live side by side as neighbours. The potential for those from one culture, holding one world view, to offend or come into conflict with those from a different culture and world view is high. The potential for the paramedic to contribute negatively or positively to this situation is also high.

There are also groups within cultures who break away from their 'parent culture' (Hebdige 1979) to form 'subcultures' holding their own unique world view which is often in conflict to the parent culture; for example: Punks and Skinheads, Goths and Emos. Most subcultures within British society have formed in reaction to, and often in opposition to, their parent culture, defining themselves and their world view around norms of fashion and musical taste. Sometimes one group can view anyone who is not part of their group as being of less value or as someone to be suspicious or mistrustful of.

153

Reflection: points to consider

How might ambulance service personnel contribute to or diffuse such mistrust among members of subcultures they interact with?

In many ways, paramedics themselves are part of a 'subculture' (having a group identity which involves a uniform, a set of customs and practices and group opinions around other members of society). Students and new graduate paramedics can quickly be 'normalised' into an ambulance culture which views some calls from the public as being less 'worthy' than others, as Case study 9.3 explores.

Case study 9.3

We were called to a 24-year-old male with knee pain. En-route my crewmate and I were less than impressed, pre-judging the situation and questioning whether this job warranted a 999 call, as often happens among weary ambulance crews. Opinions about the resilience of the younger generation and their ability to manage day-to-day life were expressed. On arrival, we put on our 'professional face' and walked into the patient's house to find a young man who was a quadruple amputee (having lost both arms below the elbow and both legs below the knee after developing sepsis from an infection). That day, while adjusting one of his prosthetic legs he had lost his balance and landed on the stump of his knee causing excruciating pain. When the pain was not managed with his normal analgesia, he had reluctantly called NHS111 for advice, and an ambulance was dispatched. Feeling very ashamed, my crewmate and I hastily adjusted our attitude and tended to our patient. We learned a valuable lesson from that job, not to let a culture of cynicism towards certain calls affect our preparation prior to arrival.

Questions to ask yourself and reflect upon:

- What cultural differences have you noticed in the area where you live/ work?
- Have they led to segregation or integration of people in that area?
- What initiatives and activities reach across cultural backgrounds and bring people together here? Is the ambulance service represented/active in these initiatives?
- Have you recognised that there is an 'ambulance culture'? How does this shape your thinking about patients, incidents, other emergency services or areas of the NHS?

Each of us will have varying views on the importance of one area of our social lives over another (such as family and work), but there can be no argument that culture is one of the areas of our lives that has an impact on subsequent education and employment opportunities (Punch et al. 2013; Giddens and Sutton 2017).

Religion

The role of religion in society is as old as society itself. As such, it is recognised in the UK as one of nine 'protected characteristics' which it is illegal to discriminate against. The vast majority of the world's population holds to a world view that includes the existence of a deity or Supreme Being. In the UK, an 'atheistic' view (non-belief in God) or 'agnostic' view (the belief that there is not enough evidence to decide either way as to whether God exists) has grown steadily since the middle of the twentieth century. However, though the numbers of those in England and Wales stating they have no affiliation to any religion have grown from 14.8 per cent in 2001 to 25.1 per cent in 2011, still 74.9 per cent of the population identify with some form of belief in God (ONS 2012).

While, in the majority of cases, religious belief may not affect the assessment or treatment a patient is willing to accept, there may be times when it does; the paramedic needs to approach such occasions with sensitivity and professionalism. A patient's view may differ from yours but the back of the ambulance is not the place to debate the issue. However strong a paramedic's own belief on the subject of faith, they should be aware that when in uniform they represent the Ambulance Service which has no formal affiliation to any particular religion, belief or non-belief system. While some patients may find comfort and reassurance in talking about faith with ambulance personnel during a traumatic situation, this needs to be handled with sensitivity, compassion and professionalism. Lazarsfeld-Jensen and O'Meara (2013) suggest that student paramedics find it easier to discuss (in classroom situations) religion than more abstract sociological concepts. Discussing religion may enable students to examine their own fundamental values and may lead to discussion about inclusiveness, prejudice and tolerance, consent and patient choice. Examination of the students' own beliefs and values can also lead to more complex sociological debate, using religion as a 'vehicle' initially. This may translate to the student becoming more sociologically aware and confident to discuss complex issues while in the practice arena. If it helps the patient, talking about faith is not 'off limits', however, if it does not help, do not do it. Let the patient bring the subject up if they wish, the paramedic should not necessarily initiate conversation in this area.

Emergency services personnel have a unique position in society in that their uniform and the meaning, respect and value society places upon those who wear it, grant them permission to act in ways that a culture, religion or custom might not afford others (Blaber 2012b), as Case study 9.4 explores.

Case study 9.4

We were dispatched to care for a female patient whose family were devout followers of a particular faith. The husband of the patient was initially concerned, that as male paramedics, both my crewmate and I should not examine his wife to assess her condition. We explained that we could request a female paramedic to attend if he and the patient would prefer, but this might take time and his wife needed urgent assessment.

The husband pointed to the ambulance crest on our shirts and said, 'Forgive me, you are medical professionals and my wife needs your help, please do all you can.' Later as we discussed what medications the patient was taking I was told I would find a prescription in the top drawer of a bureau in the couple's bedroom. While retrieving the prescription, it struck me how our uniform (and the importance society places in it) enable us to walk into strangers' houses, carry out sensitive observations on them and look into cupboards and rooms in search of medications without objection. A privileged access which should never be taken for granted and which gives the opportunity to build up or break down public trust in the service.

There is an interrelationship between many areas of our social lives. This chapter has introduced a few of these areas, others are explored in the second edition of *Foundations* (Blaber 2012c). Further sociological reading is encouraged to develop deeper insight and understanding. In addition to a sociological awareness, paramedics' working lives are dictated by government policy, which is constantly changing and evolving, according to political pressures and agendas. This results in ambulance services and other NHS organisations having to respond, change practices and adhere to current social policies. Paramedics require an understanding of how social policy develops in order to appreciate the 'bigger picture' of working within a 'national' health service.

AN INTRODUCTION TO SOCIAL POLICY

The rate of change in government and local policy means that it is more appropriate to signpost the reader to websites that are regularly updated. The speed of change means that this chapter will be out of date by the time it is published, if this approach is not taken.

The everyday practice of any healthcare professional is guided by social policy. An awareness of social policy is fundamental to ensuring contemporary practitioners are up to date with policy developments and 'move with the times' in their specific profession. Paramedics have a choice; to let policy be published and subsequent changes be implemented by their Trust without their consultation; or be aware of proposals being made about future services, ensure they have a chance to comment as professional practitioners and individually secure their future as paramedics ahead of the game and be aware of how policy shapes practice. Paramedics who work in this manner are often able to foresee changes before they happen; this in itself will put them in a much stronger position professionally (Blaber 2012b).

The Department of Health issues guidance on priorities for service development and circulars on a range of topics, explaining national policy which NHS bodies are expected to follow. Therefore, an awareness of the Department of Health organisational structure and function is useful. Go to the website: https://www.gov.uk/government/publications/the-health-and-care-system-explained/the-health-and-care-system-explained

Once you are familiar with the organisational structure you will need to know how to access the plethora of publications that are produced by the DH on a regular basis. If you visit this webpage: https://www.gov.uk/government/publications?departments%5B%5D=department-of-health, you will find all publications listed in date order, in addition to the facility to be able to filter and undertake a keyword search.

 Chapter 5 for more information about successful searching techniques.

Some of the many DH circulars are prescriptive and others are advisory in nature. The Department of Health publishes Green Papers, which enable NHS bodies and other interested parties to influence the final definitive White Paper (Box 9.2).

Box 9.2 Definition of Green and White Papers

Consultative documents can also be termed 'Green Papers'. These are published in order that comments can be submitted by members of the public and/or the professionals concerned. This is available prior to the final decisions made about service provision.

Future government policy is presented in White Papers. Some of these may go on to become Acts of Parliament.

The rate of policy production will mean that paramedics will be required to update themselves on a regular basis. During your education you will be required to examine many of the key policy documents relating to ambulance services, emergency and out-of-hospital care.

Reflection: points to consider

What do you know about recent policy documents? Can you name some? What implications do they have for your daily work?

NHS services work differently in the four devolved areas of the UK. Please see the following websites for the structure and function of the NHS where you work:

- England: http://www.nhs.uk/nhsengland/thenhs/about/pages/nhsstructure. aspx
- Wales: http://www.wales.nhs.uk/nhswalesaboutus/structure
- Scotland: http://www.scot.nhs.uk/about-nhs-scotland/
- Northern Ireland: http://online.hscni.net/home/hsc-structure/

You will find an extensive amount of information on the websites listed in this chapter. As a current, professional paramedic you have a duty to understand how the system you are working within works, from the highest level to your more local level. Most of the ways you are asked to work, meeting targets, for example, have come from a policy document that has its origins in the Department of Health. Many paramedics work with the DH in order to influence policy and are shaping your working practices.

Chapter 18 for your professional continuing professional development responsibilities.

CONCLUSION

We hope that your awareness of the importance of each of the areas mentioned in this chapter has widened your view of your own world and that of others. This chapter has asked that you reflect upon your own personal and working lives, in an attempt to make the theory more relevant to practice. It has introduced you to various sociological theorists and demonstrated the value of understanding how theory can impact practice.

An awareness of the Department of Health structure is a step towards understanding the process of policy development. An awareness of social policy proposals means that there is an opportunity to comment in a professional or personal capacity at the discussion stage. Being up to date with current social policy in relation to out-of-hospital care implies that paramedics are aware of what this may mean for them and colleagues in the future shape of ambulance services and has the potential to highlight areas of personal development and career opportunities

Chapter key points:

- The work of the classical sociologists still has resonance today.
- Our own lives and lives of others can be explored and understood through sociological theory linked to case studies.
- There are numerous areas of our lives that can be examined from a sociological perspective and you are encouraged to examine your own beliefs, judgements and behaviour.
- Most areas of our lives can be examined in sociological terms. There are areas that we cannot easily change and have 'grown up' with, such as culture, age and religion.
- All of these aspects of our lives are interdependent and inextricably linked.
- Sociology should encourage us to question and discover our own self and explore the world around us.
- The importance of government and local offices is explored.
- Signposting is provided to key websites.
- The importance of keeping up to date with policies is highlighted.

REFERENCES AND SUGGESTED READING

Blaber, A.Y. (2012a) Sociology: an introduction. In A.Y. Blaber (ed.) *Foundations for Paramedic Practice: A Theoretical Perspective*, 2nd edn. Maidenhead: Open University Press.

Blaber, A.Y. (2012b) Social factors. In A.Y. Blaber (ed.) *Foundations for Paramedic Practice: A Theoretical Perspective*, 2nd edn. Maidenhead: Open University Press.

Blaber, A.Y. (ed.) (2012c) *Foundations for Paramedic Practice: A Theoretical Perspective*, 2nd edn. Maidenhead: Open University Press.

Cohen, R. (1994) *Frontiers of Identity: The British and the Others*. London: Longman.

Coser, L.A. (1977) *Masters of Sociological Thought: Ideas in Historical and Social Context*. New York: Harcourt Brace.

Crompton, R. (2008) *Class and Stratification*, 3rd edn. Cambridge: Polity Press.

Denny, E., Earle, S. and Hewison A. (2016) *Sociology for Nurses*, 3rd edn. Cambridge: Polity Press.

Douglas, J.W.B. (1964) *The Home and the School*. London: MacGibbon and Kee.

Durkheim, E. (1956) *Education and Sociology*. New York: The Free Press.

Giddens, A. and Sutton, P.W. (2017) *Sociology*, 8th edn. Cambridge: Polity Press.

Goffman, E. (1963) *Stigma: Notes on the Management of Spoiled Identity*. New York: Prentice-Hall.

Hebdige, D. (1979) *Subculture: The Meaning of Style*. London: Routledge.

Kornblum, W. (1997) *Sociology in a Changing World*. New York: Harcourt Brace.

Lazarsfeld-Jensen, A. and O'Meara, P. (2013) Sources of wellbeing: sharpening a sociological tool for diverse populations. *Journal of Paramedic Practice*, 5(4): 206–10.

McLellan, D. (ed.) (2000) *Karl Marx: Selected Writings*. Oxford: Oxford University Press.

Mead, G.H. ([1934] 1967) *Mind, Self and Society: Works of George Herbert Mead, 1934, from the Standpoint of a Social Behaviourist*. Edited and with an introduction by Charles W. Morris. Chicago: University of Chicago Press.

NHS Confederation (2017) *Key Statistics on the NHS*. London: NHS Confederation.

NHS Employers (2017) Gender in the NHS. London: NHS Employers. http://www.nhsemployers.org/~/media/Employers/Publications/Gender%20in%20the%20NHS (accessed 9 August 2017).

ONS (Office for National Statistics) (2012) Religion in England and Wales 2011. Available at: https://www.ons.gov.uk/peoplepopulationandcommunity/culturalidentity/religion/articles/religioninenglandandwales2011/2012-12-11 (accessed 16 December 2017).

Punch, S., Harden, J., Marsh, I. and Keating, M. (2013) *Sociology: Making Sense of Society*, 5th edn. London: Pearson Education/Prentice-Hall.

Ritzer, G. (1996) *Sociological Theory*. New York: McGraw-Hill.

USEFUL WEBSITES

Age Concern: www.ageuk.org.uk

Department of Health: https://www.gov.uk/government/organisations/department-of-health

Inequality resources: www.inequality.org (organisations with inequality-related agendas)

Office for National Statistics: www.statistics.gov

The Equality Trust: www.equalitytrust.org.uk (The Equality Trust works to improve the quality of life in the UK by reducing economic inequality)

The Joseph Rowntree Foundation: https://www.jrf.org.uk/(this is an independent organisation working to inspire social change through research, policy and practice)

Psycho-social aspects of health and illness
An introduction
Amanda Blaber and Chris Storey

In this chapter:

- Introduction
- Why is this relevant?
- Models of health
- Medicalisation
- Power of the health professions
- Stigma
- The sick role
- Chronic illness and disability
- Decision-making to access healthcare
- Inequalities in healthcare
- The postcode lottery of healthcare
- Social media and healthcare
- Conclusion
- Chapter key points
- References and suggested reading

INTRODUCTION

Having briefly discussed some of the areas that affect our socialisation, experience of life and society in Chapter 9, it is important to look at our experience of health and illness in twenty-first century society.

WHY IS THIS RELEVANT?

This chapter aims to introduce how sociologists and psychologists perceive what should be the paramedic's area of *business* – ill health. This chapter assumes that the reader is familiar with definitions and meaning of health, if not, see Chapter 10 in the second edition of *Foundations*.

MODELS OF HEALTH

Paramedics are often taught to 'assess, treat, manage and refer'. This approach to patient care can be described as a 'medical' approach and sits squarely in the medical model of healthcare. This approach is that described by sociologists and is a phrase used to describe the ways doctors practised years ago.

In an attempt to address more social issues/causes of ill health, the term 'bio-psycho-social' as a model was advocated, in order to be more holistic and treat the 'whole' patient. There remains an underlying assumption and sometimes a bias that the physical body takes precedence over the mental, emotional or psychological body. This can lead to health inequalities in the way people are treated, the care they receive and the priority with which their illness is classified.

 Reflection: points to consider

Recall some of the calls that you may have attended where the reason for the call was more for mental ill health than physical illness. Before you arrived, how was the person's illness prioritised? Reflect on the attitude of your colleagues to receiving this call to attend. Was a medical model approach applied, or was the approach taken more of a bio-psycho-social one? Would you change anything, if you were called to a similar call in the future?

In reality, communities and families are more fragmented than at any time in UK history. As a result, family support is diminished. The emergency, social services and voluntary community groups are called upon to try and fulfil individual and family needs. Rather than advocate the medical model over the social approaches, it is worth considering the merits of a continuum of care.

 Reflection: points to consider

Think about your own family. Go back through the generations and examine the locations where members of your family lived three generations ago, compared to the present day. Are your family members more widely spread across the UK/world now than they were three generations ago?

Paramedics expect, quite rightly, to be sent to the scene of an emergency. Therefore, in an emergency situation the medical model is wholly appropriate. For calls where an initial assessment has been conducted and it is clear that the situation is more social in

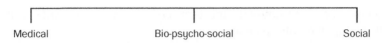

Medical	Bio-psycho-social	Social

Figure 10.1 Continuum of health models used in everyday paramedic practice

nature, the paramedic will need to be competent and confident to focus on more social issues and provide more of a holistic approach. Paramedics aim to provide holistic care for all patients, sometimes this is more medical, sometimes more social, depending on the situation they encounter. Figure 10.1 shows a proposed continuum for paramedics to consider.

Of course, the focus of the paramedic is multi-faceted and will depend on the following:

- professionalism
- how they perceive their role
- their ability to understand the patient's condition/situation
- empathy
- caring ability
- level of humanity
- own educational role preparation

This list is not exhaustive and you can add many more factors to it.

 Reflection: points to consider

Do you focus more on the physical health of patients or are you equally interested in their mental, emotional and psychological well-being?

We all have strengths and areas that we can develop both personally and professionally. By being more self-aware of your 'comfort zone', it may highlight areas of your practice where you would like to improve and develop your expertise.

MEDICALISATION

The medicalisation of health was of interest to sociologists, notably Ivan Illich (1975). The fact that the medical profession had extended their scope of practice to normal processes, such as birth, interested Illich. This extension of role also meant further development of the power of the medical profession over 'healthy' people and the power to define what is a natural process. Illich developed his thoughts and proposed that medicalisation also posed a risk to people who were at risk of 'doctor-generated illness' or the effects of medical treatment, the term he used was iatrogenesis. Illich (1975) proposed three types of iatrogenesis:

- *Clinical iatrogenesis* – unwanted side effects of medications, malpractice, neglect or ignorance, e.g. diarrhoea from antibiotics; severe sickness from chemotherapy.
- *Social (spiritual) iatrogenesis* – medicine encourages people to be health consumers and seek curative, preventative medicine, i.e. going to the doctor for the common cold; going to ED for sunburn; adding vitamins into your diet. Spiritually, healthcare professionals are commonly asked for advice and provide guidance on more social issues (see Case study 10.1).
- *Cultural iatrogenesis* – societies weaken due to over-medicalisation, as people expect medicine to be able to cure and treat all illness successfully, so people's responses to suffering, impairment and death are more profound, as they feel they have been 'let down' by medicine.

Case study 10.1

James is a 47-year-old who was referred to us from NHS111. He had phoned his GP, but was advised as it was the weekend, there was no one to see him. He had been feeling depressed and ill for a number of weeks and had mentioned to the call taker that he wondered whether it would be better if he was dead.

After assessing James' physical and mental state and listening to him describing how he felt, it became obvious that his issues stemmed from his belief that his life 'was going nowhere'. He had split up from his long-term girlfriend two months before, had not got the promotion at work that he had hoped for and found his time out of work had taken on a mundane repetition of the same activities (cooking, washing and ironing, watching television, and working on his car). While talking with him and assessing his mental state, it also became clear that though 'not being here' had been something he wondered about, he had no serious suicidal ideation.

Seeing that James' reasons for contacting us were more of a social issue, we listened and talked with him about how he was feeling and the support and help that might be available to him. While one of these was 'to make an appointment with his GP' (for an assessment of whether any medication was appropriate), we were also able to advise him of 'talking therapies' in the local area which might help, and suggest ways he could bring variety and new experiences into his free time. By the end of our conversation, James felt a lot better. He had decided to see his GP on Monday and planned to contact an old friend for a 'catch-up'. Just listening and encouraging our 'patient' had changed his outlook that day. Some people just want someone to listen to them for a while, it can make a difference.

In relation to Case study 10.1, Pink, Jacobson and Pritchard (2007: 841) suggest that 'the spiritual role that used to be the domain of the priest has been thrust into the medical sphere'. This has repercussions for paramedics as well as GPs as increasingly paramedics are acting as filters to GP services and accident and emergency units within the community. The issues of life which people face: loneliness, relationship problems, feelings of lack of fulfilment, are still very much present in society; however, with the decline in church attendance and the rise of scientism, people have to sort out alternative authorities for advice and help with their issues other than the church ministers who previously acted in this role. Increasingly the healthcare professional is seen as the person to provide such answers and, it seems, is also willing to undertake the role, or at least to acknowledge society's expectation that he or she will.

Illich persistently argued that medicine made people sick and sometimes did more harm than good. Medicalisation is one reason why paramedics get called to imminent births. Society is reliant on the medical profession, and by association, the wider health professions, midwifery and paramedics. Natural processes, such as births, would have been managed without medical assistance in years gone by across the world.

POWER OF THE HEALTH PROFESSIONS

Before power can be discussed, it is useful to explore the notion of what a 'profession' is. The first group of workers to use the term 'profession' were doctors within the medical profession. The superiority of the medical profession within the sphere of healthcare has been explored by sociologists and psychologists. They agree that a professional has distinct characteristics:

- a specialised body of knowledge;
- a monopoly of practice;
- autonomy to define the boundaries and the nature of their work;
- a code of ethics which regulates relationships both between professionals and between professionals and their clients.

Although this distinctly refers to the medical profession, some of these characteristics are common to any healthcare profession. The paramedic profession is no exception. Professions have tried to distinguish themselves from this medical ideal and create their own definitions, specific to their profession or semi-profession, a term some sociologists have used for professions other than medicine within healthcare. The intention was not to be derogatory, but to stand alone and independent from the medical profession.

Goffman (1971) suggested that in a patient–doctor relationship, the doctor was the 'expert' and the patient the 'object' of treatment. He assumed that as the medical model understands the human body scientifically, the focus is on 'fixing it', much as you would a broken-down car. Given that Goffman's (1968b) interest was mental health, it is easier to see how restrictive, and in some cases inappropriate, a purely medical model approach would seem. History has shown us that in the large Victorian asylums, residents were subjected to inhuman and experimental brain surgery to 'cure' conditions like depression. This is just one example of an extreme, severe form of power and abuse perpetrated on vulnerable adults. As a health professional we all have the potential to exert power over patients and families in our care. Your title and uniform have a large part to play here.

Reflection: points to consider

Think about entering a patient's home. Do they generally trust you with their family member who needs help? Hand over their child to you? Invite you in, trust you with their relative?

Chapter 9 and read Case study 9.4.

Of course, we are all working towards a positive outcome for patients, advocating for the best possible standards of care and striving to provide the most appropriate and timely care at all times. We do, however, all bring our prejudices, stereotypes, preconceived ideas with us prior to meeting any patient. It is a 'professional' who can 'park' these and approach each patient encounter with an open mind and fresh approach. Unfortunately, some professionals will abuse their position of power with some patients.

Reflection: points to consider

- Have you ever witnessed a colleague potentially abuse their position in a given situation?
- What could you/did you do about it?
- If it happened again, would you do anything differently?
- Refresh your understanding of the HCPC Standards of Proficiency and Guidance on Conduct and Ethics (2016).

Abuse of power does not need to be abusive or overt. It can be as simple as adopting a posture that says, 'I am not interested in caring for you'; hands in pockets are a prime example of the message you are potentially sending (Blaber 2012b).

Chapter 1 for more on communication and posture and **Chapter 4** on law and ethics.

STIGMA

Pre-existing medical or psychological conditions carry with them a 'stigma' or negativity that can form deep-seated personal opinions or beliefs. Some of these can be societal in nature.

You may have witnessed your colleagues display prejudice towards a patient. Unfortunately, some medical and psychological conditions cause the person to experience stigma from society, where they may feel different, excluded, and experience inequality in life in general, not just in health-related issues.

Goffman (1968a) identified three kinds of stigma:

- What he terms 'discrediting' or visually obvious physical deformities, such as loss of a limb or use of a wheelchair. Stigmas challenge our expectations of 'normal' social interaction and the stigmatised person is unsure of how she will be treated and how she will manage the interaction with the 'normal' person.
- Discreditable stigmas or blemishes of individual character. The stigma is not visually obvious, but may become disruptive if discovered, for example, history of mental health problems, epilepsy or having a criminal record.
- Tribal stigma of race, nation and religion.

People who are considered to have a stigma very often find it becomes dominant in their life and social role, so no matter what their other responsibilities (partner, parent, employee), they become defined by their stigmatised role, such as 'a wheelchair user', 'an epileptic'. The use of derogatory language by healthcare professionals sometimes reinforces a person's stigma – 'the stroke patient', 'the alcoholic', for example. It is important to be aware that attributes that result in stigma in some situations may not be the same in other situations; for example, being a single mother in some cultures or subcultures may be discreditable but is the norm in others, so may not result in stigma. It is also important to acknowledge that people with obvious stigmas may pose difficulty for the paramedic, especially if they have little experience of dealing with the general public and are new to healthcare. It is vital that interpersonal communication skills are practised and that difficult situations are reflected upon, in order that student paramedics can improve their interpersonal skills and approach to members of the public in a non-judgemental, confident and professional manner. The work of Goffman (1968a) identified 'stigma' as being a social concept. This is interesting to discuss, while remembering Talcott Parsons' (1951) concept of classifying illness as a 'deviance'.

Chapter 1 for more on interpersonal communication and **Chapter 4** for ethical considerations concerning paramedic practice.

THE SICK ROLE

Parsons (1951) explored the behaviour of ill people and professional responses to it as a social phenomenon, rather than a biological cause. He assumed two things: (1) that the 'patient–doctor relationship is a social system', based on appropriate behaviour and concerned with norms; and (2) that 'illness is a deviance and is potentially disruptive to social order'. Coming from a functionalist perspective, Parsons viewed illness as disrupting the functioning of society, but was intrigued to explore the role of healthcare in maintaining society's well-being. People cannot contribute to society if they are ill – health is needed to fulfil all of our normal social roles, as parents or workers, for instance. Having looked at this macro perspective, Parsons examined how individuals respond to illness (Giddens and Sutton 2017).

Reflection: points to consider

Although there have been many critiques of Parsons' theory, you still have to visit your GP to be signed off as 'sick' for more than a short period. For any type of recompense, for example, holiday insurance or government benefit, you require documents to be completed and signed by your GP to validate your claim.

The term 'sick role' was coined by Parsons (1951) to describe the way individuals and social institutions concerned with medical care (hospitals, general practitioners) socially sanctioned being ill. Parsons believed that individuals had two rights and two obligations when in the sick role:

- Individuals' rights are: sick people are allowed to give up their normal activities (going to work, school); they cannot be blamed for their incapacity.
- The two obligations are: to get well as quickly as possible and to seek competent care and cooperate with medical help.

Parsons makes a clear distinction between illness and other types of deviance (crime), as the person is not held responsible.

Contemporary sociologists (Allan et al. 2016; Nettleton 2016; Giddens and Sutton 2017) balance the discussion by noting limitations to Parsons' theory. Long-term health problems, for example, diabetes or arthritis, do not *fit* Parsons' ideology, as these

Case study 10.2

Craig is a frequent caller to the ambulance service, he has chronic obstruction pulmonary disorder (COPD), is very overweight and is alcohol-dependent. He lives alone but has a friend who sees him daily and acts as his carer. Craig lives in a very unkempt flat but he likes it that way. He does not want 'official' carers and he does not want interference from anybody.

However, Craig often slips out of his chair and cannot get up off the floor. He also regularly feels short of breath due to his COPD; whenever these situations occur, he or his friend call 999. Craig has been offered the help of support services for his conditions and situation several times but chooses not to access them. Craig is not following the 'rules' of the sick role and this leads to frustration among those healthcare professionals (HCPs) who answer his calls. Some HCPs who know Craig feel resentment towards him and speak about 'abuse of NHS services'. Craig says everyone will be happy when he is dead.

Think about the following question:

- What do you think might change things more positively for both Craig and those attending any calls that Craig might make to the ambulance service in the future?

illnesses have no cure and the individual cannot be obligated to *get well*. However, as can be seen in Case study 10.2, situations are often complex and frustrating for the individual concerned and the professional. The concept of power is also important when discussing the sick role, as doctors act in a social sense to sanction the sick role and also have legal obligations concerning long-term sick leave or controlling access to financial benefits, on behalf of the government. It seems that many individuals crave legitimisation of their illness; doctors and paramedics may be involved in the process.

Parsons (1951) viewed illness as deviance. This has been criticised as being too simple in its explanation of what can be a complex process in terms of accessing assistance, coming to terms with diagnosis and complying with treatment. If your views are similar to those of Parsons, then some illnesses will be classified as more 'deviant' than others. In the sick role and stigma sections of this chapter we have discussed the role of institutions.

For more historical and sociological information on institutions, see **Chapter 10** in the second edition of *Foundations for Paramedic Practice: A Theoretical Perspective* (Blaber 2012).

CHRONIC ILLNESS AND DISABILITY

Chronic illness is a feature of twenty-first-century Britain, as people are living longer. Many people experience the symptoms of chronic conditions; these vary widely but Giddens and Sutton (2017) suggest that chronic diseases share certain features:

- They present long-term health problems.
- They often present multiple health problems.
- There is usually no 'cure', only treatment for symptoms.
- There may be uncertainty about how illness will progress and when.
- They potentially cause major disruption to the lives of sufferers and their families.

Charmaz (1983) describes a *loss of self* as being a central feature of people who experience chronic conditions. An individual's confidence and self-worth are affected. The stigma associated with their chronic condition may mean they distance themselves from social interaction, leading to a negative vicious circle. In describing the sick role, Parsons (1951) considered the individual to be passive and seeking medical help, but many individuals with chronic illness will be 'experts' concerning their condition and a valuable source of information and learning for the paramedic. It is crucial that the paramedic respects and values the individual's expertise and uses the patient's knowledge to learn from him and provide quality care for him. It must also be remembered that people living with chronic illness often have to 'juggle' relationships with health professionals, family and friends, requiring many adaptations and adjustments. It has been argued that in our society,

> Impairment acts as a reminder of the fragility and vulnerability of the body ... Most disabled people experience their actual physical impairment as the least of their problems, it is the attitudes and reactions of others to the impairment which are felt to cause the most frustration, hurt and pain.

(Wilson 2006: 177)

Case study 10.3

Many disabled patients I have been to express the feeling that they are not wholly part of society. They felt accepted in the appropriate places, e.g. disabled sporting events and accepted when presented as 'brave victims'. But when it came to looking round the shops on a Saturday afternoon, they 'got under people's feet' or 'clogged up the High Street'. One young man, who is a wheelchair user, was applauded and praised for winning a bronze medal for Great Britain but the following day no one would help him get on a bus. 'The real kick in the teeth,' he told me, 'is that the bus stop is right outside my house; I see it every day, but the step up onto the bus is too high and no one is willing to give me a hand. My legs don't work but that's not what makes me disabled . . . it's society that disables me every day.'

When discussing disability, disability sociologists advocate the move away from a medical model where the focus is to cure or care and return the individual to *normal* – an example of the biomedical model. Disability is not a function of the physical incapacities of the individual, but is socially created, as highlighted in Case study 10.3. The focus should be on moving towards a social model, where restrictions within society that disable the individual, for example, lack of access to buildings and public transport, are addressed. The social model encourages society to reduce oppression for people with a disability, enabling them to participate in society and reduce oppression via appropriate social policies.

 Reflection: points to consider

The Paralympic movement has done much to reduce the stigma surrounding physical disability. Is this the experience of disability that people you care for have?

The vast majority of people who are physically disabled have an extremely difficult time negotiating everyday tasks such as getting to a shop, let alone shopping, due to the society and environment we have created for the able-bodied. As such, society discriminates against the disabled, when the able-bodied are capable of making adjustments. Have you ever asked yourself why door handles are not at wheelchair height? Able-bodied people have the ability to bend down to reach a door handle, something a wheelchair-dependent person cannot do.

DECISION-MAKING TO ACCESS HEALTHCARE

Sociologists have considered how and when people make the decision to seek professional help. Kasl and Cobb (1966) reviewed the literature, finding that the severity of symptoms plays only a small part in people's decision-making. There are many other factors that an individual considers before seeking help, as shown in Figure 10.2. There are other examples of such models, such as Kasl and Cobb's model, created in 1966. A person's past experience of healthcare is a crucial aspect of their decision-making. This is an area where healthcare professionals have the opportunity to make a difference. Every interaction that a person has with healthcare services, whether that be emergency or routine, will to varying extents affect their future decision-making. All of us need to be aware of this and take it seriously. The individuals and their situations described in Case studies 10.1 and 10.2 are a case in point, where attitudes and judgements made by healthcare professionals may affect future decision-making.

If we know and understand how people may make decisions and recognise that our own behaviour may have a large part to play, we can seek to modify our behaviour and image, as appropriate. If you recognise a behaviour that might have affected a

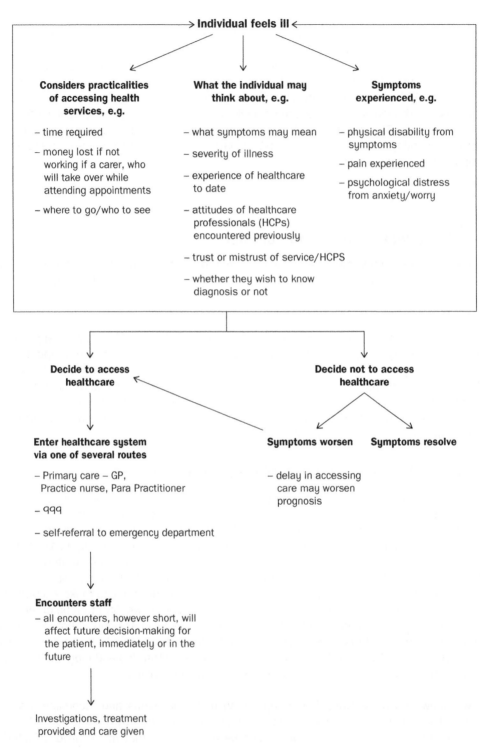

Figure 10.2 An example of a model of illness behaviour

person's past experience of paramedics, you are in a position to alter your public image and improve the client's view and experience of the out-of-hospital care service (Blaber 2012).

INEQUALITIES IN HEALTHCARE

The Office of National Statistics regularly produces statistical data on a vast array of issues, one of them being inequality. Box 10.1 details life expectancy data for 2009–2013 (ONS 2018).

The data presented in Box 10.1 clearly highlights the impact that deprivation has on health and subsequently on life expectancy in different parts of the UK (ONS 2018). Box 10.2 presents data related to the amount of years that individuals can expect to live in 'good' health or healthy life expectancy, 2009–2013 (ONS 2018).

Box 10.2 also includes statistics relating to disability-free life expectancy, this refers to the 'years of life spent free from disability'. This is slightly lower than the inequality in healthy life expectancy for both males and females. The ONS also provides regional and gender-specific statistical data for those of you who are interested in exploring

---

Box 10.1 Life expectancy inequality, 2009–2013

- Male life expectancy at birth was 79.1 years.
- Level of inequality of male life expectancy between the most and least deprived parts of England was 7.9 years.
- Female life expectancy at birth was 83 years.
- Level of inequality of female life expectancy between the most and least deprived parts of England was 5.9 years.

Box 10.2 Healthy and disability-free life expectancy, 2009–2013

- Males 63.5 years.
- Females 64.8 years.
- Level of inequality of male healthy life expectancy inequality between those living in the most and least deprived parts of the UK was 16.7 years.
- Level of inequality of female healthy life expectancy inequality between those living in the most and least deprived parts of the UK was 16.8 years.
- Inequality in disability-free life expectancy for males was 14.5 years.
- Inequality in disability-free life expectancy for females was 13.6 years.

inequality data in more detail. The data presented in Boxes 10.1 and 10.2 highlight the consistent health inequalities that exist in the UK.

There are still many areas of life where inequalities exist and affect the health of the population. Inequalities in health and premature death have become a feature of sociologists' and psychologists' work prior to, and after, the Black Report (Townsend et al. 1988), which suggested that inequalities were real and, in some areas, widening. Successive governments have attempted to develop social policy to try and reduce inequalities, but as inequalities are inextricably linked with other areas of social life, this is proving exceedingly difficult and economically expensive. Sociologists and psychologists have explored the prerequisites of good health (access to jobs, education and quality housing) and their impact on health. Racism affects the access to, and quality of, service received. Gender, as a social construction, affects what we expect of men and women in terms of health. The list continues, if you wish to read further, the texts listed here will provide a comprehensive overview (Allan et al. 2016; Nettleton 2016; Giddens and Sutton 2017).

 Chapter 9 for more information relating to social factors affecting our lives.

It is not only age and disability where inequality can be discussed. Indeed, all areas of our lives are inextricably linked, in health and in our experience of and predisposition to illness. This serves as a brief introduction to the concept of inequality; see the suggested reading for dedicated books and websites on each of the subjects.

THE POSTCODE LOTTERY OF HEALTHCARE

NHS England regularly releases data on the performance of Clinical Commissioning Groups (CCGs). The government encourages patients to examine the data on their local services in the key areas of cancer, dementia, diabetes, mental health, learning disability and maternity services. Some areas have better records of access to healthcare than others, so this is called the postcode lottery of healthcare. This data is published on MyNHS website, launched in 2014. One thing to consider is if the government is contributing to health inequality by relying on website use. What about the older generation or poorer members of society who may not own computers or have internet access?

 Reflection: points to consider

Do you always consider a person's ability/financial situation when you discuss advice or recommend technology as a means to access information?

Medication rationing

The continuing and competing demands placed upon the NHS are infinite and resources are limited. This gives rise to a basic economic problem, demand is outstripping supply. Of course, each individual patient would like the most expensive option for treatment if it promises to make the difference between them living or dying. In doing so, the cost of their individual treatment removes the options for others, as resources are not infinite and a line must be drawn somewhere. The same can be said for doctors, where they seek the best for their patients, as the result, in terms of fewer resources for other patients, when they choose expensive options for some, you could argue others suffer. So, what is at play here is 'cost versus benefit'. What the NHS strives to achieve is an efficient resource allocation. Of course, if it is you or a family member who are 'denied' a treatment option or expensive medication, it is not easy to accept such decisions.

In order to prevent these decisions being subjective and arbitrary, the National Institute for Care and Clinical Excellence (NICE) has been tasked with attempting to tackle these difficult financial and ethical issues. NICE publishes guidance about whether pharmaceuticals and other technologies should be provided by the NHS. NICE provides guidance to the NHS in England and Wales when requested to do so by the Department of Health (DH) and the Welsh Assembly. The guidance indicates whether a particular technology or medication, based on the balance of the current evidence, should be recommended as the most cost-effective use of NHS resources. Once NICE agrees to a medication being used, the NHS has 90 days within which to make it available to patients. From 2017, any medications that are likely to cost the NHS £20 million per year or more will be subject to further cost/benefit analysis as part of a government review of spending in the NHS (NICE 2017).

SOCIAL MEDIA AND HEALTHCARE

You should all be familiar with the guidance from the HCPC (2017) and CoP (2017) regarding your personal and professional use of social media. If you are not – you need to be. Many disciplinary cases have been brought against paramedics and other health professionals for inappropriate and unprofessional use of social media. This section of the chapter intends to examine the rise of social media in society and its use in healthcare from a sociological perspective.

There are huge benefits and conversely associated risks of the relatively rapid rise in 'connectedness' that has been a result of the social media 'boom'. There are risks that we all need to be mindful of in respect of the reliance on technology.

Every social connection we make personally on platforms, such as Facebook or Twitter, is logged and scrutinised and we are then targeted for products and services. Your social platforms are also often monitored by employers and potential employers who wish to examine the profile of employees or job candidates. The use of social media

Reflection: points to consider

- When you attend a patient, do you automatically set about connecting them to technology, such as lifepaks? Or do you take your time and actually 'look' at the patient first?
- Have you considered how your organisation would work if your computers were hacked and how would you get allocated to calls? Do you know the 'back-up' plan for your organisation?
- If you use electronic patient care records, what is the plan if the system fails?

can be personally and professionally risky, if you are not clear on your boundaries and professional guidance, but there are some positive uses.

There are intelligent uses, such as building virtual communities that link like-minded people across diverse geographical areas and in other parts of the world. These connections are devoid of limitations of time and place and, as such, may prove to be a useful means of support and solidarity, especially for shift and lone workers. Of course, this comes with risk. What may previously have been said in a mess room but shared in private, if put on social media, it has the potential to be eavesdropped by the public. Professionalism and codes of conduct are of major importance and boundaries need to be clear in the paramedic's mind. However, used appropriately and as a means of education, sharing ideas and developing the profession, social media is a powerful tool (Allan et al. 2016; Nettleton 2016).

We must also remember that the use of social media within our professional role has the potential to create inequalities. For example, some older people may not be knowledgeable about social media or computer 'savvy' and therefore may even find it more difficult to book an appointment with their GP; they may lose out while relying on the telephone during office hours, while others can book appointments via the internet 24/7.

Reflection: points to consider

Think about one of your shifts:

- Did you give advice, treatment or refer a patient that required the use of the internet?
- Did you take for granted that the person you cared for had access to the internet via computer or mobile phone?
- If you had thought about this, what could you have done differently?

In May 2017, the NHS suffered the most widespread hacking incident to date. This caused chaos across the country and personal misery for many patients, as operations were cancelled, ambulances diverted and departments shut down (*The Independent* 2017). This emphasises the importance of having a 'back-up plan' in all areas of health-care and being able to revert to basic, non-technologically reliant care.

There is a growing area of medical sociology that focuses purely on medical technology in healthcare. As you would expect, there is much debate on this subject, ranging from those who see technologies as discrete, inert tools to be used, abused or neglected to those who see technologies as forming part of patients' lives forever more. Nettleton (2016) provides a concise summary, if you are interested in reading further. It is beyond this chapter's ability to provide a discussion about the expensive technological equipment that is being used within the NHS. As with medications, the purchase of expensive equipment requires careful consideration and NICE is at the forefront of the appraisal of technology (NICE 2017).

CONCLUSION

There is no doubt that the discussion of health and illness is complex and subject to many sociological and psychological views/perspectives. This chapter has introduced some of the issues, but it is no substitute for further reading and investigation. We envisage that students will gain an understanding of psychology and sociology and sociological/psychological principles from this discussion and hope it will act as a cata-lyst for future enquiry.

Chapter key points:

- Some models of health, the sick role and stigma are explored.
- People react in a variety of ways to acute illness and chronic ill health.
- People's reactions and behaviour in respect of decision-making are discussed.
- All of the above are considered in terms of some sociological and psychological theories and theorists.

REFERENCES AND SUGGESTED READING

Allan, H., Traynor, M., Kelly, D. and Smith, P. (2016) *Understanding Sociology in Nursing*. London: Sage.

Blaber, A.Y. (2012) Psycho-social aspects of health and illness: an introduction. In A.Y. Blaber (ed.) *Foundations for Paramedic Practice: A Theoretical Perspective*, 2nd edn. Maidenhead: Open University Press.

Charmaz, K. (1983) Loss of self: a fundamental form of suffering in the chronically ill. *Sociology of Health and Illness*, 5(2): 168–95.

College of Paramedics (2017) *Social Media User Guidance – Summary*. Bridgwater: College of Paramedics. Available at: https://www.collegeofparamedics.co.uk/downloads/College_of_ Paramedics_Social_Media_User_Guidance_(Summary).pdf (accessed 20 December 2017).

Giddens, A. and Sutton, P. (2017) *Sociology*, 8th edn. Cambridge: Polity Press.

Goffman, E. (1968a) *Stigma: Notes on the Management of Spoiled Identity*. New York: Prentice-Hall.

Goffman, E. (1968b) *Asylums: Essays on the Social Situation of Mental Patients and Other Inmates*. Harmondsworth: Penguin.

Goffman, E. (1971) *The Presentation of Self in Everyday Life*. Harmondsworth: Penguin.

Health and Care Professions Council (2014) *Standards of Proficiency: Paramedics*. London: HCPC.

Health and Care Professions Council (2016) *Guidance on Conduct and Ethics for Students*. London: HCPC.

Health and Care Professions Council (2017) *Use of Social Networking Sites*. London: HCPC. Available at: http://www.hpc-uk.org/registrants/standards/socialnetworking/(accessed 20 December 2017).

Illich, I. (1975) *Medical Nemesis*. London: Calder and Boyars.

Kasl, S.V. and Cobb, S. (1966) Health behaviour, illness behaviour and sick role behaviour. *Archives of Environmental Health*, 12: 246–66.

Nettleton, S. (2016) *The Sociology of Health and Illness*, 3rd edn. Cambridge: Polity Press.

NICE (National Institute for Care and Clinical Excellence) (2017) *Guidance and Advice List*. Available at: https://www.nice.org.uk/guidance/published?type=ta (accessed 20 December 2017).

ONS (Office for National Statistics) (2018) Life expectancy and disability-free life expectancy statistics 2009–2013. Available at: https://www.ons.gov.uk/peoplepopulationandcommunity/ healthandsocialcare/healthandlifeexpectancies/bulletins/inequalityinhealthandlifeexpectancies withinuppertierlocalauthorities/2009to2013 (accessed 2 January 2018).

Parsons, T. (1951) *The Social System*. London: Routledge and Kegan Paul.

Pink, J., Jacobson, L. and Pritchard, M. (2007) The 21st century GP: physician and priest? *British Journal of General Practice,* 57(543): 840–2. Available at: http://pubmedcentralcanada.ca/ pmcc/articles/PMC2151827/ (accessed 20 December 2017).

The Independent (2017) NHS cyber attack. Available at: http://www.independent.co.uk/news/ uk/home-news/nhs-cyber-attack-hospitals-hack-england-emergency-patients-divert-shut-down-a7732816.html (accessed 14 September 2017).

Townsend, P., Davidson, N. and Whitehead, P. (1988) *Inequalities in Health (Black Report)*. Harmondsworth: Pelican.

Wilson, S. (2006) To be or not to be disabled: the perception of disability as eternal transition. *Psychodynamic Practice*, 12(2): 177–91.

USEFUL WEBSITES

My NHS: https://www.nhs.uk/Service-Search/performance/search (accessed 1 January 2018).

Office for National Statistics – specifically disability-free life expectancy by region: https://www. ons.gov.uk/peoplepopulationandcommunity/healthandsocialcare/healthandlifeexpectancies/ bulletins/disabilityfreelifeexpectancybyuppertierlocalauthorityengland/2014-07-24 (accessed 2 January 2018).

Child protection
Mike Brady

In this chapter:

- Introduction
- Why is this relevant?
- Legislation and guidance
- What are abuse and neglect?
- Why do abuse and neglect happen?
- Different types of abuse, neglect, and safeguarding concerns
- Management of suspected abuse and neglect
- Conclusion
- Chapter key points
- References and suggested reading
- Useful websites

INTRODUCTION

Safeguarding has always been a paramedic's responsibility, however, it has not always been considered a priority in education when compared with subjects such as trauma and resuscitation. Recent revelations about widespread historical sexual abuse and child deaths, as well as the current socio-economic climate have reiterated the need for all healthcare professionals (HCPs) not only to be aware of child protection, but also to be suitably educated in its application. This chapter aims to provide the reader with a basic understanding of child and young person protection theory, and includes information on different types of abuse, neglect, and family need which can be applied to everyday paramedic practice.

WHY IS THIS RELEVANT?

Child protection (which includes young people) is relevant to paramedic practice not only because of the deleterious effects such experiences can have on a child's later life, such as emotional difficulties, drug and alcohol addictions, and poor educational attainment (NSPCC 2017a) but also because in many cases such abuse can be recognised by HCPs and prevented.

Paramedics often encounter and treat children and families who are at risk of abuse, neglect, and failure to thrive, and they need to be able to identify and respond to these concerns. Paramedics are often invited into family homes when social workers, police officers, and health visitors are not; and they need to understand how best to use this advantage to gather information to support the reporting or referral of identified concerns (Brady 2018).

The Health and Care Professions Council (HCPC) is clear that registrants should take appropriate action to protect the rights of children (HPC 2007) and ensure that the well-being of service users is always safeguarded (HCPC 2016). For paramedics to meet their professional obligations, they require an understanding of child protection theory which they can link to practice effectively. Furthermore, to be able to practise lawfully, as expected by the HCPC (2014), paramedics require a basic understanding of the specific Acts applicable to their practice.

 Chapter 4 for more on ethics and law.

Child protection is relevant to paramedic practice, professionally, legally, and ethically – as child protection is everyone's responsibility, but especially the responsibility of those who are often the first to assess a child in an environment not always readily accessible to others.

LEGISLATION AND GUIDANCE

The United Kingdom has multiple Acts of Parliament that cover child protection, and not one single piece of overarching legislation (see Box 11.1). This approach has been

---

Box II.I UK legislation covering child protection

- Education Act 2002/2011
- Serious Crime Act 2015a
- Children Act 1989/2004
- Children and Families Act 2014
- Adoption and Children Act 2002
- Children and Adoption Act 2006
- Protection of Freedoms Act 2012
- Female Genital Mutilation Act 2003
- Children and Young Persons Act 2008
- Counter-Terrorism and Security Act 2015
- Safeguarding Vulnerable Groups Act 2006
- Borders, Citizenship, and Immigration Act 2009

argued by some to create a lack of uniformity which contributes to an incoherent public policy approach to safeguarding children (Goddard and Tucci 2008), and a lack of clear definition which can at times make identification more difficult for paramedics (Sibson and Brain 2009).

There are some laws which specifically set out the responsibilities of HCPs (such as paramedics) and which support guidance documents/frameworks. Paramedics should understand the overarching theories behind them and realise that while legislation supports and often obliges them to report and refer concerns, it will be left to those to whom they refer to decide which piece of legislation an act or omission contravenes. Explanation of the Acts and reviews is presented in chronological order, to provide the reader with a historical perspective.

Every Child Matters

Following Victoria Climbié's death in 2000 and the subsequent review in 2003, the UK government launched the initiative Every Child Matters (ECM), which set out a range of measures to dramatically reform and improve children's care. The proposals set out by ECM were:

- To support parents and carers.
- Early intervention and effective prevention.
- Accountability and integration (locally, regionally, and nationally).
- Workforce reform.

Early intervention and effective prevention are key responsibilities of paramedics. ECM was the precursor to further guidance documents which again reiterate the involvement that HCPs such as paramedics have in child protection.

The Children Act 2004

The Children Act 2004 provides a legal framework for multiple guidance documents, and provides a legislative duty on 'relevant partners' to co-operate, collaborate, collect data, and share information through multiple integrated working processes (Munro 2006; NSPCC 2017b). Such duties include the need for ambulance services and paramedics to refer and report their concerns with multiple agencies, which is important given that paramedics are often in a prime position to identify and thus prevent abuse and neglect (Brady 2018). Despite such legislation being in place, however, there is still recent evidence that the data sharing responsibilities incumbent upon ambulance services and paramedics are not being fulfilled (Kirtley 2013).

Section 11.2a of the Children Act (2004) specifically places duties upon ambulance services and thus paramedics to ensure that they consider the need to safeguard and promote the welfare of children when carrying out their functions. The Act recognises that HCPs are in a strong position to identify welfare needs or safeguarding concerns and, where appropriate, can provide support and safety. The fact that ambulance services are mentioned within legislation highlights the role that paramedics play in protecting children and families, and should encourage individual paramedics and ambulance services to ensure that training and support are adequate, effective and accessible.

Working Together to Safeguard Children

This emphasis on expanding and including all potential partners in safeguarding is reiterated in a later government initiative: Working Together to Safeguard Children (WTSC) (2006), revised in 2010, 2013 and 2015. WTSC sets out how organisations and individuals should work together to safeguard and promote the welfare of children and young people in accordance with the Children Act (1989/2004).

Importantly for paramedicine, all four versions of WTSC cite the role of ambulance services, and thus paramedics. WTSC 2006 and 2010, for example, state that ambulance staff may be in a position to identify initial concerns regarding a child's welfare, and will have access (by phone or in person) to family homes, and be involved with individuals at times of crisis. Each WTSC publication argues that it is important for all to understand fully their responsibilities and duties as set out in primary legislation. Given that paramedics are included in such government initiatives, aspects of which have basis in legislation, they need to understand their role in child protection.

The Munro Reviews

A review of child protection systems was undertaken in 2010, the first of three annual consecutive reviews chaired by Professor Eileen Munro. The Munro Reviews analysed, criticised, and made recommendations to all those working in child protection and further afield, such as education and healthcare.

The reviews make mention of frontline practitioners within the community, and so its findings are applicable to paramedic practice. The first report was deliberately analytical, and made no major recommendations. The following two reports, however, set out proposals for reform which were intended to create the conditions that enable professionals to make the best judgements about the help to give to children, young people and families. Munro's Reviews criticise the over-bureaucratisation of simple services aimed at protecting and nurturing children and young people. Munro (HM Government 2012) concluded that by decreasing the bureaucracy within current systems and supporting professional development of staff, the quality, management, accountability, and shared learning within child and family social work can all increase.

Such support and development for paramedics could include:

- Regular up-to-date training and education.
- Access to senior clinical support and advice 24/7.
- Receiving regular feedback or audit of their CP referrals.

- Having access to safeguarding polices and guidance via portable tablet/ toughbook.
- Being able to submit safeguarding referrals from electronic patient care records (EPCRs).

Each review cites a wide range of research evidence and often recommends undertaking further research to better understand practice. There is relative paucity, however, in research related to paramedics' involvement in child protection, and, as such, more is needed both to understand their involvement and the barriers they face to recognising abuse, neglect, and need, which we continue to explore.

The Serious Crime Act

The Serious Crime Act 2015 (HM Government 2015b) is an Act which builds upon current criminal and civil law to ensure that enforcement agencies can continue to effectively and relentlessly disrupt, pursue, and prosecute serious and organised criminals. While it may appear to be an Act which predominantly focuses upon the management of crime, it has implications for how paramedics carry out their work; and specifically, how they manage female genital mutilation (FGM) and domestic violence.

 Chapter 4 for the differences between criminal and civil law and **Chapter 13** for more detail regarding domestic violence and human trafficking.

The introduction of the Serious Crime Act (HM Government 2015b) saw a mandatory legal obligation for HCPs to report evidence of, disclosures of, or suspicions of FGM. This not only bolstered HCPs' position to break confidentiality where needed but made paramedics among many more professionals legally accountable. Given this legal accountability, it is important for paramedics to be able to recognise signs, symptoms, and causal factors of FGM, which will be explored later.

While domestic violence is currently included within legislation such as the Domestic Violence, Crime and Victims Act 2004, Section 76 of the Serious Crime Act created a new offence of 'controlling or coercive behaviour in an intimate or family relationship'. This new offence closes a gap in the existing law around psychological and emotional abuse that stops short of physical abuse (CPS 2017), and prohibited behaviours include:

- enforcing rules and activity which humiliate, degrade, or dehumanise;
- proliferating themes of family 'dishonour';
- depriving someone of their basic needs;
- threats to harm a child.

Such behaviours affect children and young people who witness domestic violence, suffer emotional abuse, and sexual abuse or exploitation. Paramedics are in a prime position within the community to recognise these behaviours as they enter houses and gather information.

Various pieces of legislation underpin many guidance documents to help support HCPs to carry out their legal and professional responsibilities to protect children and young people.

WHAT ARE ABUSE AND NEGLECT?

It is impossible to provide worldwide uniformed definitions of child abuse and neglect, given the anthropological differences in race, religion, culture, and gender emphasis. Even within the same discipline, there is debate about whether definitions should be based on the behaviour of the perpetrator, the experience of the child, or some combination of these.

Unless those working with children and young people have a clear definition of what constitutes abuse and neglect, they are unlikely to be able to identify those potentially at risk and those at risk of perpetrating it. For example, it is important that paramedics understand that the terms paedophile and sex offender are often used interchangeably – incorrectly (Richards 2011). Not all child sex offenders are paedophiles and conversely, not all paedophiles are child sex offenders. This pre-, mid-, and post-pubescent distinction is relevant because while a young person may be physically (anatomically) able to have a sexual relationship (thus not paedophilic), it does not mean that they are cognitively ready to have one and or that the relationship is not coercive, exploitative, or an abuse of a position of trust. Thus, when managing possible abuse, paramedics must consider not only the age of a person (Box 11.2), but their intellectual capacity, their emotional vulnerability, the relationships involved, and much more. Although at times complex, this section will outline various definitions, and signs for the paramedic to consider.

Neglect is somewhat less complex to define, however does not come without its considerations. Neglect is defined as:

> The persistent failure to meet a child's basic physical and/or psychological needs, likely to result in the serious impairment of the child's health or development. Neglect may occur during pregnancy, or once a child is born, and can involve lack of food, protection and appropriate medical treatment.

> (HM Government 2010: 39)

It is important to understand that while both abuse and neglect can be carried out purposely and with malicious intent, neglect can also result from socio-economic deprivation or an inability to cope for various reasons. Recognising these differences is important for those working with children and young people, as the emphasis can be either one of protection or removal of a child or one of guidance, support, and financial assistance.

> ## Box II.2 The actual age of a child
>
> In the UK, there is no single law that defines the actual age of a child:
>
> - The Children Act (1989) and (2004) respectively define a child as: 'Anyone who has not yet reached their 18th birthday.'
> - The Child Poverty Act (2010), however, defines a child as: 'A person under the age of 16.'
> - From an international perspective: the World Health Organisation (WHO 2017a) defines the maltreatment of a child as: 'The abuse and neglect that occurs to children under 18 years of age.'
> - Not all sources focus on the chronological age of a child. UNICEF (2005), for example, refers to childhood as being much more than just the space between birth and the attainment of adulthood, but rather the state and condition of a child's life and the quality of those years as having time to play, grow confident, to be free from fear, violence, and exploitation.

Failure to thrive, for example, is a term that has been used to describe 'a failure of expected growth (usually weight) and well-being' (Forfar 1984), and has more recently been termed weight faltering. While weight faltering is indeed an indicator of abuse, neglect, and deprivation, however, the assertion that abuse, neglect, and deprivation are the only causes has been questioned in recent years, leading to the proposal that its management should be less aggressive (Shields et al. 2012). Differentials for failure to thrive include organic disease, maternal depression, feeding and eating difficulties, in addition to more sinister causes. This highlights how complex defining child abuse and neglect can be, and further highlights how paramedics should remain open-minded to possible causes, while still reporting and referring all their concerns.

WHY DO ABUSE AND NEGLECT HAPPEN?

The causes of child abuse and neglect are often complex and multifaceted. Child protection is a relatively modern concept and is thought to have resulted from the changing nature of childhood itself (Munro 2006). Childhood has historically only been available to those from the higher echelons of society, with poorer children forced into work by necessity as soon as they were able. Various socio-political movements moulded childhood, such as: challenges to the patriarchal family model, changing roles of women within the family, and the introduction of child rights. There is a level of interchangeability between the terms safeguarding and protection. Although views differ, child protection is thought to outline the responsibilities of public agencies and private organisations to ensure children are protected against physical, emotional, and sexual abuse, and neglect. The term safeguarding is more conceptual and has a wider impact on a child's ability to thrive. Safeguarding refers to the overall health, development, and growth of a child, and what can be done to ensure they reach their full potential.

Box 11.3 outlines some of the possible causes of abuse and neglect, which are not exhaustive. Understanding risk factors can help the HCPs predict children at risk and children in need (Whitnell 2012). While there are possible links or causal factors of

Box II.3 Some of the factors that could lead to the risk of abuse and neglect

Parent/carer

- Stress
- Aggression
- Low self-esteem
- Substance misuse
- Mental health needs
- Lack of parenting skills
- Poor coping mechanisms
- Isolation and lack of support
- Domestic violence or coercion
- Normalised self-injurious behaviour
- Unrealistic expectations of what a child can do
- Physical and/or emotional dependence on others
- Poor communication or communication difficulties
- History of violent relationships within the family or social networks

The environment/location

- Overcrowding
- Geographical isolation
- Opportunistic (e.g. School/Social Club)
- Other children with challenging behaviour
- Poor or insecure living conditions, homelessness

Relationships

- Financial difficulties/power
- Self-gain (sexual exploitation)
- Domestic violence or coercion
- Unequal power relationships (controlling, coercive or threatening behaviour)
- Lack of understanding about the child's condition, resulting in inappropriate care
- Challenging behaviour by the person which the carer finds intolerable or stressful
- Isolation due to the demands of caring, and a lack of practical and emotional support
- History of abuse in the family, either being abused or responsible for previous abuse

abuse and neglect, professionals need to understand that they do not necessarily pre-determine its likelihood. A family living in poverty, for example, are not necessarily neglectful, and a parent once abused themselves does not always necessarily go on to abuse their own children.

Parents can often be socially isolated, and more so when single and on low incomes – as housing, transport, and the cost of social participation are often prohibitive. This isola-tion can often result in poor mental health, high levels of stress, inadequate coping mechanisms, and thus emotional abuse, physical abuse, or neglect. Although it must be noted that social isolation can occur in affluent families also.

Abuse can often be caused by a poor understanding and unrealistic expectations of what a child can and cannot do. Bed wetting or poor toilet use, for example, can be viewed by some parents as insolence – as opposed to normal development. A child fail-ing to pass an exam or win a competition can be viewed as laziness or disobedience. Parents can find such behaviour difficult to manage and this can result in them feeling incompetent as a parent, leading them to be angry at their child (Whitnell 2012). In addition to this perception of challenging behaviour – children often do display behaviour that is challenging to manage, which can also lead to parental impotence, and thus anger. Such displays of poor coping mechanisms and inadequate parenting styles can lead to emotional and physical abuse and often neglect and are often made worse by parental mental health problems, learning difficulties and intellectual limitations.

It is important for paramedics to understand the risk factors to children and young people being abused or neglected, as they may heighten their awareness and contrib-ute to clinical decision-making when considering a safeguarding referral. Knowledge of such risk factors need to be used alongside knowledge of the different types of abuse, neglect, and social concerns.

 Reflection: points to consider

You do not need proof that a child is being abused or neglected, just reasonable grounds to suspect. If in doubt, seek support or refer.

DIFFERENT TYPES OF ABUSE, NEGLECT AND SAFEGUARDING CONCERN

There are many types of abuse, neglect, and safeguarding concern that the paramedic should be aware of (see Box 11.4). Categories listed in Box 11.4 are perhaps the most widely known and talked about; however, there are certain categories of abuse that are

Box 11.4 Types of abuse

- *Physical abuse* may involve hitting, shaking, throwing, poisoning, burning or scalding, drowning, suffocating, the deliberate induction of illness, or otherwise causing physical harm to a child.
- *Domestic abuse* is any incident or pattern of incidents of controlling, coercive or threatening behaviour, including violence or abuse between those aged 16 or over who are or have been intimate partners or family members regardless of gender or sexuality.
- *Witnessed domestic violence* is child abuse and involves a child or young person inadvertently or forcibly witnessing any recognised definition of domestic violence.
- *Youth intimate partner/dating violence* is defined as the physical, sexual, psychological, or emotional violence within a dating relationship, including stalking. It can occur in person or electronically and might occur between a current or former dating partner.
- *Emotional abuse* is the persistent emotional maltreatment of a child such as to cause severe and persistent adverse effects on the child's emotional development. It may involve conveying to children that they are worthless or unloved, inadequate, or valued only as far as they meet the needs of another person.
- *Sexual abuse* involves forcing or enticing a child or young person to take part in penetrative and non-penetrative sexual activities, or in the production of sexual images not necessarily involving a high level of violence, whether the child is aware of what is happening. The perpetrators can be both men and women.
- *Child sexual exploitation* includes situations involving contexts and relationships where young people receive 'something' (e.g. food, alcohol) as a result of performing, and/or others performing on them, sexual activities; in which persons have power over them by virtue of their age, gender, intellect, physical strength and/or economic or other resources.
- *Forced marriage* (which differs from an arranged marriage) is when someone faces physical pressure to marry (for example, threats, physical violence, or sexual violence) or emotional and psychological pressure (e.g. family dishonour), and is illegal in the UK.
- *Children missing in education (CME)* are considered those who by their own actions or the inactions of their parents do not receive efficient full-time education – as set out in the Education Act (2011). CME are at significant risk of underachieving and becoming NEET (not in education, employment, or training) later in life, and are likely (although not always) to be victims of abuse, neglect, and at risk of physical, emotional, and psychological harm.
- *Self-harm* describes a range of behaviours, including but not limited to: cutting, scalding, hair pulling, breaking bones, overdoses, drinking to excess, stabbing, and strangling.

more difficult to identify, are still considered taboo, or due to socio-political climates at the time of writing, require more explanation.

Fabricated (induced) illness

Other causes for concern may be recurrent emergency department attendances, failure to thrive and induced or fabricated illness (RCPCH 2002; DCSF 2008). Fabricated or induced illness – previously known as Munchausen Syndrome by Proxy (MSBP) – is a rare condition, in which a parent or carer fabricates or induces illness or injury in others, most usually a child, with no obvious motive or gain. Recognising, identifying and accepting fabricated or induced illness is not easy and may require clinicians to suspend their disbelief, maintaining the welfare of the child as a priority (Whitnell 2012).

Female genital mutilation (FGM)

Female genital mutilation is also known as female genital cutting, sewing, or female circumcision. This procedure includes any partial or total removal of the external female genitalia or injury to the female genital organs for non-medical reasons (WHO 2017a) (Box 11.5) and is illegal in the UK (Female Genital Mutilation Act 2003).

FGM is predominantly practised in 28 countries worldwide on females between infancy and the age of 15. It is believed to be associated with cultural ideals of femininity and modesty, including the notion of beauty and cleanliness, with the removal of all body parts considered male or unclean. Such procedures are often carried out by untrained community leaders and are a breach of a woman's human rights. FGM can happen in any country and can be undertaken by anyone of any religious affiliation but is more closely associated with, for example, the Central Africa Republic, Ghana, Nigeria and Somalia (UNPF 2017).

Peate (2014) states that the paramedic as a front-line member of staff is well placed to identify girls and women in need of treatment to deal with the consequences of

---

Box II.5 Types of FGM

- *Clitoridectomy*: this is the partial or total removal of the clitoris.
- *Excision*: this is the partial or total removal of the clitoris and the labia minora.
- *Infibulation*: this is the narrowing of the vaginal opening through the cutting and repositioning the labia minora, or majora, and sometimes through stitching.
- *All other harmful procedures to the female genitalia* for non-medical purposes.

FGM and to identify and protect those at risk – a view supported by the UK House of Commons Home Affairs Committee's (2014) report on FGM.

Paramedics need to remain aware of such abuse when visiting or examining female children and young people and be suspicious if:

- Young females are taken out of the country, without other siblings or parent.
- Young females are taken to high-risk countries without sufficient explanation.
- Young females have difficulty urinating or frequent incontinence or urinary infections.
- Young females have menstrual problems or kidney failure or cysts or abscesses.
- Young females have relatives who are FGM victims.
- Young females are in the company of an older unfamiliar leader (the cutter).

The introduction of the Serious Crime Act (HM Government 2015b) saw a legal obligation for HCPs, such as paramedics, to report actual or suspicions of FGM. For this reason, among others, it is important for paramedics to understand the risk factors and signs of FGM and to request update training from their employers and additional teaching from their higher education institutes if they are not confident in recognising such features.

Child trafficking

Child trafficking is a complex multifaceted crime caused by many factors, not least because of socio-economic inequality, geopolitical destabilisation, and greed. There is a misconception that child trafficking is solely the movement of a child or young person from one country to another, however, trafficking can mean the movement of a child or young person from any location to another – such as from town to town.

Although definitions of human trafficking in general exist, child trafficking is defined as the 'recruitment, transportation, transfer, harbouring or receipt of a child, whether by force or not, by a third person or group, for different types of exploitation' (The Department of Health, Social Services, and Public Safety 2011: 4). Such exploitation may include:

- child sexual exploitation;
- forced marriage;
- forced labour (domestic, industrial, agricultural);
- criminal activity (drugs transportation, pickpocketing/burglary).

Many children are conned, persuaded, or even forced to leave their homes, as traffickers use grooming, coercion, or exploitative techniques to gain the trust of families or as a collection of debts. Paramedics form a group of healthcare staff that should be able to recognise signs of child trafficking (RCPCH 2014), given their position within the community and often as first HCP on scene. Signs include children and young people who:

- spend a lot of time doing household chores and have no time for play;
- are living apart from their family, in unregulated private foster care;
- are not sure which country, city, or town they are in;
- are unable or reluctant to give personal details;
- might not be registered with a school or a GP practice;
- have no access to their parents or guardians;
- are seen in inappropriate places such as brothels or factories;
- have injuries from workplace accidents;
- give a prepared story which is very similar to stories given by other children.

Child radicalisation and the Prevent Strategy

Much like child trafficking, child radicalisation is a complex and multifaceted safeguarding concern, and can itself be indicative of neglect and abuse. Radicalisation can be caused by many factors, including high unemployment, reactions to terror attacks, disillusion and disengagement from mainstream society, and grooming.

Signs of possible radicalisation include:

- change in friendship groups;
- converting to new religion (especially a change of appearance);
- new argumentative behaviour and unwillingness to listen to other points of view;
- expressions of sympathy or justification for extremist ideologies and groups.

Paramedics will encounter children and young people who may be vulnerable to being drawn into terrorism (violent and non-violent extremism) through their everyday practice (Home Office – Counter Terrorism 2016). HCPs such as paramedics and the organisations for whom they work have statutory responsibilities under the Counter-Terrorism and Security Act 2015 not only to identify those at risk from radicalisation, but also to refer them to appropriate agencies for the support they require.

The Prevent Strategy (2011), which has not been without its valid critics, aims to prevent people from being drawn into terrorism and ensure that they are given appropriate advice and support through working with sectors and institutions where there are risks of radicalisation that need addressing. Paramedics can complete a PREVENT referral through their normal safeguarding means and do not require proof, only a reasonable suspicion or concern.

MANAGEMENT OF SUSPECTED ABUSE AND NEGLECT

Adequate education is one of the most important elements of identification, management, and prevention of child maltreatment – and all ambulance services have statutory duties to ensure their staff are adequately trained in child protection. Paramedics need to approach their learning and development departments if they think they require more training and education, the lack of which is a significant barrier to child protection (RCPCH 2014). Box 11.6 offers indicators of child abuse and neglect.

Box II.6 Indicators of child abuse and neglect

Physical abuse

- Multiple unusually shaped bruises of different ages
- Bruises in hard-to-reach areas
- Withdrawal from physical contact
- Anxious when other children cry
- Fear of returning home/history of running away
- Reluctance to undress/attend Physical Education classes/swimming/ seeing the school nurse
- Aggressive towards others
- Kept at home by parents a lot
- Parents unable to proffer reasonable explanations for bruises/behaviour

Sexual abuse

- Bruising or scratching to genital areas, chest, abdomen, or neck
- Blood-stained clothing/underclothing
- Soreness and discomfort around mouth and in vaginal/anal areas causing pain and discomfort when walking or sitting
- Swollen or infected penis or vaginal discharge (consider sexually transmitted diseases, and repeated thrush/urinary infections)
- Child may display inappropriate sexual behaviour/knowledge for their age and development (may draw sexual organs)
- Cry hysterically when underclothing is removed
- Regress interpersonally and have low self-esteem (poor personal hygiene or bathe excessively)
- Nightmares, bed wetting, and insomnia
- Talk about a 'friend' being abused
- Become depressed
- Have large amounts of money or products of monetary value (presents) beyond their means (child sexual exploitation)

Emotional abuse

- Low self-esteem, lack of confidence, poor personal hygiene
- Extremes of aggression or passivity
- Self-harm
- Lying, stealing, and hoping to get caught (for additional attention)

- Poor social relationships/inability to have fun/inability to understand others' upset or sadness
- Inability to react rationally to making simple mistakes
- Poor language skills/developmental delay

Physical neglect

- Nappy rash/poor personal hygiene (urine smell, unbrushed hair)
- Underweight for their age (conversely can be morbidly obese)/lack of muscle tone
- Always hungry (stealing/scavenging food) – distended abdomen – gorging on food when offered
- Unwell often – no GP involvement
- Often late for school/nursery – unprepared for the day
- Under-dressed for the time of year/clothes do not fit
- Clingy to other parental figures
- Developmental delay/poor educational attainment

Emotional neglect

- Developmental delay/poor educational attainment
- Inability to express emotion normally
- Signs of stress/pressure
- Fear of new social situations/environments/unwilling to risk-take
- Lack of confidence/low self-esteem
- Parents may have uncaring/abrasive attitude
- Parents may have a lack of interest in child's landmarks, goals, and progress
- Parents may assume a passive responsibility or complete lack thereof (forgetting to collect child from school/sending a stranger)

(Whitnell 2012)

 Reflection: points to consider

You cannot rely on someone else completing a safeguarding referral. If you don't do it, no one will.

A further barrier to effective child protection for paramedics is a misconception that definitive proof of maltreatment is required before reporting or referral can occur (Brady 2018). It is the responsibility of the paramedic to document *possible* evidence of maltreatment, however, only reasonable grounds for suspicion, or 'serious levels of concern about the possibility of child maltreatment but no proof of it' (NICE 2013) are needed for a referral/report to be made to agencies such as:

- the police
- social services
- Prevent Strategy
- the general practitioner
- child/family health visitor

Paramedics are in a prime and unique position to do the following:

- Observe if a child's needs are being met.
- Observe interactions between children and carers.
- Observe if a child is being adequately safeguarded from harm in the home environment.
- Gather information on the home environment.
- Provide sufficient witness evidence to referring agencies (feelings, observations, concerns) (Whitnell 2012).

Best practice dictates that children and families should be made aware of any referral, and even asked for a permission for referral to be made; however, this is often not practical (or safe) in clinical practice – and the safety and welfare of the child must be the key consideration. Paramedics may share information against the will of a parent or guardian, or without consent from the child, when there is an overriding public interest in the disclosure, or when a young person does not have the maturity or understanding to decide about disclosure, or when disclosure is required by law (HM Government 2015a). Consideration needs to be given to when and how information is shared, as well as what is necessary, proportionate, and relevant to share – in an adequate, timely, and secure manner.

Trust between the paramedic and child cannot be underestimated, and the paramedic must treat the child/ren with dignity, respect and honesty. An allegation of abuse by a child is an important indicator and it is important to listen to what the child is saying. If a child's first language is not English, family members must not be used as interpreters in cases of suspected abuse. Care must be taken not to directly accuse the parents, as this can often cause difficulty in immediate communication, cooperation, and ultimately patient care and safety (Brown, Kumar and Millins 2016).

Paramedics often work alone but can gain support from their senior clinical advisor on call, their clinical support desk, the emergency social team – or a call can be placed to the nearest children's emergency department for advice (on a recorded line). The method of referral differs between different ambulance services and clinical commissioning areas, and can be made online, over the phone, or more recently via the electronic patient care record. If transporting a child, then the paramedics must make a verbal handover to the senior nurse in charge and document to whom they spoke – ensuring shared professional responsibility (Brown, Kumar and Millins 2016).

Various frameworks exist for health and social care practitioners, however, there is little specifically for paramedics to use to support their practice. Frameworks such as the Assessment Framework (HM Government 2015a) and the Graded Care Profile (NSPCC 2015) are useful sources of information for paramedics; however, most commonly it is high-quality training, access to adequate support 24/7, and easy-to-follow accessible processes that best support paramedics apostrophe everyday practice.

Read Case study 11.1 to reflect on the main points covered in this chapter.

Case study 11.1

You are called to the home of Angela – a 36-year-old female with abdominal pain. You enter Angela's home and find her house to have little furniture, with no visible food in the kitchen, and sections of carpet missing in the living room. Angela is clearly living on a very limited budget. As you assess Angela, you meet her 14-year-old daughter Grace who is keen to show you her brand new smartphone. Angela asks Grace where she got the new phone from, to which she replied, 'Oh, I found it when hanging out with my new friends.' Angela tells the paramedics that Grace and her friends have been hanging around with a group of males in their early twenties after school; she doesn't approve. Grace also appears to be wearing an expensive necklace. When asked where she got it from, she responds in a secretive and vague manner before leaving abruptly to go hang out with her new friends, despite Angela being in pain.

1 Is there a possible problem here?
2 What would you do immediately?
3 Would you record the event, and if so where?
4 Do you need permission to report your concerns?
5 From whom could you take further advice?

Having read Case study 11.1 and thought about questions 1–5, read the answers below in the reflection: points to consider box, to see if, on reflection, your thoughts and potential actions are similar:

Reflection: points to consider

1 Yes. Grace appears to have possessions which are beyond the financial ability of Angela to provide and appears to have an inappropriate friendship with a group of males with an unsuitable age gap. These are signs of possible *Child Sexual Exploitation (CSE)*.

2 Ask where Grace goes with these 'new' friends and call the duty social team to report your concerns. Consider also calling the police on 101 and reporting your concerns to the duty child protection officer.

3 Yes. Complete a child protection referral as normal, but remember that these can often take time to process, especially over the weekend, so speak to the duty social team as well.

4 It is usually best to speak to families before making a referral to include them in decision-making. You don't need permission to report concerns over CSE, however, which is covered under the Serious Crime Act 2015.

5 You can call your operational officer, clinical support desk, or duty social team to gain advice and support. Remember that you do not need proof to report your concerns. Share the decision with others by gaining advice.

CONCLUSION

Paramedics unarguably have a key role to play in child protection. Embedded within the community, called on in times of emergency, and having access to a child's home environment, paramedics have the chance to fundamentally change the lives of the children and young people with whom they come into contact.

Paramedics are no longer considered to be protocol-driven, stretcher-bearing ambulance drivers, but rather highly educated HCPs with a speciality in emergency and unscheduled community care. With this change in professional status comes a change in responsibility – and one which paramedics must continue to live up to.

From child sexual exploitation, FGM, trafficking, to children missing in education, child protection is a dynamic and ever-changing area of health and social care practice. It is up to both individual paramedics and the organisations for whom they work to ensure that training is adequate, support is effective and accessible, and learning takes place from mistakes. Paramedics legally, professionally, and morally have a duty of care, not necessarily to undertake in-depth investigations but rather to recognise, report, refer, and support children, young people, and families.

Chapter key points:

- Paramedics have an integral role to play in child protection.
- Paramedics are in a unique position within the community to identify those at risk.
- Paramedics are legally and professionally obligated to protect children and young people.
- HEIs need to ensure their students feel confident and competent in this area.
- Ambulance services need to ensure that their paramedics' training and support are adequate, effective, and accessible.

REFERENCES AND SUGGESTED READING

Brady, M. (2018) An investigation of the role of paramedics in child protection. PhD thesis. Swansea University.

Brown, S.N., Kumar, D. and Millins, M. (eds for JRCALC and AACE) (2016) *UK Ambulance Service Clinical Practice Guidelines*. Bridgwater: Class Professional Publishing.

CPS (2017) *Controlling or Coercive Behaviour in an Intimate or Family Relationship: Legal Guidance*. London: The Crown Prosecution Service.

DCSF (Department for Children Schools and Families) (2008) *Safeguarding Children in whom Illness is Fabricated or Induced*. London: DCSF.

Female Genital Mutilation Act (2003) London: The Stationery Office.

Forfar, J. (1984) Failure to thrive, in *Textbook of Paediatrics*, 3rd edn. Edinburgh: Churchill Livingstone.

Goddard, C. and Tucci, J. (2008) *Responding to Child Abuse and Neglect in Australia. A Joint Submission to the Australian Government Responding to Australia's Children. Safe and Well – A National Framework for Protecting Australia's Children*. Melbourne: Monash University.

Health and Care Professions Council (2014) *Standards of Proficiency. Paramedics*. London: HCPC.

Health and Care Professions Council (2016) *Paramedics. Standards of Conduct, Performance and Ethics*. London: HCPC.

Health Professions Council (2007) *Standards of Conduct, Performance and Ethics*. Consultation document. London: HPC.

HM Government (2003) *Every Child Matters*. London: The Stationery Office.

HM Government (2004) *Children Act*. London: The Stationery Office.

HM Government (2006) *Working Together to Safeguard Children 2006: A Guide to Inter-Agency Working to Safeguard and Promote the Welfare of Children*. London: The Stationery Office.

HM Government (2010) *Child Poverty Act*. London: The Stationery Office.

HM Government (2012) *The Munro Review of Child Protection Progress Report: Moving Towards a Child-Centred System*. London: The Stationery Office.

HM Government (2013) *Working Together to Safeguard Children 2013: A Guide to Inter-Agency Working to Safeguard and Promote the Welfare of Children*. London: The Stationery Office.

HM Government (2015a) *Information Sharing. Advice for Practitioners Providing Safeguarding Services to Children, Young People, Parents and Carers*. London: HM Government.

HM Government (2015b) *Serious Crime Act*. London: The Stationery Office. Available at: https://www.gov.uk/government/collections/serious-crime-bill (accessed 19 June 2017).

HM Government: Department for Education (2010) *Working Together to Safeguard Children 2010: A Guide to Inter-Agency Working to Safeguard and Promote the Welfare of Children*. London: The Stationery Office.

HM Government: Department for Education (2011) *Munro Review of Child Protection: Final Report – A Child-Centred System*. London: The Stationery Office.

HM Government: Department for Education (2015) *Working Together to Safeguard Children 2015: Statutory Guidance on Inter-Agency Working to Safeguard and Promote the Welfare of Children*. London: The Stationery Office.

Home Office (2016) *Mandatory Reporting of Female Genital Mutilation. Procedural Information*. London: Home Office.

Home Office: Counter-Terrorism (2011) *Prevent Strategy*. London: Home Office.

Home Office: Counter-Terrorism (2016) *Prevent Duty Guidance for Scotland and England and Wales*. London: Home Office.

House of Commons Home Affairs Committee (2014) *Female Genital Mutilation: The Case for a National Action Plan*. London: Her Majesty's Stationery Office.

Kirtley, P. (2013) *If You Shine a Light, You Will Probably Find It: Report of a Grass Roots Survey of Health Professionals with Regard to Their Experiences in Dealing with Child Sexual Exploitation.* Derby: NWG Network.

Munro, E. (2006) *Child Protection*. London: SAGE Publications Ltd.

NICE (National Institute of Clinical Excellence) (2013) *When to Suspect Child Maltreatment.* Manchester: National Institute of Clinical Excellence.

NSPCC (2015) *Graded Care Profile 2*. Available at: https://www.nspcc.org.uk/services-and-resources/services-for-children-and-families/graded-care-profile/ (accessed 30 December 2017).

NSPCC (2017a) *Signs, Symptoms and Effects of Child Abuse and Neglect*. NSPCC. Available at: https://www.nspcc.org.uk/preventing-abuse/signs-symptoms-effects/ (accessed 30 December 2017).

NSPCC (2017b) *Legislation, Policy and Guidance: Children Act 2004*. Available at: https://www.nspcc.org.uk/preventing-abuse/child-protection-system/england/legislation-policy-guidance/ (accessed 30 December 2017).

Peate, I. (2014) FGM: The role of front-line staff (Editorial). *Journal of Paramedic Practice*, 6(5): 221.

RCPCH (Royal College of Paediatrics and Child Health) (2002) *Fabricated or Induced Illness by Carers*. London: Royal College of Paediatrics and Child Health.

RCPCH (Royal College of Paediatrics and Child Health) (2014) *Safeguarding Children and Young People: Roles and Competences for Health Care Staff*. London: Royal College of Paediatrics and Child Health.

Richards, K. (2011) *Trends and Issues in Crime and Criminal Justice: Misperceptions About Child Sex Offenders*. Canberra: The Australian Institute of Criminology.

Shields, B., Wacogne, I. and Wright, C. (2012) Weight faltering and failure to thrive in infancy and early childhood. *BMJ*, 345: e5931.

Sibson, L. and Brain, L. (2009) Safeguarding children: role of health professionals. *Journal of Paramedic Practice*, 1(12): 493–500.

The Department of Health, Social Services and Public Safety and The Police Service for Northern Ireland (2011) *Working Arrangements for the Welfare and Safeguarding of Child Victims of Human Trafficking*. Belfast: The Department of Health, Social Services, and Public Safety.

UNFPA (United Nations Population Fund) (2017) Female genital mutilation (FGM): frequently asked questions. Available at: https://www.unfpa.org/resources/female-genital-mutilation-fgm-frequently-asked-questions#practice_origins

UNICEF (2005) The state of the world's children 2005: Childhood under threat. UNICEF. Available at: https://www.unicef.org/publications/index_24432.html

Whitnell, J. (2012) Safeguarding children. In A.Y. Blaber (ed.) *Foundations for Paramedic Practice: A Theoretical Perspective*, 2nd edn. Maidenhead: Open University Press, pp. 153–73.

WHO (2017a) *WHO Child maltreatment*. Available at: http://www.who.int/topics/child_abuse/en/ (accessed 19 June 2017).

WHO (2017b) *Classification of Female Genital Mutilation*. World Health Organisation. Available at: http://www.who.int/reproductivehealth/topics/fgm/overview/en/ (accessed 19 June 2017).

USEFUL WEBSITES

Childline: www.childline.org.uk

Children's Society: www.childrenssociety.org.uk

Department for Education: https://www.gov.uk/government/organisations/department-for-education

Department of Health: https://www.gov.uk/government/organisations/department-of-health

Families in Society journal: http://familiesinsocietyjournal.org/

Independent Safeguarding Authority: http://www.safeguardingmatters.co.uk/uk-safeguarding-approach/isa-barring/

Joseph Rowntree Foundation: www.jrf.org.uk

National Society for Prevention of Cruelty to Children (NSPCC): www.nspcc.org.uk

The Hideout – a Women's Aid created space for children and young people to understand more about domestic violence: http://thehideout.org.uk/

UK Government: www.gov.uk/collections/statistics-looked-after-children

UK Government: www.gov.uk/government/collections/statistics-children-in-need

Women's Aid (charity organisation): www.womensaid.org.uk

World Health Organisation for the United Kingdom: http://www.who.int/countries/gbr/en/

12

Public health from a paramedic perspective
Gemma Chapman and David Rea

In this chapter:

- Introduction
- Why is this relevant?
- Public health development
- Public Health Outcomes Framework
- Allied health professionals (paramedics) and public health
- Conclusion
- Chapter key points
- References and suggested reading
- Useful websites

INTRODUCTION

This chapter provides an introductory overview of how paramedics represent an integral role in the field of public health. With 6.6 million face-to-face interactions with the public throughout the United Kingdom (UK) during 2015–2016, paramedics have the opportunity to positively impact on and improve the health and well-being of individuals within our society. The ability to prevent injury and disease, prolong life and promote health through the organised efforts of society as a whole (Acheson 1988) is naturally becoming more demanding with the significant rise in life expectancy that brings multiple associated challenges. An increase in long-term and chronic conditions, including individuals suffering multiple co-morbidities, requires greater input from health and social care services, which, as a nation, are already working to capacity with stretched financial and physical resources. As a result and by the very nature of ambulance services providing a round-the-clock service, paramedics are more frequently faced with complex cases and incidents exacerbated by multiple underlying factors infringing on health and social care needs. Alternatively, they are also faced with a multitude of incidents where admission to emergency departments is not required and the ability to use and draw upon other services and resources is now becoming a central part of the paramedics' role. While needing to be confident and competent in the clinical skills and underpinning knowledge of the profession, student paramedics, as well as those qualified, also need to develop an understanding of what public health is, how it is portrayed throughout society and how the role of the paramedic can improve public health and aid in supporting the public to become healthier by reducing risk factors, which in turn will assist in preventing ill health and premature death.

WHY IS THIS RELEVANT?

In recent years, focus has been placed on health professionals providing a preventative approach to public health. Ambulance clinicians responding to the public's urgent and emergency care needs are frequently the first point of contact that someone has with the health and social care system. Additionally, unlike many other disciplines, paramedics provide a service that interacts with society across the whole life course not one specific population group, in a range of settings, most frequently their own home and at any given time. As such, this enables paramedics to develop a full and detailed picture of an individual's overall circumstances. This then identifies a range of opportunities whereby paramedics can draw upon other appropriate services that can positively support and assist individuals in improving their overall health. Additionally, the developing education and scope of practice of paramedics are encouraging detailed and focused patient examination of all bodily systems in both adults and children. In turn, this allows paramedics to identify causes for ill health and open doorways to services that can support individuals and aid in bringing about change, treatment and cure. A multitude of common underlying factors causing ill health exist, such as obesity, drug and substance misuse, alcohol binging, smoking, mental health, social factors (loneliness, isolation, poor housing), however, through widespread public health initiatives, and early recognition, the overall health and well-being of society can be improved.

Reflection: points to consider

Have you ever come away from an incident wishing you could have done more? Wondering what impact your actions may have? Or simply wondering if anything will change? Think of some prominent public health initiatives and campaigns and consider how your interactions with a patient may have been related to these and worked towards improving the health and well-being of our society.

PUBLIC HEALTH DEVELOPMENT

Historically, the notion of population health was known whereby individuals looked at incidences of illness and their relationship to social conditions and class. This identified that conditions such as peptic ulcers, rheumatic heart disease and juvenile rheumatism were more prevalent in those who were unemployed and in a lower social class. Over time into the late eighteenth century, this thought and debate developed further into the notion of 'diseases of civilisation'. Other epidemics of disease were being seen, such as gout and tuberculosis, however, those in the privileged classes were avoiding these illnesses and were exceeding average life expectancies, yet experiencing chronic and mental disease associated with luxury. Between 1832 and 1966, Great Britain was struck with four cholera epidemics as part of the pandemic outbreaks that were seen across the globe. Again, this affected the poor ill-defined middle classes. These developing relationships ultimately then posed the question of what the future was for the health of civilisation and how this would ultimately impact on the economic strength of the nation (Gilbert 2017).

It was also during the eighteenth century that the beginnings of democratisation and expanding commerce in Europe and America saw the introduction of a new rationalist and democratic agenda to see equality for all citizens to ensure protection from disease and positive health. However, this came at the same time as the first Industrial Revolution that saw high redundancy levels in rural communities and an increase in population size in urban industrial towns and locations. As a result, disease and ill health started to increase rapidly in these environments instead. Furthermore, many injuries were beginning to be seen in factories, at sea and in agriculture. This continued until protective legislation was introduced, such as the Factory Act of 1833 which aimed at improving the working conditions and health and well-being of those who worked in factories and mines. The nineteenth century saw the first public health and social epidemiology disciplinary school in France. Initially the same theories and thoughts applied, with wealth, sanitary facilities and employment all dividing the health outcomes of the population.

Edwin Chadwick first introduced the Public Health Act 1848 in England, his idea of improvement was to ensure clean water and sewage works be installed in cities, however, this went unnoticed and was completed when the Royal Sanitary Commission of 1869–1871 was reviewed. Many believe the reason for this going unnoticed was because the doctors of the time were unable to agree on the causes of cholera. John Snow in 1854 published his findings to suggest cholera was in fact conveyed by water. This was the beginning of epidemiology, proving that scientific knowledge is beneficial in the development of health and well-being development.

With no positive change being noted, yet significant disaster from disease evident in the years following the Industrial Revolution, it was only when political voices and independent organisations started to appear that significant health improvements started to be seen. By the first decade of the twentieth century, major British cities had started to become miniature welfare states. In the years following, the wealthier classes agreed to greater taxes on their wealth and property, which led to the investment in sanitary systems, paved and clean roads and health promotion services, such as food inspectors and education. These reforms started to show positive results by a reduction in ill health and injury. Continuing through the twenty-first century, democratic and industrialised nations started to apply the approach of the public health movement, seeing the benefits of tax-funded preventative health, educational and social services, which have continued to develop to today. Along with this, policy and practice are also developing. However, we are now frequently faced with dilemmas of compromising individuals' independence and choice, by admitting them to hospital instead of providing services at home due to the limited availability of these services at any specific time (Gilbert 2017).

Public health development never appears to be complete; while massive positive changes have been achieved by the work completed so far, new and developing challenges continue to emerge. Fire-related deaths caused as a result of smoking products have dropped by 15 per cent in the last decade following smoking cessation promotion, yet research is developing in areas such as globalisation and health, new infections and disease, and the impact of air quality as a result of pollution released in today's environment from vehicles and factories.

More recently, many continue to seek to define 'Public Health', with multiple definitions appearing in a Google search. In the main, a common theme continually shows, in that public health is seen as both an art and a science aiming broadly to support, manage and increase the health of the population to ensure the continuity of a sustainable society. Over the last two centuries, the public health movement has been more commonly seen as a means to measure the state of the population's health locally, nationally and internationally. It is heavily reliant upon the tax-funded and state-driven census systems providing the data and intelligence required to be able to make sense of the changes seen within public health. Dependent also on this data are the academic disciplines of public health, epidemiology and demography to be able to provide an analysis and understanding of the data collected to further understanding, research and development.

 Chapters 9 and 10 for relevant sociological theory and social issues.

Activity

Public health has developed into its own discipline, with health professionals compiling an annual calendar of campaigns, initiatives and events. Have a look at the campaigns in Box 12.1 and consider incidents you either attended or that you could attend where you could draw on these campaigns to promote public health and assist in improving the health and well-being of our society. Write down your ideas.

Box 12.1 Some public health initiatives

Dry January	Epilepsy Awareness Purple Day	Death Awareness Week	World Blood Donor Day
National Obesity Awareness Week	World Health Day	Mental Health Awareness Week	International Overdose Day
Sun Awareness Week	Action on Stroke Month	Diabetes Week	World Suicide Prevention Day
No Smoking Day	World Asthma Day	Carers Week	Movember: men's health awareness month
COPD Awareness month	National Stress Awareness Day	International Day for the Elimination of Violence Against Women	National Personal Safety Day

Now take a look at the following link to see what other national campaigns occur throughout the year: http://www.nhsemployers.org/your-workforce/retain-and-improve/staff-experience/health-work-and-wellbeing/sustaining-the-momentum/calendar-of-national-campaigns-2016

PUBLIC HEALTH OUTCOMES FRAMEWORK

Public Health England (PHE) developed the Public Health Outcomes Framework, identifying four overarching domains to improve public health as a whole. These are:

1 improving the wider determinants of health;
2 health improvement;
3 health protection;
4 healthcare: public health and preventing premature mortality.

Each domain discusses specific and targeted areas in society, identifying the rationale as to why they are significant and what data can be collected and used as measures to identify improvement through targeted work streams and initiatives.

While not all sections discussed within the PHE Outcomes Framework may appear specifically relevant to the paramedic profession, associations and relevancies can be made. This section discusses a broad overview of the links that can be made within the areas noted in each domain and how they are relevant to the paramedic profession.

Domain 1: Improving the wider determinants of health

This discusses the differences seen in life expectancy and healthy life expectancy between communities, looking at how long we live and how well we live. It is identified as a key high-level health inequality outcome that is core to the aims of the Department of Health. Paramedics work in both urban and rural environments, in areas of poverty and areas of affluence, paramedics attend many pre-hospital cardiac arrests, witnessing end of life frequently. Data for this outcome is collected through death registrations, while paramedics do not specifically register the deaths, pre-hospital cardiac arrests resulting in the recognition of life extinct will contribute towards this data collection. More specifically, multiple areas are discussed within the domain of improving the wider determinants of health. Emphasis is on life expectancy and a variety of reasons that influence this. With paramedics working within communities, a lot of incidents they attend and the information they gather will impact on this data collection and aid in the development of research in specific areas. Children in low-income families can be helped by the quality of information documented on the patient clinical record, when any child is attended within the community. Paramedics have the chance to see children in their natural family surroundings, and are privileged to document social circumstances, schooling, family networks, smoking in the home, diet – all of which provide a range of information that can impact on increasing children's health and well-being. Additionally, adults with long-term health conditions, learning disabilities and mental health conditions are individuals who are frequently seen by paramedics in a wide range of environments. While mainly non-time-critical events and requiring social support and guidance, paramedics have the opportunity to obtain and document a thorough history, identifying if these patients are in employment, absent from work, living independently or within the social care network, their contact with other allied health professionals and services. This information is passed on to public health initiatives and research to improve the health of society inadvertently through areas such as 'working well', developing structures to aid in the support given to individuals to remain in the work place when managing long-term and chronic conditions.

A more specific relationship can be seen between the impact paramedics can have from a public health perspective on those patients killed or seriously injured in road traffic collisions (RTCs). RTCs are an area of expertise for the emergency services (paramedics), yet are a major cause of preventable deaths and morbidity, especially within younger age groups. Significant evidence suggests many road traffic collisions are preventable and could be avoided if there was significant high-level education, awareness, infrastructure and vehicle safety. Multiple public health strategies and initiatives exist for road safety with the aim of reducing the mortality figures. For those accidents attended by paramedics where the outcome of the patient is not as negative, the chance to discuss and highlight road safety in collaboration with other emergency services is possible. Furthermore, paramedics can get involved with campaigns aimed at educating those young people at an optimum age of being legally old enough to obtain a driving licence, by presenting real-life stories, and this could have a positive impact on the next generation of licence holders.

Other areas of consideration discussed in domain 1 where paramedics have contact and can interact is domestic abuse, by considering and submitting Domestic Abuse, Stalking and Harassment (DASH) referrals, or the regional equivalent. This is an example of a public health initiative where paramedics can play a part in the wider healthcare professional network by reducing the incidences of domestic violence and supporting individuals affected to improve their health and well-being. Paramedics working in more urban environments interact with many individuals affected by homelessness, educating and signposting these people to services, hostels and centres where they can access healthcare and maintain and improve their general health.

 Chapter 11 for more details regarding child protection and **Chapter 13** about safeguarding adults.

Domain 2: Health improvement

Each of the points discussed can be influenced by paramedics taking the time to observe behaviour and gather a patient history, then using this information to work with multiple other services and healthcare providers, in addition to signposting individuals to various campaigns, allowing them to make positive individual choices to improve their overall health. Diet, smoking, self-harm, substance misuse are poignant examples of where paramedics can help educate individuals about lifestyle choices and the changes they can make to benefit them in the longer term. Signposting people to smoking cessation services, local leisure centres, groups such as Alcoholics Anonymous or arranging appointments with GPs or practice nurses are some examples of how this may be done.

Domain 3: Health protection

This is an area arguably less relevant to the work of paramedics. However, vaccination coverage is widely discussed and this is something paramedics can be open to discussing with patients if and when the need arises. Additionally, from an organisational perspective, having an approved sustainable development management plan to aid with the reduction in carbon emissions by 2050 will benefit the health of society by preventing premature mortality and improving ill health as a result.

Domain 4: Public health and preventing premature mortality

While cases of infant mortality are something no paramedic ever wants to attend, sadly these do occur and carefully detailed and thorough documentation can pay dividends to other services in understanding the reasons for this and supporting research into how these events can be avoided. Paramedics are increasingly being invited to attend child death review panels, and can work collaboratively with representatives from public health organisations and professionals to prevent future deaths.

Mortality rates from causes considered preventable include many causes of death where paramedics have been involved. The most common way that paramedics have a link to this is again through the thorough documentation they complete, including statements for coroners when required. This can enable others with a more focused approach in this area to be able to understand each situation as a whole and identify anything that might have been a contributory cause. Or identify an area that requires more attention in the future to prevent re-occurrence and this will ultimately aid in the overall improvement of a healthy society. Preventing Suicide in England (HM Government 2012) is a strategy to save lives. Paramedics are often called to people who have committed suicide. The inclusion of this within the Public Health Outcomes Framework (Public Health England 2016a) is to ensure all services are making sustained efforts to keep suicide rates below recently seen levels.

The full Department of Health document entitled *Improving Outcomes and Supporting Transparency* (2016) provides more detail on each of the domains and shows how each domain can be implemented within the paramedic's daily practice.

ALLIED HEALTH PROFESSIONALS (PARAMEDICS) AND PUBLIC HEALTH

The Allied Health Professionals Federations (AHPf) with Public Health England and each of the supporting colleges (College of Paramedics 2015) have produced a strategy, demonstrating a vision of how allied health professionals will work within the field of public health. The four overarching indicators are as discussed above and have led to AHPf identifying their four strategic goals (Allied Health Professionals Federation (2018):

1. Reducing service costs through prevention (via public health) and efficient treatment, thus improving outcomes for adult patients, including mental health.
2. To seek clarity on strategic planning, in light of student funding reforms, development of apprenticeships and student placement issues.
3. AHP leaders need to be represented in Sustainability and Transformations Partnerships (STPs).
4. For people who have health and social care needs to be met, a funding settlement requires agreement.

AHPf discuss how they foresee the achievement of each of these goals. The success of the goals identified above relies on ensuring public health is included in education, broadening the development of public health opportunities post graduating and in the workplace. Also working alongside organisations to develop methods of measuring the impact their profession is having on public health and how this can be evidenced. The emphasis is also on developing stronger relationships between AHPs and public health leaders; to continue the development of public health and share best practice within all healthcare disciplines. The overall aim is to improve patient outcomes.

However, what is expected of the paramedic profession and how does this affect the ambulance service specifically?

The AHPf strategy requires each of the professional bodies (College of Paramedics 2015) to ensure organisations within their own profession have implementation plans to embed this strategy. Within the ambulance services of the United Kingdom, the Association of Ambulance Chief Executives (AACE) and the College of Paramedics work together supporting each ambulance service Trust, providing and guiding them on the implementation and achievement of specific clinical quality indicators and development opportunities to ensure strategies such as this can be implemented. Current documented evidence suggests that over 80 per cent of the incidents (National Audit Office 2017) that paramedics attend are non-time-critical and the development of pathways allows paramedics to make a full assessment of the needs of each patient and engage in conversation to educate them on health advice and supply links to other services. Referring to the four domains of public health, examples of the contributions paramedics can specifically make are within areas such as falls prevention, infection control, early diagnosis and interventions. Early diagnosis and intervention can ultimately be seen in relation to conditions such as strokes, trauma patients and myocardial infarctions. There is increased emphasis within ambulance Trusts on getting those patients to the correct hospital and facility within that hospital in nationally agreed time frames, to receive definitive care and have the best chance of survival and healthy discharge. The volume of calls received for patients who have fallen makes up a large proportion of the ambulance services' work. Through re-attendance to an individual or from obtaining a thorough history and understanding in the time spent with them, especially with the older generations, recommendations and referrals to investigate conditions such as depression and dementia may also be identified. While some individuals do experience injury, there is also a high number of calls that are for 'assistance only' and 'non-injury'. As such, ambulance services can impact on falls prevention by offering advice within an individual's home to reduce risk, and can contact the falls referral teams to encourage health assessments and the introduction of aids in the home to reduce the likelihood of re-occurrence. Infection control is embedded in every AHP and correct procedures are practised, following set organisational policy. The lack of RIDDOR reportable diseases and infections and the reduction in sickness levels of infectious conditions prove positively that organisations are contributing to this example.

The AHPf have worked with organisations to identify how they foresee success being measured. Emphasis is placed on undergraduate programmes to ensure public health education is being delivered to students. Organisations must publish work evidencing their impact on two additional public health priorities and provide case studies showing how they impact on public health. Finally, AHPf require allied health professionals to recognise and agree that public health is part of their substantive role and should be delivered consistently throughout their practice.

The full strategy can be accessed at: http://www.ahpf.org.uk/files/AHP%20Public%20Health%20Strategy.pdf

Case study 12.1 provides a practical link between the public health theory discussed in this chapter and the potential application that a paramedic has the capability to implement with patients in their care.

Case study 12.1

You are working nights over a Bank Holiday payday weekend, the weather has been hot and sunny and performance is expected to be high. You receive an emergency call in the early hours of Saturday morning to the city centre to a patient collapsed outside a popular nightclub. On arrival you find a patient medically well with no injuries, however, vulnerable and intoxicated with no means of getting home.

Let us look at the burden of alcohol and think about what could be done from a public health perspective, considering initiatives and work already completed.

Facts

- Alcohol is the leading risk factor of ill health, early mortality and disability within the 15–49 age group and the fifth leading risk factor for ill health across all age groups.
- There has been a 4 per cent rise in licensed establishments with 210,000 licensed premises in England and Wales alone.
- There are over 1 million alcohol-related hospital admissions every year with specific alcohol-related mortality at 54.3 years, a cost to the NHS of £3 billion (Public Health England 2015b).
- The public health burden of alcohol can be seen through health, social and economic harms, tangible, direct and indirect costs, and intangible ones, such as pain and suffering, emotional distress.

Individual considerations and vulnerability factors

- The volume of alcohol consumed
- The frequency of drinking
- The quality of alcohol consumed
- Age
- Gender
- Familial factors
- Socio-economic status

Current campaigns and initiatives

- 'Drink responsibly'
- Dry January
- Drink Driving campaigns
- Drunk tanks

What could you do?

- Avoid unnecessary hospital admission.
- Contact friends or family who have not been drinking to take responsibility for the individual and collect them.
- Transport the individual to a 'drunk tank' to sober up and be monitored safely.
- Provide information regarding health and well-being related to alcohol.
- Educate and spread awareness of the risks associated with excessive alcohol consumption.

Chapter 1 for suggestions about communication strategies; **Chapter 4** for more about ethical and legal considerations; **Chapter 2** for reflection suggestions.

CONCLUSION

Having an awareness of the development of public health helps to build on the knowledge, understanding and practices of how paramedics today can positively influence the health of society. The education of paramedics now being degree-led offers the ideal opportunity to educate early and embed these practices and thought processes, while increasing the appetite for individuals to look deeper into the field of public health and lead their own learning into this area.

The collaboration of the Allied Health Professionals Federation in conjunction with Public Health England is an integral point in the history of the public health discipline, and is included and encouraged within each profession to ultimately increase the health and well-being of our society as a whole.

Chapter key points:

- The development of the public health discipline was discussed.
- Education about public health is paramount to the practice of undergraduate paramedics.
- The development of public health within allied health professions is emphasised.
- The chapter provides a foundational overview of the more detailed public health documents, policies and strategies with reference to a broad array of literature that can be accessed for more specific detail.

REFERENCES AND SUGGESTED READING

Acheson, D (1988) *Public Health in England: The Report of the Committee of Inquiry into the Future Development of the Public Health Function*. London: HMSO.

Allied Health Professionals Federation (AHPf) (2018) *Allied Health Professionals Federation Current Main Objectives*. Available at: http://www.ahpf.org.uk/ (accessed 27 February 2018).

Association of Ambulance Chief Executives (2014) *Future National Clinical Priorities for Ambulance Services in England*. Available at: http://aace.org.uk/wp-content/uploads/2014/05/Future-national-clinical-priorities-for-ambulance-services-in-England-FINAL-2.pdf

College of Paramedics (2015) *Allied Health Professionals (AHPs) in Public Health Reports*. Available at: https://www.collegeofparamedics.co.uk/news/allied-health-professionals-ahps-in-public-health-reports

Department of Health (2016) *Improving Outcomes and Supporting Transparency Part 2: Summary Technical Specifications of Public Health Indicators*. Available at: https://www.gov.uk/government/uploads/system/uploads/attachment_data/file/545605/PHOF_Part_2.pdf

Faculty of Public Health (2010) *The UK's Faculty of Public Health: Working to Improve the Public's Health*. Available at: http://www.fph.org.uk/what_is_public_health (accessed 17 December 2017).

Fenton, K. and Hindle, L. (2017) *Ambulance Services on Board to Promote Public Health*. London: Public Health England.

Gilbert, P. (2017) *On Cholera in Nineteenth-Century England*. Available at: http://www.branchcollective.org/?ps_articles=pamela-k-gilbert-on-cholera-in-nineteenth-century-england

HM Government (2012) *Preventing Suicide in England: A Cross-Government Outcomes Strategy to Save Lives*. Available at: https://www.gov.uk/government/uploads/system/uploads/attachment_data/file/430720/Preventing-Suicide-.pdf (accessed 17 December 2017).

National Audit Office (2017) *NHS Ambulance Services*. Available at: https://www.nao.org.uk/wp-content/uploads/2017/01/NHS-Ambulance-Services.pdf (accessed 17 December 2017).

NHS Employers (2017) *Calendar of National Campaigns 2016/17*. Available at: http://www.nhsemployers.org/your-workforce/retain-and-improve/staff-experience/health-work-and-wellbeing/sustaining-the-momentum/calendar-of-national-campaigns-2016 (accessed 17 December 2017).

Public Health England (2015) *A Strategy to Develop the Capacity, Impact and Profile of Allied Health Professionals in Public Health 2015–2018*. Available at: http://www.ahpf.org.uk/files/AHP%20Public%20Health%20Strategy.pdf (accessed 17 December 2017).

Public Health England (2016a) *Strategic Plan for the Next Four Years: Better Outcomes by 2020*. Available at: https://www.gov.uk/government/uploads/system/uploads/attachment_data/file/516985/PHE_Strategic_plan_2016.pdf (accessed 17 December 2017).

Public Health England (2016b) *The Public Health Burden of Alcohol and the Effectiveness and Cost-Effectiveness of Alcohol Control Policies*. Available at: https://www.gov.uk/government/uploads/system/uploads/attachment_data/file/583047/alcohol_public_health_burden_evidence_review.pdf (accessed 17 December 2017).

Safe Lives (2017) *Safe Lives: Ending Domestic Abuse*. Available at: http://www.safelives.org.uk/about-us (accessed 1 December 2017).

WHO (2017) *Public Health Services*. Available at: http://www.euro.who.int/en/health-topics/Health-systems/public-health-services (accessed 17 December 2017).

USEFUL WEBSITES

Allied Health Professionals Federation: http://www.ahpf.org.uk

Department of Health: https://www.gov.uk/government/organisations/department-of-health

Faculty of Public Health: http://www.fph.org.uk
HSC Public Health Agency: http://www.publichealth.hscni.net
Public Health England: https://www.gov.uk/government/organisations/public-health-england
Royal Society for Public Health: https://www.rsph.org.uk
Safe Lives: http://www.safelives.org.uk/about-us
World Health Organisation: http://www.euro.who.int/en/health-topics/Health-systems/public-health-services

13

Safeguarding adults
Dave Blain

In this chapter:

- Introduction
- Why is this relevant?
- Legislation and guidance
- What are abuse and neglect?
- Types of abuse
- Handling suspected abuse/neglect and raising concerns
- Conclusion
- References and suggested reading
- Useful websites

INTRODUCTION

This chapter relates to people aged 18 years of age or over. The term 'safeguarding adults' possibly means many things to healthcare professionals. Ideally this concept should mean that an adult should be free from abuse and neglect, and to be able to live safely without the risk or threat of abuse and neglect. This area of work can provide a challenging dichotomy for healthcare professionals as adults with 'capacity' will sometimes make unwise decisions regarding their own safety. Often they place themselves at risk of abuse and neglect, without consideration for the advice and support offered by the attending healthcare professionals. Schwappach (2010: 119) suggests that 'Although evidence demonstrates patients can have a positive attitude to being involved in making decisions about their own safety, involvement in these processes varies.' There are many social, physical and psychological factors that affect vulnerability and the context in which these factors are based. To merely term someone as vulnerable requires very careful consideration as there are many types of vulnerability that healthcare professionals will observe and experience during their roles.

Regardless of what kind of environment paramedics find themselves working in, safeguarding adults awareness and training should be a fundamental element of all induction and ongoing educational processes. There has been far greater focus historically on ensuring protective legislation is in place to protect children, especially via the Children Act 1989/2004. The Care Act gained royal assent in 2014 and the subsequently published guidance includes updated references to safeguarding adults and is beginning to redress the balance between safeguarding children and safeguarding adults.

 Chapter 11 for safeguarding children's well-being.

This chapter will provide the essential knowledge to enable paramedics to practise with a suitable level of responsibility and routine enquiry when appropriate and necessary. Paramedics and healthcare professionals of all grades and roles must consider the Care Act 2014 as essential reading to maintain currency of their knowledge on safeguarding adults.

WHY IS THIS RELEVANT?

Safeguarding adult issues may be highlighted at any time by paramedics both in a professional capacity and via personal non-work exposure to neglect and abuse. Issues may be identified during call handling, attendance at 999 and urgent calls, or primary care consultations, for example. Safeguarding adults issues may also be identified through single or integrated governance processes such as frequent caller audits, risk reporting processes, legal requests or clinical audits.

Paramedics are sometimes in a very privileged and unique position to identify safeguarding adult issues due to the nature of working in the out-of-hospital emergency care setting. These situations can dictate that sometimes paramedics are the only professionals who enter the premises or speak to victims of abuse and neglect. 'What don't I know about this patient' should be considered at the same level as the available information that informs any treatment regime or care pathway for health professionals.

The Joint Royal Colleges Ambulance Liaison Committee (Brown, Kumar and Millins 2016: 24) suggests, 'The trainee and named supervisor must be aware of their professional obligation, under the duty of candour, in particular the duty to report incidents of harm or potential harm.'

Any concerns about or suspicion of abuse and neglect of adults must be addressed by either sharing information with the police or social care, or if paramedics are unsure of how to respond to circumstances, an initial discussion should take place with more senior colleagues in their own organisation. There are many other internal and external routes that are available to raise concerns or access help and support for victims of poor care that perhaps does not reach the threshold of abuse and neglect for safeguarding processes. Consideration of risk reporting mechanisms, NHS Serious Incident

(SI) processes or complaints procedures also offers health professionals other options in ensuring the safety of patients. It is often very difficult to distinguish between wilful neglect or ill treatment or basically not doing what should be done and doing what should not be done. As healthcare professionals experience such issues, clear legislation and guidance are available to address these breaches in patient care. The College of Paramedics (CoP) further supports this and requires registrants to be aware that they have a professional obligation, under the duty of candour, to report incidents of harm or potential harm (CoP 2017: 35–6).

As well as being involved in cases of abuse and neglect by people unknown to professionals, there may be occasions when allegations or observations of abuse or neglect involve the professionals working alongside paramedics. This would understandably be a real challenge and potentially be a difficult situation to deal with, but ultimately the responsibility to report these cases falls within the role of a registered professional.

Caroline (2014) acknowledges that having an understanding of why certain abuse and neglect issues evolve will be beneficial to the paramedic who is caring for the patient and family. To think that human beings abuse and neglect each other in such ways may be distressing or disturbing for healthcare professionals, regardless of their role and function in the sector and maybe was not considered at the beginning of a paramedic's career. This provides a timely reminder about personal resilience and seeking self-help, as safeguarding issues may be immediately upsetting or emotionally corrosive over time. Involvement in incidents causing such distress must be acknowledged by individuals and organisations, prompting them to seek and provide welfare and support for all involved. Hopefully paramedics can recognise when high levels of physiological stimulation of their own sympathetic nervous system are apparent and manage the situation accordingly with coping skills. This may even be applied to such events as legal hearings or other anxiety-causing court appearances regarding incidents of a safeguarding nature.

Paramedics also have patient safety responsibilities that may overlap with safeguarding concerns and systems. These are also referenced within current professional registration and guidance from the Health Care Professions Council (HCPC).

LEGISLATION AND GUIDANCE

Although paramedic practice is governed by many acts of legislation and national guidance, the main documents impacting on safeguarding adult processes are:

- The Care Act 2015
- The Mental Capacity Act 2005
- The Mental Capacity Act Code of Practice 2005
- The Mental Health Act 2007
- The Modern Slavery Act 2015
- The Counter-Terrorism and Security Act 2015.

This is not an exhaustive list but captures the main elements of legislation currently influencing adult safeguarding practice.

The Care Act 2014

The Care Act 2014 supersedes previous safeguarding adult guidance referenced in 'No Secrets' (2000) and establishes a clear legal framework for how local authorities and other partner agencies should work collaboratively to protect adults at risk of or suffering from abuse or neglect. The Care Act (2014) also stated that each area must establish a multi-agency Safeguarding Adult Board (SAB) with representation from the local authority, clinical commissioning group and the police service. Other partners are also invited as per each local SAB arrangement. NHS organisations and private health providers have safeguarding leads who will be aware of how to raise concerns with local SAB processes in each area.

The Act established six principles for safeguarding adults explained in Box 13.1.

Box 13.1 The six principles for adult safeguarding

1   *Accountability – Accountability and transparency in delivering safeguarding.* For paramedics, this emphasises the requirement to adhere to current clinical guidelines and ensure that actions are commensurate with professional registration.
2   *Empowerment – People being supported and encouraged to make their own decisions and provide informed consent.* Paramedics must implement the practice of making safeguarding personal (MSP) at all times. It is essential that paramedics assess and record time-specific mental capacity status as part of all assessments and treatment regimes with consent status fully documented. The Mental Capacity Act Code of Practice (2007: 15) suggests, 'The Act also states that people must be given all appropriate help and support to enable them to make their own decisions or to maximise their participation in any decision-making process.'
3   *Partnership – Local solutions through services working with their communities.* Paramedics must share their concerns with local partner agencies and professionals to address and resolve any safeguarding adult issues that are identified or suspected. This may be a simple telephone call to share information about a 999 call, or escalation of concerns about a patient or professional.

   Communities also have a part to play in preventing, detecting and reporting neglect and abuse. As practitioners who predominantly spend the majority of duty within the community, paramedics hold a vast amount of knowledge about the community in which they work and the people who live in that community. Concerns could be shared with a Community Safety Partnership (CSP), for example, to consider and address the issues.

---

4   *Prevention – It is better to take action before harm occurs.* Paramedics and the organisations they work for also possess information regarding individuals and addresses that highlight cause for concern. This may be through high volumes of calls, flags placed on addresses for various reasons and repeated non-conveyance following 999 calls, for example. A Serious Case Review (SCR) by the Cornwall Adult Protection Committee in 2007, following the death of Steven Hoskin, provides an example of missed opportunities that ambulance staff did not take to raise concerns of a safeguarding nature. A large proportion of information is available through ambulance Emergency Operation Centres (EOC) and can be accessed by paramedics who may have suspicions following involvement with such issues. Early help by paramedics in preventing further escalation and abuse may be the only opportunity that any professional has to intervene and prevent abuse and neglect continuing.

5   *Proportionality – The least intrusive response appropriate to the risk presented.* It is essential that paramedics adhere to guidance regarding dignity and respect values. Enquiring exactly what vulnerable individuals would like to happen during and following contact with paramedics takes primacy over attempts to make a patient fit an organisation's processes. When faced with safeguarding adult challenges, it is important that paramedics consider all the options that must also include what the patient wants to happen and their desired outcomes, as within MSP guidance within the Care Act 2014. Patients must be given control of how they want to live and be supported to make safe choices.

6   *Protection – Support and representation for those in greatest need.* It is essential that paramedics act swiftly to protect vulnerable individuals when abuse and neglect are clearly identified. This may even dictate that the attendance of the local constabulary is requested so that police protecting vulnerable people units (PVPU) receive early information and their engagement is immediate. The HCPC guidance (2016: 8) for registrants suggests that, 'You must report any concerns about the safety or well-being of service users promptly and appropriately.'

Paramedics are often found in very challenging safeguarding situations especially when a differential diagnosis is required between abuse, neglect or poor standards of care, to dictate decision-making. These situations are often very complex with paramedics sometimes only in possession of minute medical histories and social backgrounds of the people they are dealing with. Paramedics must not deal in isolation when involved in such cases and must consider which other agencies or professionals may be involved and are available to help and support actions and decision-making processes. Understandably this is a real challenge for everyone at certain times of the day, but intelligence gathering can start with further information from the EOC historical data or clinical notes, where held.

WHAT ARE ABUSE AND NEGLECT?

The Care Act 2014 provides the following description of when safeguarding duties apply to an adult who:

- has need of care and support (whether or not the local authority is meeting any of those needs); and
- is experiencing, or at risk of, abuse or neglect; and
- as a result of those care and support needs is unable to protect themselves from either the risk of, or the experience of, abuse or neglect.

The Association of Directors of Adult Social Services (ADASS) also offers the following definition: 'Abuse is the violation of an individual's human or civil rights by a person or persons' (ADASS 2005: 4). As the paramedic role progresses further into urgent and unscheduled care rather than complete focus on emergency care, consideration must be given to implementation of these principles during all episodes of patient contact, whether face-to-face or as part of call handling. Patients may have care and support needs at all times by definition, however, all of the three above descriptors must be met prior to concerns being raised with safeguarding adult teams within local authorities. Even when all three are not met, it does not negate the requirement for provider agencies to maintain high standards of care or investigate any concerns that professionals have. When paramedics are unsure, then a conversation must take place with senior colleagues, the organisation's safeguarding lead or local authority safeguarding staff working in local safeguarding hubs.

TYPES OF ABUSE

Incidents of abuse and neglect may be singular or historically repeated over a long period of time. The abuse may also affect only one person or groups of people. Such examples may affect those individuals living in a care setting where there is evidence of organisational abuse and neglect. The cases such as those revealed following investigations in the Winterbourne View abuse scandal that highlighted both poor standards of care and deliberate wilful neglect, resulted in six members of staff receiving custodial sentences for abuse and neglect of vulnerable individuals. In concluding, Flynn (2012: 143) stated: 'Although person-centred care, participation and empowerment characterise national policy priorities, these were alien to the experiences of Winterbourne View Hospital patients and their families. Their silencing was scandalous.'

Other large-scale safeguarding investigations have also highlighted that sometimes one perpetrator is responsible for multiple acts of abuse and neglect, as seen in the case of Dr Harold Shipman, who killed at least 215 patients over a 24-year period. The Shipman Inquiry (HM Government 2002: 200) into the deaths of the patients killed concluded:

> It is deeply disturbing that Shipman's killing of his patients did not arouse suspicion for so many years. The systems which should have safeguarded his patients against his misconduct, or at least detected misconduct when it occurred, failed to operate satisfactorily.

Paramedics must remain vigilant and raise concerns whatever the environment or situation is when suspecting or witnessing abuse and neglect of adults. The small piece of information that paramedics hold may trigger reviews of all sizes and nature, ranging from low-level risk reports to full national inquiries. It is essential that paramedics are familiar with local inter-agency processes and feel confident to raise concerns when the need arises.

Within the Care Act (2014), one of the local SAB's functions is that they are required to conduct Safeguarding Adult Reviews (SAR) as part of learning lessons to improve practice and working together to protect vulnerable individuals. The process is not to develop a blame culture or administer punitive sanctions against individuals or organisations. Very often the employing organisations of paramedics are represented at SAR panels in order to participate in the process as part of creating strong learning partnerships. This engagement enables the fostering of a positive learning culture, and recommendations for paramedics and their organisation may be the result of such reviews. These may be wide-ranging and include review of policies, updating of training resources and improving information-sharing processes as examples.

Discriminatory abuse

Discriminatory abuse may include any forms of bullying, harassment, derogatory remarks or similar due to any of the current nine protected characteristics within the Equality Act 2010. This type of abuse may also overlap with hate incidents and hate crimes which are reportable to the local constabulary, either via 101 or 999 services. There is later reference in the chapter to acts of extremism, but some hate incidents may include elements of extremist behaviour that impacts on an individual's safety and well-being.

Domestic abuse

Domestic abuse is pervasive to all cultures, communities and social backgrounds in our society. The Domestic Violence, Crime and Victims Act 2004 definition of domestic abuse was changed in the 2012 amendment to also include vulnerable adult references. The domestic abuse definition, adapted from the Care Act (HM Government 2014) includes:

- Any incident or pattern of incidents of controlling, coercive or threatening behaviour, violence or abuse . . . by someone who is or has been an intimate partner or family member regardless of gender or sexuality.
- Includes: psychological, physical, sexual, financial, emotional abuse; so-called 'honour'-based violence; Female Genital Mutilation; forced marriage.
- Age range extended down to 16.

Currently the Office for National Statistics (ONS) (2015) reported that there are circa 2.1 million cases of domestic abuse reported in England and Wales each year. The statistics suggest that 1.4 million of these are against females and 700,000 against males. The perpetration of domestic abuse affects all age groups, and paramedics must always consider the impact on the whole family when dealing with such incidents. Please 'THINK FAMILY' to ensure that all concerns are included as part of dynamic risk assessments and ongoing care plans for patients calling paramedics for help and support. This also includes carers, relatives and other household members who may be living in the residence. Consider if children are living at the address and what the risk and impact of the abuse is doing to them, what is it like for them to live in this house?

 Chapter 11 to read more on the subject of domestic violence.

Fairly recent research is suggesting that vulnerable older people are also being subjected to domestic abuse and violence in the same way as younger generations. Some of the statistics provided by Safe Lives (2016) reported the following;

- Victims aged 61+ are much more likely to experience abuse from an adult family member than those 60 and under.

  61+ years old   ≤ 60 years old
  44%   6%

- Victims aged 61+ are much more likely to experience abuse from a current intimate partner than those 60 and under.

  61+ years old   ≤ 60 years old
  40%   28%

- Older victims are less likely to attempt to leave their perpetrator in the year before accessing help.

  61+ years old   ≤ 60 years old
  27%   68%

- Older victims are more likely to be living with the perpetrator after getting support.

  61+ years old   ≤ 60 years old
  32%   9%

- Older victims are significantly more likely to have a disability – for a third, this is physical (34%).

61+ years old   **≤ 60 years old**

48%   13%

Adapted from Safe Lives (2016).

When paramedics witness or receive disclosures regarding domestic abuse, then these concerns must be documented and reported via current arrangements. It may be also necessary to involve the local constabulary in the incident even if the victim does not want to press charges, then a victimless prosecution can still be considered and pursued by the criminal justice system.

Financial or material abuse

There are many methods that perpetrators of financial or material abuse will use to access money and/or possessions. These may range from simple opportunistic thefts to large multi-million pound internet-based scams. Paramedics may be tasked to attend victims of assault and robbery where further disclosures of ongoing financial abuse are shared by the vulnerable individual. These allegations must be taken seriously and may also involve close family and relatives. There may also be disclosures that suspicion or allegations are aimed at other professionals or carers working with the victim. These issues must be raised immediately that should include referral to professional registration bodies where necessary and appropriate. Although not always regarding money and possessions, financial abuse could also be related to properties, inheritance, wills and lasting power of attorney (LPA) arrangements.

Evidence of such abuse may potentially be suggested by some of the following indicators;

- Poor living conditions as unable to invest in maintenance and repairs.
- Poor self-care as lack of money to purchase new clothes and toiletries.
- Accruement of bills as unable to pay utilities, etc.
- Cold and poorly heated properties.
- Unable to locate debit/credit cards or money.
- Unusual activity and withdrawals from bank accounts.
- Unknown callers to the address.
- Changes to financial documents such as wills and LPA.
- Frequent telephone calls from unknown persons.
- Lack of food and drink in the home leading to weight loss.

Modern-day slavery

Modern-day slavery is an illegal trade where humans are treated like commodities being bought and sold for large amounts of money. Current government statistics predict there are currently between 10,000–13,000 victims of modern slavery in the UK. Paramedics at any time may find themselves involved in cases of modern-day slavery and must be equipped to recognise indicators, how to raise concerns and what services can be offered to such victims. The Modern Slavery Act published in 2015 provides clear information on offences, prevention orders, enforcements and protection of victims. The Act specifically addresses the current challenges faced to interrupt and end trafficking and slavery in the UK.

Modern slavery is an umbrella term that includes human trafficking, forced or compulsory labour, and domestic servitude. Human trafficking has three elements:

- The act – what is done, for example, recruitment, harbouring or transportation of a person/people.
- The means – how it is done, for example, threat of force, coercion or abduction of a person/people. N.B. For a child under 18 years of age there does not need to be the element of means present due to child protection legislation.
- The purpose – why it is done, for example, sexual exploitation.

Slavery, servitude, forced or compulsory labour has two elements:

- The means – *how* it is done
- The purpose – *why* it is done
- N.B. For a child under 18 years of age, only the purpose needs to be present.

There are currently four main types of slavery recognised by agencies and these are organ harvesting, sexual exploitation, forced labour and domestic servitude. Organ harvesting is particularly concerning as medical/clinical professionals potentially would have to be involved in any surgical procedures either directly or in an advisory capacity.

Paramedics must be aware of the local arrangements to report and support potential victims of modern slavery. Currently, any concerns regarding victims of modern slavery must be reported by paramedics via the National Referral Mechanism (NRM) process. The NRM was first established in 2009 to support victims of trafficking, but was extended in 2015 with the introduction of the Modern Slavery Act. To access the NRM, concerns must be raised with one of the agencies recognised as a first responder in the process. The current list of first responders can be seen in Box 13.2.

Once completed by the first responder agencies (see Box 13.2), the NRM referral form is then forwarded to one of the current Competent Authorities (CAs) for consideration. The CAs currently are the NCA's Modern Slavery Human Trafficking Unit (MSHTU) and the Home Office Visas and Immigration (UKVI) team. If accepted into the NRM process, a victim is granted a 45-day period of reflection, recovery and support. Decisions will be made as to whether the individuals are victims of trafficking or modern slavery. Support and information regarding the NRM process are available at: http://www.nationalcrimea-gency.gov.uk/about-us/what-we-do/specialist-capabilities/uk-human-trafficking-centre/national-referral-mechanism.

Box 13.2 List of first responders

- National Crime Agency (NCA)
- Police forces
- UK Border Force
- Home Office Immigration and Visas
- Gangmasters Licensing Authority
- Local Authorities
- Health and Social Care Trusts (Northern Ireland)
- Salvation Army
- Poppy Project
- Migrant Help
- Medaille Trust
- Kalayaan
- Barnardos
- Unseen
- TARA Project (Scotland)
- NSPCC (CTAC)

In 2017, the NCA recorded data suggests a steady increase each year of referrals that identifies potential victims of modern slavery, see Table 13.1.

The data in 2016 demonstrates there was one referral relating to organ harvesting, 429 relating to domestic servitude, 487 referrals were unknown or could not be classified, 1313 were for sexual exploitation and 1575 were for labour exploitation (Figure 13.1).

The NCA also provides a breakdown of nationalities of victims of modern slavery in the UK. Figure 13.2 identifies the top five nationalities reported in 2016. It is interesting to note that the UK was the third highest nationality in the collected data.

Table 13.1 NRM referrals, 2013–2016

Year	NRM referrals
2013	1746
2014	2340
2015	3266
2016	3805

Source: National Crime Agency (2017).

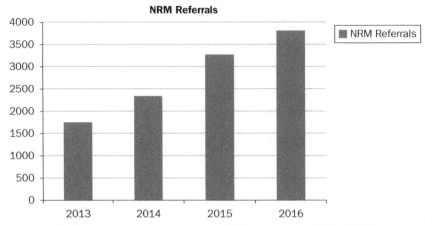

Figure 13.1 Visual presentation of NRM referrals, 2013–2016

Source: National Crime Agency (2017).

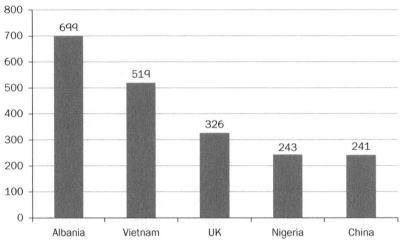

Figure 13.2 Top 5 nationalities of slavery in the UK, 2016

Source: National Crime Agency (2017).

There are some general indicators that victims of modern slavery may display during contact with paramedics, and vigilance is key in noticing these. Some things to look out for are:

- Fear of police/authorities.
- Fear of the trafficker and belief that their lives or family members' lives are at risk.
- Signs of physical and psychological trauma.
- Limited freedom of movement.

- Someone else has possession of their passport/ID.
- Unaware they are victims of trafficking.
- Seem to be in debt to someone.
- Total reliance on someone accompanying the victim to translate everything.

Victims may be living in cramped and squalid conditions that paramedics often observe when entering houses and residences. There may be multiple occupants living at the address with poor or no English spoken.

Currently many areas of the UK are establishing multi-agency modern slavery partnerships that raise awareness and provide training for professionals. Paramedics must be aware of the local arrangements to report and support potential victims of modern slavery. NRM forms are available to download from https://www.gov.uk/government/publications/human-trafficking-victims-referral-and-assessment-forms

Neglect and acts of omission

It is sometimes a real challenge for professionals to decide what is neglect and what is poor standards of care. It is essential that such cases are discussed with other professionals engaged in the care of individuals or groups of people when paramedics have such concerns. The opinions of professionals may also vary, leading to multi-agency safeguarding meetings called strategy meetings or case conferences. Paramedics should be familiar with any local safeguarding escalation procedures that exist that may address complex cases and incidents.

Organisational abuse

Paramedics are very familiar working in the environment of out-of-hospital care and therefore are ideally placed to witness or raise suspicions of abuse and neglect in an organisational setting. These may be nursing, care or residential homes of disparate provision, with varying standards of care offered to service users and residents. The events may be singular in nature or a series of incidents of ongoing poor care or ill treatment.

This issue may also be prevalent in a hospital or other clinical settings. Factors to consider may be poor clinical practice, lack of procedures, paucity of staff training, no safe staffing levels or incorrect placements of residents. These issues are often very complex but paramedics who have such concerns must consider the appropriate route for raising these issues. If not through the safeguarding route, then consideration must be given to other processes such as risk reporting, Care Quality Commission (CQC), local authority contracts and commissioning teams or Clinical Commissioning Groups (CCG) safeguarding leads for discussions about those concerns. Organisational safeguarding leads will be able to advise on these processes.

Physical abuse

This type of abuse considers anything physical that is done to an individual that may cause actual or potential harm such as punching, kicking, slapping, biting, scratching or beating with objects as examples.

It must also be known that this type of abuse also includes the use of inappropriate and excessive restraint and intentional incorrect administration of medication.

Psychological abuse

Previously known as emotional abuse, this issue has been extended to capture many of the other acts perpetrated against adults with care and support needs who are at risk of abuse and neglect. These may include:

- forced isolation and threat of abandonment;
- deprivation of support and lack of contact;
- intimidation through fear leading to emotional abuse;
- persistent embarrassment and humiliation that may be face-to-face or via social media;
- controlling or coercive behaviour aimed at disempowering and undermining an individual;
- threats of physical violence;
- imposing a false sense of fear of what authorities and organisations will do if not compliant with requests.

 Chapter 11 to compare the similarities and differences between safeguarding children and adults.

Self-neglect

Self-neglect is nothing new for paramedics to witness or hear during incidents, telephone calls or consultations. However, the Care Act now recognises this as a type of abuse and neglect. This is potentially a huge area of concern for paramedics when visiting homes and houses and consulting with patients.

A starting point may be the environment in which a patient may be living when paramedics are attending 999 calls. Some factors to consider:

- external state of the property including cluttered gardens,
- poor security;
- lack of locks on doors and windows;
- dangerous animals;
- poor state of repair to the property.

Consider the internal environment of the property and be empathetic to what is it like for the people living there. Hoarding is now also referenced in the Care Act as a type of self-neglect.

Chapter 8 to read more about the issue of hoarding.

Fire and Rescue Services (FRS) nationally have cluttering tools that can be used to assess the risk from the possessions and rubbish in the property. Paramedics may consider contacting their local FRS and share information about such risks if the resident consents to this. Paramedics may also consider a discussion with the local authority environmental health team, who also possess legislative powers to assist in such situations. Look out for some indicators such as:

- Signs of hoarding?
- Cluttering that may be considered a fire risk?
- Signs of vermin and infestation?
- Unsafe or out-of-date utility fittings?
- Any evidence to suggest the resident is a victim of hate crime/incidents?
- Sanitation and drainage systems effective and working?
- Can the property be secured when you leave?

Self-neglect also includes an individual who fails to self-care by keeping clean and looking after themselves. Paramedics will observe such things during face-to-face 999 calls and lack of poor hygiene will be evident for all the senses to detect! Please consider what other agencies or professionals may be or are already involved in the care and support of the patient and who else could help. Also consider if there are any multi-agency procedures in place locally between partner agencies for such cases.

Sexual abuse

Sexual abuse may occur in combination with some of the afore-mentioned references especially linked with modern slavery and domestic abuse and paramedics may find these situations extremely distressing. Sexual abuse may take many forms and have a significant psychological and physical impact on individuals. Paramedics must be patient, understanding and provide a cathartic opportunity for victims to tell their story when appropriate.

This type of abuse may include:

- allegations of rape or actual injuries resulting from the attack;
- forced sexual acts to which the adult did not consent;
- involvement in pornography;
- indecent exposure;
- sexual harassment claims;
- sexual assaults involving so-called date rape drugs;
- inappropriate touching or groping.

Conveyance to the ED may not always be the most appropriate care pathway for victims of sexual abuse and close working with the police is necessary. Paramedics must make themselves familiar with the local procedures for dealing with cases of sexual abuse and this should include processes for accessing the local Sexual Assault Referral Centre (SARC) or similar in the area.

Paramedics also need to be aware that individuals with learning disabilities or intellectual disabilities are at increased risk of sexual abuse/violence, due to a number of factors:

- lack of understanding that it may be sexual abuse;
- total dependence on caregiver(s)/services;
- lower communication skills and abilities to report;
- lack or reduced mental capacity to consent;
- shame and feelings of guilt preventing reporting.

Balderian (1991) suggests that 97–99 per cent of perpetrators in this type of abuse against individuals with disabilities are known and trusted by their victims. This must be a further consideration for paramedics when attending such incidents and the associated enhanced risks for this cohort of patients.

Adults who are vulnerable to radicalisation and extremism

There are also responsibilities to safeguard individuals who may be vulnerable or suscep- tible to radicalisation and extremism. In 2011, the Department of Health published the guidance 'Building Partnerships, Staying Safe' to assist the health sector to contribute to the national counter-terrorism strategy (CONTEST). The strategy has four work streams:

- Prevent
- Pursue
- Protect
- Prepare

The prevent element is driven by multi-agency working and provision of training for pro- fessionals who are able to raise concerns about potential victims of radicalisation to local multi-agency processes known as Channel Panels. Health professionals can com- plete prevent referrals to Channel Panels following local processes within organisations and prevent partnerships. NHS organisations contractually must have prevent leads, so any queries can also be raised with them when required for support and guidance. The Channel Panels meet monthly and collate intelligence and information from agen- cies, decide on any supportive actions to protect, support and safeguard the individual. Channel panels consider all types of extremism that may include, for example, right- wing, extreme right-wing, animal rights, and radical Islam.

 Chapter 11 to read more about this type of vulnerability.

HANDLING SUSPECTED ABUSE/NEGLECT AND RAISING CONCERNS

There are many terms used relating to safeguarding adults processes for reporting actual or suspected cases of abuse and neglect. Each local authority has their own process for raising concerns and paramedics must be familiar with local procedures for raising any safeguarding adults concerns.

CONCLUSION

Safeguarding adults is everyone's responsibility and any concerns should be raised via the appropriate and professional routes available to paramedics at all times. Numerous safeguarding reviews continue to demonstrate that paramedics are involved in many contacts with subjects of such cases, so it is essential that safeguarding adults training is firmly embedded within all curricula for personal development and any corporate inductions. Information recorded during telephone calls can sometimes be different to the information provided to attending paramedics, so it is always worth contacting EOCs about the content and nature of the 999 call if there are any suspicions of abuse and neglect.

Chapter key points:

- Paramedics must be aware of current safeguarding adults legislation.
- Safeguarding adults must be treated with the same importance as safeguarding children.
- Safeguarding adults cases may be more complex than safeguarding children cases due to consent and mental capacity issues.
- Safeguarding adults begins with dignity and respect for the patient(s).

REFERENCES AND SUGGESTED READING

Association of Directors of Adult Social Services (2005) *Safeguarding Adults: A National Framework of Standards for Good Practice and Outcomes in Adult Protection Work.* London: ADASS.

Balderian, N. (1991) Sexual abuse of people with developmental disabilities. *Sexuality and Disability,* 9(4): 323–35.

Brown, S.N., Kumar, D. and Millins, M. (eds for JRCALC and AACE) (2016) *UK Ambulance Service Clinical Practice Guidelines.* Bridgwater: Class Professional Publishing.

Caroline, N. (2014) *Emergency Care in the Streets,* 7th edn. London: Jones and Bartlett Learning.

College of Paramedics (2017) *Paramedic Post Graduate Curriculum Guidance.* Bridgwater: College of Paramedics, pp. 35–6.

DH (Department of Health) (2000) *No Secrets: Guidance on Developing and Implementing Multi-Agency Policies and Procedures to Protect Vulnerable Adults from Abuse.* London: TSO.

DH (Department of Health) (2011) *Building Partnerships, Staying Safe: The Health Sector Contribution to HM Government's Prevent Strategy: Guidance or Healthcare Workers.* London: TSO.

DH (Department of Health) (2014) *Care and Support Statutory Guidance.* Issued under the Care Act 2014. London: Department of Health.

Flynn M. (Chair) (2012) *Winterbourne View Hospital Serious Case Review. South Gloucestershire Safeguarding Adults Board.* Available at: http://sites.southglos.gov.uk/safeguarding/adults/i-am-a-carerrelative/winterbourne-view/ (accessed 1 August 2017).

Health and Care Professions Council (2016) *Paramedics. Standards of Conduct, Performance and Ethics.* London: HCPC.

HM Government (2002) *The Shipman Inquiry.* London: TSO.

HM Government (2005) *The Mental Capacity Act.* London: TSO.

HM Government (2007a) *Mental Capacity Act – Code of Practice.* London: TSO.

HM Government (2007b) *Mental Health Act.* London: TSO.

HM Government (2010) *The Equality Act.* London: TSO.

HM Government (2014) *The Care Act.* London: TSO.

HM Government (2015a) *The Care Act 2014. Care and Support Statutory Guidance.* London: TSO.

HM Government (2015b) *Modern Slavery Act.* London: TSO.

Home Office (2011) *Counter-Terrorism: Prevent Strategy.* London: TSO.

Home Office (2012) *Domestic Violence, Victim and Crime Act.* London: TSO.

Home Office (2015) *Counter-Terrorism and Security Act.* London. TSO.

Mark, J., Millins, M., Kumar, D. and Brown, S. (eds) (2016) *UK Ambulance Services Clinical Practice Guidelines 2016.* Joint Royal Colleges Ambulance Liaison Committee. Association of Ambulance Chief Executives (Great Britain). Bridgwater: Class Publishing.

National Crime Agency (2017) *NRM Referrals and Nationalities.* Available at: http://www.nationalcrimeagency.gov.uk/publications/national-referral-mechanism-statistics (accessed 11 September. 2017).

ONS (Office for National Statistics) (2015) *Crime Survey England and Wales 2013–14.* London: Office for National Statistics.

Safe Lives (2016) *Safe Later Lives: Older People and Domestic Abuse.* Available at: http://safelives.org.uk/sites/default/files/resources/Safe%20Later%20Lives%20-%20Older%20people%20and%20domestic%20abuse.pdf (accessed January 2018).

Schwappach, D.L.B. (2010) Engaging patients as vigilant partners in safety: a systematic review. *Medical Care Research and Review,* 67: 119–48.

USEFUL WEBSITES

Association of Directors of Adult Social Services (ADASS): https://www.adass.org.uk/home

Care Act (2014): https://www.gov.uk/government/publications/care-act-2014-part-1-factsheets

Care Quality Commission (CQC): http://www.cqc.org.uk/what-we-do/how-we-do-our-job/safeguarding-people

Department of Health (DH): https://www.gov.uk/government/publications/safeguarding-adults-the-role-of-health-services

Domestic Abuse Victim Support: https://www.victimsupport.org.uk/crime-info/types-crime/domestic-abuse

Modern Slavery Helpline: https://www.modernslaveryhelpline.org/

Modern Slavery Partnership: http://www.humberantislave.com/

National Referral Mechanism (NRM): http://www.nationalcrimeagency.gov.uk/about-us/what-we-do/specialist-capabilities/uk-human-trafficking-centre/national-referral-mechanism

National Referral Mechanism NRM Forms: https://www.gov.uk/government/publications/human-trafficking-victims-referral-and-assessment-forms

NHS England: https://www.england.nhs.uk/ourwork/safeguarding/

Social Care Institute for Excellence (SCIE): http://www.scie.org.uk/adults/safeguarding/

The Prevent Strategy: https://www.gov.uk/government/uploads/system/uploads/attachment_data/file/97976/prevent-strategy-review.pdf

14

Caring for people with dementia

John Krohne and Vicky Milburn

In this chapter:

- Introduction
- Why is this relevant?
- Alzheimer's dementia
- Vascular dementia
- Dementia with Lewy bodies
- Fronto-temporal dementia
- Common medications in dementia
- Visual-perceptual deficits
- Communication
- Dementia and pain
- Delirium
- Stigma and ethics
- Conclusion
- Chapter key points
- References and suggested reading

INTRODUCTION

Dementia is a general term for a number of organic brain diseases (Holmes and Amin 2016), usually of a chronic or progressive nature, in which there is disturbance of multiple higher cortical functions, including memory, thinking, orientation, comprehension, calculation, learning capacity, language and judgement (WHO 2015). Over 20 per cent of paramedic call-outs to those aged over 75 are likely to be related to dementia (Buswell et al. 2016).

In order to provide the best individualised, holistic care, it is important for paramedics to have an understanding of the different symptoms associated with the main types of dementia, rather than assuming that all patients with dementia will present in the same way. When medical professionals are considering diagnosing dementia, patients should undergo a series of comprehensive assessments; this includes taking the history from the patient and their family, cognitive and mental state examinations, a review of their medications and a physical examination which may include blood tests and often a urine test (NICE 2006). On occasion when the diagnosis may be in doubt, magnetic resonance imaging (MRI) or computed tomography (CT) scans are used to detect early subcortical vascular changes (NICE 2006).

Although there are many different types of dementia, the most commonly seen in paramedic practice will be Alzheimer's dementia (approximately 60 per cent), vascular dementia (20 per cent), dementia with Lewy bodies (5 per cent) and fronto-temporal dementia (2 per cent) (Holmes and Amin 2016). Many cases of dementia may have mixed pathology, for example, Alzheimer's with vascular dementia.

Which parts of your brain did you use to get to work today? Remembering to go to work, deciding what to have for breakfast, coordination and emotional control to drive to work. Now consider if you lost the ability to do one of these things. This does not mean you would not be able to get to work, but you would need to develop alternative strategies and support mechanisms to ensure you arrived at the destination. This is the same when living with dementia, particularly those types with slower onset such as Alzheimer's and fronto-temporal dementia. The individual can spend several years still able to function independently with support, so it is important for paramedics to include the person living with dementia in the decision-making process as much as possible. This approach is referred to as 'person-centred care', first developed by Kitwood (1997), where we look past the label of dementia and consider the individual 'living with dementia' as a way of highlighting the person rather than the disease. Literature surrounding dementia refers to 'person', 'patient' and 'service user' which are used interchangeably in this chapter.

Reflection: points to consider

- Do you tend to refer to your patients/service users by their diagnosis?
- Consider how this may make a person feel.
- Could you use a more person-centred approach?

WHY IS THIS RELEVANT?

Dementia and, in particular, Alzheimer's dementia, are recommended key areas of study in the College of Paramedics' curriculum guidance (2015; 2017). Attending an older person in the pre-hospital environment can pose many challenges, which are further complicated when the patient is cognitively impaired by dementia (Harvey 2014). This may result in people with dementia being more likely to be taken to hospital because ambulance crews cannot assess them properly (Buswell et al. 2016).

In a highly pressurised, busy pre-hospital environment, it is important to remember that taking a few extra moments to consider the person living with dementia will improve the patient's experience. The actions you take at the start of the interaction can make a big impact on how the situation will play out, both positively and negatively. Think of the ripples spreading out in a pond when you drop a stone in it; taking a few moments at the start of your interaction to review the approaches you need to take will improve patient care in the long run, stopping some of these 'ripples' from forming. This chapter will give you the underpinning theory on dementia, including assessment and communication strategies, which will make a significant difference when attending patients who have dementia. Case study 14.1 at the end of the chapter will help you to assess what you have learnt.

Reflection: points to consider

- 850,000 people in the UK have a diagnosis of dementia, of which 42,000 are under the age of 65 (Alzheimer's Society 2014).
- One in three people aged over 65 will develop dementia before they die (NHS England 2014).
- Between 60–80 per cent of people with dementia experience a fall (Alzheimer's Society 2016).

ALZHEIMER'S DEMENTIA

Alzheimer's dementia is characterised by a progressive decline in memory and intellect (Teten et al. 2015) and is the dementia most commonly seen by paramedics in practice. Those with an Alzheimer's dementia diagnosis live an average of eight years after their symptoms become noticeable to others, but survival can range from four to 20 years, depending on age and other health conditions (Alzheimer's Association 2017). Symptoms range considerably from those which may present earlier in the disease progression and those later (Table 14.1).

Table 14.1 Potential symptoms of Alzheimer's dementia

Earlier symptoms	Later symptoms
Forgetting recent events/misplacing items	Unable to recognise family members
Forgetting places, object names and faces	Hallucinating and suffering delusions
Repetition of speech	Problems with speech and language
Mood swings and increased anxiety	Aggressive and demanding behaviour
Restlessness	Disturbed sleep
Problems with concentration	Physical issues – incontinence, difficulty eating and swallowing, weight loss or significant weight gain

VASCULAR DEMENTIA

Vascular dementia is the second most prevalent dementia you are likely to encounter in paramedic practice. It is a progressive disease caused by impaired blood flow to the brain (Box 14.1). Risk factors for vascular dementia are shown in Box 14.2.

Box 14.1 Potential symptoms of vascular dementia

- Impaired memory
- Reduction in cognitive abilities
- Paralysis on one side of the body
- Balance issues
- Swallowing issues
- Pain and extreme tiredness
- Incontinence
- Vision issues
- Speech and language problems

Box 14.2 Risk factors for vascular dementia

- Stroke
- Cardiac disease
- High blood pressure
- High cholesterol
- Smoking
- Male
- Diabetes
- Depression
- Obesity

 Reflection: points to consider

Controlling these risk factors can reduce the chances of getting vascular dementia. For example, 30 minutes of moderately intense exercise five times per week can reduce the risk of developing heart disease, stroke, dementia, diabetes and some cancers by at least 30 per cent (Academy of Royal Medical Colleges 2015).

DEMENTIA WITH LEWY BODIES

Dementia with Lewy bodies is less prevalent than Alzheimer's dementia and vascular dementia but unlike other dementias, memory impairment is not usually a symptom in the early stages (Box 14.3).

Box 14.3 Main symptoms of dementia with Lewy bodies

- Parkinsonism-type symptoms (including slowing of movement, tremor, stiffness)
- Visual hallucinations
- Fluctuating levels of alertness
- Reduced ability to smell
- Sleep disturbance

FRONTO-TEMPORAL DEMENTIA

Although only accounting for 2 per cent of dementia diagnoses (Holmes and Amin 2016), fronto-temporal dementia (FTD) is the second most common neurodegenerative dementia in people under the age of 65 (Pressman and Miller 2014). FTD is classified into three clinical variants: (1) behavioural-variant FTD; (2) non-fluent variant primary progressive aphasia; and (3) semantic-variant primary progressive aphasia (Bang et al. 2015). Two-thirds of FTD diagnoses will be of behavioural variant FTD (Alzheimer's Society 2017a) (Box 14.4).

Box 14.4 Main symptoms of behavioural variant FTD

- Disinhibition
- Impulsive behaviour
- Inability to grasp consequence of actions
- Apathy
- Loss of empathy
- Loss of planning, organising and decision-making abilities

The patient is likely to be unaware of these symptoms.

For the other two types of FTD (non-fluent variant primary progressive aphasia and semantic-variant primary progressive aphasia), the main symptoms are linked to speech and language issues.

 Reflection: points to consider

People with mild deficits who do not meet the criteria for dementia are considered to have mild cognitive impairment (MCI). MCI involves subtle changes in memory or other cognitive abilities that are greater than would be expected with normal ageing but less severe than with a dementia diagnosis. These changes are generally not serious enough to significantly interfere with the person's daily life and independence (Alzheimer Society of Canada 2014), however, more than 50 per cent of people with MCI develop dementia in later life (NICE 2006).

Table 14.2 Common medications in dementia

	Acetylcholinesterase inhibitors	NMDA (N-methyl-D-aspartate) receptor antagonist	Antipsychotics**
Example	Donepezil Galantamine Rivastigmine	Memantine	Risperidone Haloperidol (short term only <1 week) (Lorazepam***)
Intention of action	Reduce symptoms do not cure	May slow progression	Help reduce symptoms of severe psychosis/agitation
Alzheimer's dementia	Yes (mild to moderate severity) see above examples	If ineffective/intolerant to Acetylcholinesterase inhibitors OR Suffering severe Alzheimer's dementia	Yes but increases risk of cerebrovascular events and decreases memory
Vascular dementia	Not usually beneficial	No evidence	Yes but increases risk of cerebrovascular events
Lewy bodies	Yes if agitated, see above examples	No evidence	No increased risk of severe adverse events Only used in exceptional circumstances
Fronto-temporal dementia	The focus is mainly on reducing symptoms, there is some evidence that specific antidepressant drugs can help with certain behavioural issues. Acetylcholinesterase inhibitors/NMDA receptor antagonists are NOT commonly used as there is no evidence as to their effectiveness and some trials reported they worsened symptoms.		

** Only if severe psychosis or agitated behaviour is resulting in substantial distress.

*** Lorazepam is a benzodiazepine (not an antipsychotic) but occasionally used in the short term instead of an antipsychotic.

Sources: NICE (2006), Alzheimer's Research UK (2016) and Alzheimer's Society (2017a).

COMMON MEDICATIONS IN DEMENTIA

Table 14.2 list the common medications in dementia.

VISUAL-PERCEPTUAL DEFICITS

Paramedics interacting with patients living with dementia need to be aware of the impact of potential vision and perception changes (Box 14.5). These changes will vary dependent on the type of dementia diagnosis.

Box 14.5 Visual and perceptual deficits that may impact on the paramedic's interaction and care of the person living with dementia

- Depth perception, e.g. unable to judge distance when transferring from chair to stretcher.
- Peripheral vision acuity/narrowing of the visual field, e.g. inability to see the paramedic who approaches from the side of the patient.
- Misperceptions, e.g. shiny flooring mistaken for water or dark carpet mistaken for a hole in the ground.
- Hallucinations: although people living with dementia do experience hallucinations, this is not common. Often it is the person's visual and perceptual deficits that are interpreted as hallucinations when the person is actually just mistaking what they have seen.

 Reflection: points to consider

Hold your hands up to your eyes like a pair of binoculars. How does this restrict your peripheral vision? As a paramedic, how would you need to approach this person? Peripheral vision issues are common in persons living with dementia, but they will not be obvious to you.

If you were asked to walk across a big hole in the road, would you do it? So why is it 'difficult' or 'unhelpful' behaviour when a patient with perceptual deficit refuses to cross a dark carpet if they think it is a hole?

COMMUNICATION

The person living with dementia cannot be assumed to be incapable of making decisions on the basis of their diagnosis alone (Smebye et al. 2012) and they should have the opportunity to be involved in decisions about their care. To enable this, good communication between paramedics and the patient/family/carer is vital.

The carer/family member can often compensate for the impaired person's inability to stay focused on one topic (Teten et al. 2015) but it is important, as much as possible, to ensure that the individual patient is included in conversations. Paramedics and other healthcare professionals are responsible for facilitating decision-making and ensuring the participation of the person with dementia wherever possible. This can be done by using adapted communication strategies (Table 14.3).

Table 14.3 Common dementia communication issues and possible solutions

Problem	Possible solution
Building relationships	• Smile • Open body language • Calm tone of voice • Orientate the person by informing them where they are, who they are with and what is going on • Use names rather than he/she • Refer to the dementia personal information record/ people who know the patient well • Take an interest in objects in the patient's personal environment to establish rapport, e.g. pictures, ornaments and pets
Understanding language	• Avoid using complex language • Use gestures/demonstrations • Use pictures when possible
Physical assessment	• Explain each step of the procedure, e.g. 'I am going to place a blood pressure cuff around your arm, it will feel tight for a few seconds.' • Avoid making the person feel rushed
Maintaining conversation threads	• Offer verbal prompts about topic of conversation • One point at a time
Visual and perceptual deficits	• Interacting one-on-one • Slow down your movements
Making decisions	• Use closed rather than open questions • Involve family members
Environment	• Reduce distractions, e.g. background noise, consider moving to a quiet room • An unfamiliar environment may be unsettling

---

Chapter 1 to read more about various communication strategies.

Personal information records in dementia care are increasing in prevalence, for example the Alzheimer's Society (2017b) have produced the support tool 'This is me'. Paramedics should review these documents in order to provide person-centred care. Topics such as family background, likes and dislikes, routines and personality may be included; having an awareness of such information can aid communication and enable a more positive experience for the patient.

Reflection: points to consider

The singular most important thing in communicating with people who are cognitively impaired is **PATIENCE!!!**

DEMENTIA AND PAIN

Lord (2009) specifies that a paramedic's ability to effectively manage pain depends on their capacity to identify the nature and severity of pain from the clinical information. The Joint Royal Colleges Ambulance Liaison Committee (JRCALC) ambulance practice guidelines (Brown, Kumar and Millins 2016) recommend that paramedics use the Verbal Numeric Rating Scale (VNRS) to guide decisions relating to pain management and analgesia administration. Using the VNRS, patients are asked to self-report and score their pain from 0–10. Paramedics should attempt to facilitate this for patients with cognitive impairment when possible. Although this approach is encouraged as part of patient-centred care, the process of assessing pain in cognitively impaired patients is a difficult and complex process. Reynolds et al. (2008) found that the prevalence of recorded pain rates and amount of analgesia administered decreased as the level of cognitive impairment increased, suggesting that pain in patients with dementia is not being assessed or managed correctly. With this knowledge, paramedics need to give careful consideration to assessing pain and administering analgesia to dementia patients.

Paramedics are often called to patients with dementia who are believed to be suffering acute pain. Lord (2009) found that the majority of pain assessment tools for cognitively impaired patients were designed to assess chronic pain and suggest that they may not be practical for use in the pre-hospital arena. Reasons for their impracticality include a reliance on observation of the patient over a period of time performing a variety of tasks. The most popular pain assessment tool designed specifically for cognitively impaired patients in paramedic practice is the Abbey Pain Scale as it considers both acute and chronic pain and can be completed in a timely manner. Table 14.4 presents commonly used pain assessment tools in paramedic practice.

Table 14.4 Commonly used pain assessment tools in paramedic practice and their application for cognitively impaired patients

Pain assessment tool	Description	Application for cognitively impaired patients
Verbal Numeric Rating Scale (VNRS)	• Self-report score of pain from 0–10	• Difficult for patients with moderate–severe cognitive impairment
Verbal Rating Scale (VRS)	• Self-report ranking of pain – mild, moderate or severe	• No discrete pain score • Potentially patients who are unable to perform VNRS may have the cognitive ability to perform VRS
Wong-Baker FACES	• Visual aid • Patients identify which face best describes their pain	• Can be used in non-verbal patients • Difficult for patients as cognitive impairment increases • Originally designed for children
FLACC scale	• Considers face, legs, arms, cry and consolability • Scored 0–2 for each giving a score out of 10	• Questions over its reliability and validity • Difficulties arise if the clinician assessing does not know the patient
The Abbey Pain Scale	• Observation for six areas including physiological and physical changes, vocalisation, facial expressions, body language and behaviours	• Designed specifically for cognitively impaired patients • Relatively quick to complete • Considers acute and chronic pain

---

> ## Box 14.6 Recommended steps in pain assessment and management for cognitively impaired patients
>
> - Physical assessment – indication of injury
> - Patient's behaviour – agitation, facial expressions, body language, etc.
> - Information from others – information from dementia personal information record/people who know patient well
> - Consider the use of a pain assessment tool
> - Consider an analgesic trial to see how the patient's behaviour changes
>
> Adapted from Lord (2009)

JRCALC (Brown, Kumar and Millins 2016) state that patients who are cognitively impaired may not be able to score their pain and that behavioural cues should be considered and assessed in these patients (Box 14.6). Paramedics need to be more aware of physical cues and changes in behaviour in order to assess pain, as well as considering the injury or potential acute medical pain that is being suspected. Having a greater appreciation of these communication challenges will allow paramedics to give more thought and consideration to assessing pain and administering analgesia for potentially painful injuries or conditions.

DELIRIUM

Dementia is a chronic confusional state in direct contrast to delirium which is an acute confusional state (Inouye 2006). Delirium is a common and serious problem among acutely unwell people (European Delirium Association 2014). The prevalence of delirium

Table 14.5 Potentially modifiable risk factors in delirium

Risk factor	Comment
Physical factors	- Infection - Vascular compromise (e.g. stroke, myocardial infarction) - Urinary catheterisation - Constipation - Pain - Dehydration - Malnutrition
Environmental factors	- Sleep deprivation - Physical restraint/immobilisation - Emotional distress - Unfamiliar/change in environment

Source: Adapted from Anand and MacLullich (2017).

Table 14.6 Malignant social psychology behaviours/traits and the potential impact on paramedic practice

Behaviour/trait	Description	Links to Health and Care Professions Council (2016) Standards of Conduct, Performance and Ethics
Accusation	Blaming a person for their lack of ability/ understanding	• Standard 1.1: Treat service users as individuals, respecting their privacy and dignity
Infantilisation	Communicating with a person as a parent would to a young child	
Labelling	Treating the person as a diagnosis rather than as an individual with an illness	
Disempowerment	Not recognising a person's abilities	• Standard 1.2: Work in partnership with service users to involve them, where appropriate in decisions about their care and treatment
Ignoring	Treating the person as if they were not there	
Imposition	Forcing a person to go against their preferred choice	• Standard 1.4: You must have consent from service users or other appropriate authority before you provide care, treatment or other services
Stigmatisation	Treating a person as if they were a diseased object/ outcast	• Standard 1.5: Do not discriminate against service users by allowing personal views to affect the care provided
Disruption	A sudden intrusion that disturbs the individual	• Standard 2.1: Be polite and considerate
Objectification	Treating a person as if they were an object rather than a person	• Standard 2.2: Listen to service users and take account of their needs and wishes
Invalidation	Not recognising how a person might be feeling about a situation	
Outpacing	Presenting information at a rate too fast for the person to understand	

Banishment	Physically or psychologically excluding a person from a situation	• Standard 6.2: Do not put the health or safety of service users at risk
Treachery	Use of deception to manipulate, distract or control the person	• Standard 9: Be honest and trustworthy
Disparagement	Verbal or psychological messages that tell a person they are incompetent or worthless	• Standard 9.1: Conduct must justify public trust and confidence
Intimidation	Inducing fear through threats or intimidation	
Mockery	Making fun of the person, teasing or humiliating them	
Withholding	Refusing to give attention/ treatment	

Sources: Adapted from Kitwood (1997) and Health and Care Professions Council (2016).

in community settings increases with age, rising to 14 per cent among those over 85 years old (Inouye 2006). It is likely that previous episodes of delirium increase the risk of a diagnosis of dementia (Vardy et al. 2014).

Delirium can lead to poorer outcomes if untreated, yet it is often missed. It can be difficult to distinguish between delirium and dementia and some people may have both conditions. If clinical uncertainty exists over the diagnosis, the person should be managed initially for delirium (NICE 2010).

In contrast to dementia, delirium is likely to have a quick onset and a duration usually lasting from hours to days. Depending on the type of delirium, the person may display hyperactive or hypoactive symptoms (or a mix of both) (Table 14.5). There is likely to be significant impairment to the person's ability to stay focused and symptoms can fluctuate rapidly during the day. Unlike dementia, hallucinations are common in delirium.

With treatment, the person is likely to recover from delirium. Paramedics will often be called to dementia patients with vague or non-specific conditions, for example, increased confusion or drowsiness. It is important that you consider a possible cause for this change in behaviour rather than attributing it solely to the dementia.

STIGMA AND ETHICS

Kitwood (1997) referred to the concept of 'Malignant Social Psychology' in dementia. He identified 17 behaviours and traits in the delivery of care which can intensify a patient's sense of loss of independence and feeling devalued (Read et al. 2016) (Table 14.6).

Case study 14.1

Betty is an 88-year-old lady with a diagnosis of Alzheimer's dementia. Her cognitive function has slowly declined over a period of time and she is now non-verbal. She lives at home with her husband Harry and cat Toby. It is 03.30 and you have been called to attend Betty at home after Harry was woken by Betty screaming as she has fallen in the kitchen. On arrival you find Betty on the floor of the kitchen unable to get up and clearly in some distress, agitation and discomfort.

 ## Reflection: points to consider

Based on the points discussed in this chapter, what strategies could you employ to ensure that Betty is assessed and treated appropriately?

Communication

This chapter has discussed the value of effective communication strategies when interacting with people living with dementia. With this in mind, when interacting with Betty ensure that you smile, refer to 'Betty' and 'Harry' by name and make friends with Toby the cat who is sitting nearby. You know Harry is an important person in Betty's life, so consider involving him in the assessment. Use simple language, verbally explain, step by step, your actions and demonstrate the procedures you would like to carry out. An example could be putting the oxygen saturation probe on Harry's finger before attempting to put it on Betty's finger. You should consider slowing down your movements and doing one thing at a time, for example, taking the oxygen saturations reading before attempting to record a blood pressure.

Pain assessment

Using Lord's (2009) suggested steps in pain assessment for cognitively impaired patients, you make a physical assessment of the injury, a fracture is suspected to Betty's hip as she has shortening and rotation to her left leg. Consider Betty's behaviour, she is agitated, upset and tearful. Harry may be able to advise if this is normal behaviour for Betty, but it is also important for you to try and involve Betty in the pain assessment if possible. How might you do this? Using a pain assessment tool could be advantageous to help support your decision to consider an analgesic trial. There is evidence that pain in severely cognitively impaired patients is poorly managed, so having an appreciation of some of the issues surrounding this complex area will help overcome some of these challenges.

Stigma and ethics

Paramedics have a moral and professional duty to ensure they treat Betty as an individual and that they respect her privacy and dignity. Paramedics should work with Betty to involve her in decisions surrounding her care, using her husband Harry to support her when required. Table 14.6 outlines some of the potential areas you may need to consider in this situation.

> **Chapter 4** to read more about ethical and legal considerations; **Chapters 9 and 10** for sociological perspectives; and **Chapter 13** for detail on safeguarding adults.

CONCLUSION

It is important to use a person-centred approach and consider the person rather than the dementia diagnosis. Paramedics need to take a few extra moments at the beginning of their interaction and during assessment to review their approach. This chapter has demonstrated how an increased understanding of dementia-related issues will have a significant impact on the experiences of both the person with dementia and the attending paramedics.

Chapter key points:

- The four main types of dementia are Alzheimer's dementia, vascular dementia, dementia with Lewy bodies and fronto-temporal dementia.
- Main symptoms are disturbances of multiple higher cortical functions.
- Dementia may also cause visual and perceptual deficits.
- Considering and tailoring communication when interacting with dementia patients are vital.
- When assessing pain, consider how you can enable patients to score their own pain.
- Assessing behavioural traits and physical cues is a crucial part of pain assessment for dementia patients.
- Delirium should be considered if an acute behavioural change is reported.
- Paramedics need to have an awareness of their own behaviour and its potential impact on the patient.

REFERENCES AND SUGGESTED READING

Academy of Royal Medical Colleges (2015) Exercise: The miracle cure and the role of the doctor in promoting it. Academy of Royal Medical Colleges. Available at: http://www.aomrc.org.uk/wp-content/uploads/2016/05/Exercise_the_Miracle_Cure_0215.pdf (accessed 2 January 2018).

Alzheimer Society of Canada (2014) *Mild Cognitive Impairment.* Available at: http://www.alzheimer.ca/~/media/Files/national/Other-dementias/other_dementias_MCI_e.pdf (accessed 2 January 2018).

Alzheimer's Association (2017) *What Is Alzheimer's?* Available at: http://www.alz.org/alzheimers_disease_what_is_alzheimers.asp (accessed 27 December 2017).

Alzheimer's Research UK (2016) *Treatments Available.* Available at: http://www.alzheimersresearchuk.org/about-dementia/helpful-information/treatments-available/ (accessed 8 July 2017).

Alzheimer's Society (2014) *Dementia UK*, 2nd edn overview. Available at: http://eprints.lse. ac.uk/59437/1/Dementia_UK_Second_edition_-_Overview.pdf (accessed 2 January 2018).

Alzheimer's Society (2016) *Exercise Therapy in Early Dementia.* Available at: https://www.alzheimers. org.uk/info/20200/care_and_cure_magazine_archive/518/exercise_therapy_in_early_dementia (accessed 28 December 2017).

Alzheimer's Society (2017a) *Frontotemporal Dementia.* Available at: https://www.alzheimers. org.uk/info/20007/types_of_dementia/11/frontotemporal_dementia (accessed 2 January 2018).

Alzheimer's Society (2017b) 'This Is Me'. Available at: https://www.alzheimers.org.uk/download/ downloads/id/3423/this_is_me.pdf (accessed 21 July 2017).

Anand, A. and MacLullich, A.M.J. (2017) Delirium in hospitalized older adults. *Medicine*, 45(1): 47–50.

Bang, J., Spina, S. and Miller, B.L. (2015) Frontotemporal dementia. *The Lancet*, 386(10004): 1672–82.

Brown, S.N., Kumar, D., Millins, M., Mark, J. and Joint Royal Colleges Ambulance Liaison Committee, Issuing Body (2016) *UK Ambulance Services Clinical Practice Guidelines 2016.* Bridgwater: Class Professional Publishing.

Buswell, M., Lumbard, P., Fleming, J., Ayres, D., Brayne, C. and Goodman, C. (2016) Using ambulance service PCRs to understand 999 call-outs to older people with dementia. *Journal of Paramedic Practice*, 8(5): 246–51.

College of Paramedics (2015) *Paramedic Curriculum Guidance*, 3rd edn revised. Bridgwater: College of Paramedics.

College of Paramedics (2017) *Paramedic Curriculum Guidance*, 4th edn revised. Bridgwater: College of Paramedics.

Dementia UK (2015) Tips for better communication with a person living with dementia. Available at: https://www.dementiauk.org/wp-content/uploads/2015/10/tips-for-communication4.pdf (accessed 1 January 2018).

DH (Department of Health) (2009) *Living Well with Dementia: A National Dementia Strategy.* London: Department of Health.

European Communities (2005) *Rare Forms of Dementia. Final Report of a Project Supported by the Community Rare Diseases Programme 2000–2002.* Luxembourg: European Commission. Available at: http://ec.europa.eu/health/archive/ph_threats/non_com/docs/raredementias_ en.pdf (accessed 30 December 2017).

European Delirium Association (2014) The DSM-5 criteria, level of arousal and delirium diagnosis: inclusiveness is safer. *BMC Medicine*, 12: 141.

Harvey, C. (2014) Is there scope for an observational pain scoring tool in paramedic practice? *Journal of Paramedic Practice*, 6(2): 84–8.

Health and Care Professions Council (2016) *Standards of Conduct, Performance and Ethics.* London: Health and Care Professions Council.

Holmes, C. and Amin, J. (2016) Dementia. *Medicine*, 44(11): 687–90.

Inouye, S.K. (2006) Delirium in older persons. *The New England Journal of Medicine*, 354: 1157–65.

Kitwood, T.M. (1997) *Dementia Reconsidered: The Person Comes First.* Buckingham: Open University Press.

Lord, B. (2009) Paramedic assessment of pain in the cognitively impaired adult patient. *BMC Emergency Medicine*, 9(20).

NHS England (2014) *Five Year Forward View.* Available at: http://www.england.nhs.uk/wp-content/ uploads/2014/10/5yfv-web.pdf (accessed 1 January 2018).

NICE (National Institute for Health and Clinical Excellence) (2006) *Dementia: Supporting People with Dementia and Their Carers in Health and Social Care (Updated 2016).* Available at: https://

www.nice.org.uk/guidance/cg42/resources/dementia-supporting-people-with-dementia-and-their-carers-in-health-and-social-care-pdf-975443665093 (accessed 31 December 2017).

NICE (National Institute for Health and Clinical Excellence) (2010) *Delirium: Prevention, Diagnosis and Management.* Manchester: National Institute for Health and Clinical Excellence.

Pressman, P.S. and Miller, B.L. (2014) Diagnosis and management of behavioural variant fronto-temporal dementia. *Biological Psychiatry*, 75: 574–81.

Prince, M. et al. (2014) *Dementia UK: Update*, 2nd edn report produced by King's College London and the London School of Economics for the Alzheimer's Society.

Read, S.T., Toye, C. and Wynaden, D. (2016) Experiences and expectations of living with dementia: a qualitative study. *Collegian*, 36(10).

Reynolds K., Hanson L., Devellis, R., Henderson, M. and Steinhauser, K. (2008) Disparities in pain management between cognitively intact and cognitively impaired nursing home residents. *Journal of Pain and Symptom Management*, 35(4): 388–96.

Smebye, K., Kirkevold, M. and Engedal, K. (2012) How do persons with dementia participate in decision making related to health and daily care? A multi-case study. *BMC Health Services Research*, 12(1).

Teten, A.F., Dagenais, P.A. and Friehe, M.J. (2015) Auditory and visual cues for topic maintenance with persons who exhibit dementia of Alzheimer's type. *International Journal of Alzheimer's Disease*, 2015 (126064).

Vardy, E., Holt, R., Gerhard, A., Richardson, A., Snowden, J. and Neary, D. (2014) History of a suspected delirium is more common in dementia with Lewy bodies than Alzheimer's disease: a retrospective study. *International Journal of Geriatric Psychiatry*, 29: 178–81.

WHO (World Health Organisation) (2015) *International Statistical Classification of Diseases and Related Health Problems (ICD-10) 10th Revision*. Available at: http://apps.who.int/classifications/icd10/browse/2015/en#!/F00-F09 (accessed 3 January 2018).

15 End of life care

Ann French and Gary Vale

> **In this chapter:**
>
> - Introduction
> - Why is this relevant?
> - History of palliative care
> - Policy and guidance
> - Gold Standards Framework (GSF)
> - Advance Care Planning (ACP)
> - The Mental Capacity Act
> - Do Not Attempt Cardiopulmonary Resuscitation (DNACPR)
> - Preferred priorities of care
> - Breaking bad/significant news
> - Conclusion
> - Chapter key points
> - References and suggested reading

INTRODUCTION

Since the early 2000s, a number of policies and frameworks have been developed which provide structure and guidance for everyone involved in the care of patients at the end of their lives. This chapter will introduce you to the history of palliative care and the key policies which have emerged to underpin end of life care for patients and their families. As paramedics you all too often attend patients who are in the end stages of life with or without clear directives in place. This chapter will encourage you to think about your role and your contribution in meeting the challenge of providing optimum end of life care for individuals.

WHY IS THIS RELEVANT?

As people approach the end of their life, their health needs generally increase, requiring more frequent access to healthcare providers. In England, approximately 500,000 people die each year; this number is expected to rise by 17 per cent from 2012 to 2030

(NHS England 2014) with the percentage of deaths occurring in the group of people aged 85 years or more rising to 32 per cent in 2003 to 44 per cent in 2030. Currently there are 15 million people in England with a long-term condition (LTC); by 2025, this is expected to rise to 18 million (DH 2013; 2015). Since 2008, people dying in their 'usual place of residence', i.e. at home or in care homes has risen from 38 per cent to 44.5 per cent (NELCIN 2014); this is due to the increasing awareness of the importance of end of life care and the implementation of policies to ensure patients have more involvement in their treatment plans and more choice over where they are cared for at this phase of their life.

However, the National Council for Palliative Care (2010) state that more than 50 per cent of people would prefer to die at home. Thomas et al. (2004) conclude that for many, the place of death is by default rather than by choice, due to lack of planning or service provision, problems with symptom control or carer support. As a paramedic or healthcare professional you will be actively involved in the care of patients at the end of their life and this can be challenging, emotionally demanding as well as rewarding and immensely satisfying when everything goes well. You need to be able to communicate effectively with family and carers, understand the legal obligations and know when to withhold unwanted interventions. Knowledge and understanding of the policies and frameworks underpinning end of life care and how they should be applied will support your decision-making and provide you with the tools to ensure the care you provide meets the needs and preferences of the individual.

Chapter 1 for more on communication skills and **Chapter 4** for legal and ethical issues.

Definition of end of life care (EoLC)

The Department of Health has given a definition of end of life care:

> Helps all those with advanced progressive, incurable illness to live as well as possible until they die. It enables the supportive and palliative care needs of both patient and family to be identified and met throughout the last phase of life and into bereavement. It includes management of pain and other symptoms and provision of psychological, social, spiritual and practical support.
>
> (DH 2010b: 47)

Reflection: point to consider

Before reading on, do you know of any important policies, frameworks or guidelines nationally or locally related to end of life care?

HISTORY OF PALLIATIVE CARE

Caring for people at the end of life has always been seen as an important part of healthcare, from nursing nuns who cared for the dying many years ago to the development of the hospice movement. Dame Cicely Saunders, founder of the modern hospice movement, has been credited with the development of palliative care. As a nurse, social worker and latterly a physician, she explored not only the best way to care for the holistic needs of a patient but also to learn more about what the patient was experiencing. Through her work at St Joseph's Hospice in Hackney, the concept of total pain evolved (Clark et al. 2005). She aspired not only to provide excellent clinical care but emphasised the importance of education and research. Dame Cicely Saunders founded St Christopher's Hospice in Sydenham, South London, in 1967 following eight years of fundraising and planning (Saunders 2005). This independent organisation which focused on the care of people when they were dying became a source of inspiration around the world and the modern hospice movement began. The concept of 'palliative care' was devised by the Canadian surgeon Balfour Mount who visited St Christopher's in 1973 and then explored how the idea of hospice care could be combined with hospital medicine. By 1987, the Royal College of Physicians and of General Practitioners recognised palliative care as a specialty which was seen as a turning point in palliative care history. The World Health Organisation (WHO 2010) defines palliative care as:

> an approach that improves the quality of life for patients and their families facing the problems associated with life-threatening illness, through the prevention and relief of suffering by means of early identification and impeccable assessment and treatment of pain and other problems, physical, psychosocial and spiritual.

WHO (2010) clarifies this further in a number of points. Palliative care does the following:

- provides relief from pain and other distressing symptoms;
- affirms life and regards dying as a normal process;
- intends neither to hasten or postpone death;
- integrates the psychological and spiritual aspects of patient care;
- offers a support system to help patients live as actively as possible until death;
- offers a support system to help the family cope during the patient's illness and in their own bereavement;
- uses a team approach to address the needs of patients and their families, including bereavement counselling, if indicated;
- will enhance quality of life, and may also positively influence the course of illness;
- is applicable early in the course of illness, in conjunction with other therapies that are intended to prolong life, such as chemotherapy or radiation therapy, and includes those investigations needed to better understand and manage distressing clinical complications.

One of the major criticisms of palliative care over the years has been the focus on patients with cancer. The House of Commons Health Committee (2004) suggested that the greatest inequality was the lack of provision of palliative care services for patients with a non-cancer diagnosis. In the same year, Dame Cicely Saunders suggested to the WHO that 'the next stage is surely the introduction of palliative care into mainstream medicine'. Since then there have been many major policies and drivers that have advocated the provision of palliative care for all, regardless of where the patient is being cared for or what their diagnosis is. The Department of Health addresses the need for palliative care in several National Service Frameworks; end of life care was a main theme of the Darzi Report (DH 2008a) and finally the Department of Health produced the long-awaited End of Life Care Strategy (DH 2008b). However, focus on end of life care has not always been positive. In 2012, a series of articles were published in the media that raised concerns over the use of the Liverpool Care Pathway (LCP) once recommended as good practice by the End of Life Care Strategy (DH 2008b). The LCP was originally developed by the Royal Liverpool University Hospital and the Marie Curie Hospice in Liverpool to guide the care of patients within the last few days of life. The aim of the LCP was to ensure that wherever a person died, the care they received in the last days of life was uniformly good. The main concerns raised in the media related to the appropriate use of the pathway and the withdrawal or withholding of medication, nutrition and hydration. This led to an independent inquiry into the use of the pathway by Baroness Julia Neuberger (DH 2013a).

The recommendation of the inquiry was that the Liverpool Care Pathway should be phased out and instead there should be more emphasis on the individual care of the patient and their family. The inquiry highlighted the need for open and honest communication between healthcare professionals, patients and families and the need to ensure both patients and their families are involved in discussions relating to care. Indeed, the review made 44 recommendations, including calls for more guidance on how to diagnose dying, along with guidance for healthcare professionals on decision-making at this stage of life.

In the last few years since the review of the LCP, there have been a number of key documents to help guide healthcare professionals to provide end of life care, some of which are discussed below; however, the controversy about the pathway has shown that end of life care cannot be reduced to merely following a number of guidelines. All healthcare professionals need to be able to respond to a person and their family with compassion, using a variety of skills and above all treating them as a unique individual.

POLICY AND GUIDANCE

The *End of Life Care Strategy: Promoting High Quality Care for All Adults at the End of Life* (DH 2008b) was the first for the UK and covers adults in England. The strategy recognised the excellent innovative work of the hospice movement and the experience of the National End of Life Care Programme (2004–2007).

The overall aim of the End of Life Care Strategy was to provide a 10-year vision for the provision of end of life, ensuring access to high quality care for all people approaching the end of their life, irrespective of age, gender, ethnicity, religious belief, disability,

---

> **Box 15.1 The six ambitions for the Palliative and End of Life Care, 2015–2020 framework**
>
> - Everyone is seen as an individual and should be treated as such.
> - Each person gets fair access to care.
> - Comfort and well-being of the individual should be maximised.
> - Care is coordinated.
> - All staff are prepared to care.
> - Each community is prepared to help.

sexual orientation, diagnosis or socio-economic status. It encompasses all adults with advanced, progressive illness and care delivered in all settings, including the home environment. Since the launch of the strategy in 2008, public awareness of end of life care has increased, partly owing to the work of *Dying Matters* (2015) and the need to plan for the end of life has become more of a priority. Since 2008, other policies and guidance have shaped the provision of care for the dying, such as the NICE Quality Standards (2011), however, the emphasis now is on local decision-making and delivery. The National Palliative and End of Life Care Partnership (2015) built on the work of the End of Life Care Strategy with the publication of the *Ambitions for Palliative and End of Life Care, 2015–2020*. This framework encourages organisations to develop more effective ways of working and promotes the effective and creative use of resources (see Box 15.1). The framework recognises that successful provision of good end of life care lies in working in partnership, and working collaboratively. Examples of this include: shared record keeping, 24/7 access to services and effective leadership.

To realise these ambitions, building blocks must be in place such as having honest conversations, clear expectations, an integrated approach to care and the opportunity for people to take control of their own care. The focus of this framework is to create an impetus for better care at the end of life.

 Reflection: points to consider

The objectives above set many challenges for all healthcare providers and organisations. What would you envisage these to be for you in your role as a paramedic?

GOLD STANDARDS FRAMEWORK (GSF)

The GSF is a systematic approach to formalising best practice, so that quality end of life care becomes standard for every patient. It is concerned with helping people to live

> ## Box 15.2 Five goals of GSF
>
> These are to provide for patients with any final illness with:
>
> 1 consistent high-quality care;
> 2 alignment with patients' preferences;
> 3 pre-planning and anticipation of needs;
> 4 improved staff confidence and teamwork;
> 5 more home-based, less hospital-based care.

well until the end of life and includes care in the final years of life for people with any end-stage illness in any setting.

According to the GSF, the majority of people will spend 90 per cent of the final year of their life at home, yet over half of the population do not die where they choose. It has been previously stated there is a significant gap between preferred and actual place of death with too many people dying in hospital and too few in their own home, care home or hospice. A key goal of the GSF is to enable more people to die in their preferred place, reducing unnecessary hospital admissions and the numbers who inappropriately die in acute hospital wards. Over 90 per cent of GP practices in the UK have a palliative care register (GSF 2009). This ensures that patients who have palliative care needs are identified and information related to their illness, preferred priorities of care and choices are known to all the members of the primary healthcare team and out of hours services. Box 15.2 highlights the five goals of the GSF.

As a paramedic, you are a key advocate for patients and carers, reducing the need for admission by mobilising other services, advising how to access services and calming difficult situations (GSF 2009). Patients at the end of their life frequently need care from multiple services and transfer between locations, such as home and hospital for treatment, investigations or respite care. This in itself will increase the amount of contact that you as ambulance personnel will have with them. They need access to care and support 24/7 to avoid being admitted to hospital as an emergency rather than being cared for in their home or normal place of residence. The End of Life Care Strategy (DH 2008b) identifies that as a society we do not talk openly about death and dying. It is suggested that relatively few adults, including older adults, have discussed their preferences for care with a close family member or friend. This makes it difficult or impossible for ambulance personnel and all healthcare professionals to ensure patients' wishes are met. The introduction of advanced care planning has provided structure and advice to ensure individuals are in a position to make their wishes known.

ADVANCE CARE PLANNING (ACP)

The NHS End of Life Care programme defined ACP as follows:

> Advance care planning is a voluntary process of discussion and review to help an individual who has capacity to anticipate how their condition may affect

them in the future, and if they wish, set on record: choices about their care and treatment and/or an advance decision to refuse a treatment in specific circumstances, so that these can be referred to by those responsible for their care or treatment (whether professional staff or family carers) in the event that they lose capacity to decide once their illness progresses.

(DH 2010a: 4)

These discussions might include the preferences for their treatment, such as how and where they would like to be cared for. Some local areas have addressed issues in planning for the end of life, one example is Deciding Right (Northern England Clinical Network 2014), a Northern England Clinical Network Initiative to ensure the same approach is taken to advance care planning and Do Not Attempt Cardiopulmonary Resuscitation by using the same recognisable documentation across the area.

An Advance Care Plan can have three outcomes:

1. *Advance statement*: this is a verbal or written statement of a person's wishes and preferences, beliefs and values. It must be stated by someone who has capacity for those care decisions, and only becomes active when that person loses capacity for those decisions. It is not legally binding but all carers are required to take it into account if the person loses capacity and a care decision has to be made according to the best interests process on the Mental Capacity Act (DH 2005a). An example of this is a preferred priorities of care document.

2. *Advance Decision to Refuse Treatment (ADRT)*: this is a verbal or written refusal of treatment. It must be stated by someone who has capacity for those care decisions, and it only becomes active when that person loses capacity for those decisions. It must be written if refusing life-sustaining treatment, it must state that the treatment is being refused 'even if my life is at risk'. An ADRT is legally binding if it is valid and applicable to the situation. The National End of Life Programme (2013) lists several key elements relating to the making of an ADRT:
   - An advance decision should be made voluntarily.
   - The individual needs to be over 18 years of age.
   - The individual must have capacity to make an ADRT.
   - The advance decision should specify the treatment which is to be refused and the circumstances in which refusal applies.
   - The decision must be valid.
   - The decision must be in writing, signed and witnessed for it to apply.
   - An advance decision can only be used to refuse treatment and not to demand treatment or request any procedure that is against the law such as euthanasia.
   - A copy should be retained in the relevant patient records.

3. *Lasting Power of Attorney (LPA)*: when an individual has capacity, they can legally nominate a person to make decisions on their behalf should they lose capacity for those decisions in the future. A Property and Affairs LPA cannot make healthcare decisions. These can only be made by a Personal Welfare

LPA, and such an LPA can only make life-sustaining treatment decisions if this is authorised in the original LPA order. An LPA is bound by the same Mental Capacity Act (MCA) process of Best Interests.

THE MENTAL CAPACITY ACT

The Mental Capacity Act (DH 2005a) was implemented in 2007 and all health and social care professionals have a duty to abide by the code of practice within this. The Mental Capacity Act gave individuals the right to make an advance decision to refuse treatment (ADRT).

The Mental Capacity Act (DH 2005b) has five main principles:

- A person must be assumed to have capacity unless it is established that they lack capacity.
- A person is not to be treated as unable to make a decision unless all practicable steps to help him to do so have been taken without success.
- A person is not to be treated as unable to make a decision merely because he makes an unwise decision.
- An act done or decision made, under this Act for or on behalf of a person who lacks capacity must be done, or made, in his best interests.
- Before the act is done, or the decision made, regard must be had to whether the purpose for which it is needed can be as effectively achieved in a way that is less restrictive of the person's rights and freedom of action (DH 2005b: 5).

Brady (2014) expresses the importance of the patient's voice and the recording of their wishes, what they wish to receive and the setting or location where they wish to be cared for. He suggests that there needs to be a clear understanding of the MCA (DH 2005a) as it is an integral part of end of life care.

 Chapters 4 and **13** for more details on the Mental Capacity Act.

 Reflection: points to consider

As a paramedic, think about how the management of some of your patients might change if they have an advance care plan. Have you considered this yourself?

DO NOT ATTEMPT CARDIOPULMONARY RESUSCITATION (DNACPR)

DNACPR orders have been a cause of significant concern to professionals, patients and their families in addressing their wishes at the end of their life (NHS National End of Life

Care Programme 2007). DNACPR decisions are an important element of care and a clear example of when advance decisions documenting the patient's wishes must be known in relation to future care and treatment. This will result in informed decisions being made in what can be stressful and emergency situations following calls from distressed relatives, carers or the general public. Stone et al. (2009) interviewed paramedics and questions were asked related to DNACPR. It concluded that almost all participants had used advanced cardiac life support on patients they thought were terminal and then wondered if the interventions they performed were right for the patient. Rosenberg et al. (2013) stated it is important to understand that 'do not resuscitate orders' (DNROs) do not equal 'do not treat'; discussions with the family, friends and carers are critical to help understand the patient's wishes along with the specific instructions where time allows.

The British Medical Association (Resuscitation Council UK 2016) offers guidance on decision-making for a person who is nearing their end of life from a terminal illness, when death is imminent and cardiopulmonary resuscitation (CPR) would not be successful, and there is no formal decision made and recorded. In such circumstances, any healthcare professional who makes a carefully considered decision not to start CPR should be supported by their senior colleagues, employers and professional bodies (Resuscitation Council UK 2016). But nonetheless these are sensitive and distressing discussions. Education for paramedics on patient-centred EoLC is essential to help increase confidence in DNACPR, which is only applicable to CPR.

Every Moment Counts (NCPC 2015) proposes a person-centred coordinated approach to care and describes critical outcomes and success factors in end of life care, support and treatment, from the perspective of the patient and their carers. The overall objective is to make the last stages of life as good as it can be for the patient and those closest to them. All those involved would need to be honest, confident and consistent in this approach. This means having honest and confident conversations as to what the patient's goals and plans might be during this time, also who are those people most important to the patient. By using a consistent approach this will allow for appropriate and timely support to be put in place. As part of these conversations explore the patient's needs with regard to any emotional, spiritual, physical and practical support they might need. This patient-centred approach can help to ensure coordinated care for all concerned.

Brady (2014) suggests that the legal and ethical responsibility for initiating or withholding CPR falls to the most senior clinician in charge (DH 2008), and given the frequency of this type of call, this will often fall to a paramedic.

Verbal wishes expressed by family or caregivers at the scene of resuscitation are difficult to validate and are not recognised as legitimate evidence against active resuscitation (Stone et al. 2009). Consequently, invasive treatments and resuscitation procedures can be initiated in situations when death is expected or imminent.

The final decision regarding the application or not of the CPR decision in an emergency rests with the healthcare professionals responsible for managing the patient's immediate situation. These healthcare professionals may, on attending an arrest, make a clinical assessment resulting in a different decision from the one on the CPR decision form. As with any clinical decisions, healthcare professionals must be able to justify their decision, in particular, clinicians should be cautious of overriding a DNACPR decision where the CPR decision form records that the patient has expressed a clear wish not to receive attempted CPR (Resuscitation Council UK 2016: 26).

In addition, patients who have valid DNACPR orders may undergo unwanted resuscitation if their documents are questioned or unknown by family members, friends and healthcare providers. To ensure paramedics and healthcare providers are aware of the needs and wishes of individuals, information systems must facilitate the sharing of information. The NHS publication *Promoting Innovative End of Life Care Practice within Ambulance Trusts* (DH 2007) provides excellent examples of practice initiatives across the country to meet the needs of patients at the end of their life, one of which is a DNACPR policy implemented by North West Ambulance NHS Trust.

Clinical guidelines issued by the Association of Ambulance Chief Executives advise paramedics that in the presence of cardiopulmonary arrest they should always initiate CPR unless the patient has a condition unequivocally associated with death, specifically massive cranial and cerebral destruction, hemicorporectomy or similar massive injury, rigor mortis, hypostasis, decomposition/putrefaction or incineration. The Ambulance Service guidelines state also that resuscitation can be discontinued where there is a formal DNACPR 'order' or an Advance Decision that states the wish of the patient not to undergo attempted resuscitation, or where a patient is in the final stages of a terminal illness where death is imminent and unavoidable and CPR would not be successful, but for whom no formal DNACPR decision has been made. Readers are urged to read the full Ambulance Service guidelines if more detailed information on ambulance clinicians' response to cardiorespiratory arrest is required. To ensure that paramedics do not start CPR against the recorded wishes of the patient, it is important that ambulance services have robust systems in place to record ADRTs and decisions about CPR, and to communicate these immediately to the paramedics who respond to an emergency call to a patient for whom such a document exists. With increasing use of electronic records such documents may be stored centrally. As paramedics have to satisfy themselves that the document exists and is valid in the circumstances encountered, an agreed method of emergency communication of any such decision, and of the basis for it, is necessary and should be subject to clinical governance (Resuscitation Council UK 2016: 29). Where documentation does not exist, the advice offered by the JRCALC guidelines (Brown, Kumar and Millins 2016) suggests that CPR may be discontinued or not even started, 'A patient in their final stages of a terminal illness where death is imminent and unavoidable and CPR would not be successful, but for whom no DNACPR decision has been made' (Brown, Kumar and Millins 2016: 46).

Another initiative is the 'Message in a Bottle' scheme. This scheme encourages healthcare professionals to leave information which is vital for paramedics in a labelled container in the fridge. A sticker is placed on the back of the patient's front door alerting them to the fact that they are part of the scheme.

PREFERRED PRIORITIES OF CARE

The Preferred Priorities of Care document is one example of an advance care plan. Originally known as the Preferred Place of Care (PPC) document, it was designed by Lancashire and South Cumbria Cancer Network and first introduced into practice in 2001 by Storey et al. (2003). The document is intended to be a patient-held record that follows the patient through their trajectory of care. The document enables patients and carers to discuss their main priorities at the end phase of life and promotes honest and open communication. Prompts include:

- In relation to your illness, what has been happening to you?
- What are your preferences and priorities for your future care?
- Where would you like to be cared for in the future?

Many patients express a wish to die at home (Resuscitation Council UK 2016) and as a result it will mean ambulance staff and paramedics will come into contact with patients who are nearing the end of their life, either as a result of planned transfers or where a sudden crisis occurs (Brown, Kumar and Millins 2016). These contacts may be due to a sudden change in their health or as the result of something completely unrelated to their main illness. Current JRCALC guidelines (Brown, Kumar and Millins 2016) offer robust advice regarding the management of this type of patient alongside clear guidance for dealing with any exacerbation of the underlying condition. The paramedic may find themselves attending a patient in the dying phase due to a sudden deterioration of the condition or unexpected complications that family members might not yet be prepared for. It is crucial that the paramedics respect all concerned, however, they must attempt to establish the patient's wishes, while acknowledging the possibility of differing views between family members and carers (Box 15.3). The competent patient's right to make an autonomous decision to stay at home and to receive palliative care must be supported by the practitioner, liaising with the GP to arrange that the patient receives the right care at the right time.

The National Ambulance Service Medical Directors (NASMeD 2014), when considering the future clinical priorities for ambulance services in England, acknowledged the involvement of the ambulance service in end of life care. Paramedics are frequently at the scene or shortly after the point of death and have to make decisions on whether resuscitation is required or would be futile, often based on limited knowledge of the patient's wishes. JRCALC (Brown, Kumar and Millins 2016) suggested key priorities, which were informed by the National End of Life Care Programme (2013), see Box 15.4.

Box 15.3 Pain management in end of life stage

- Pain relief is a duty of all clinicians when attending a patient at the end of their life.
- Similarly, a DNACPR does not mean any other appropriate care will be withheld.

Box 15.4 JRCALC (2016) suggested key end of life care clinical priorities for ambulance services in England

- Ensure that there is generic documentation regarding Do Not Resuscitate orders and when and when not to resuscitate policies.
- Ensure ambulance systems are linked to patient-specific end of life care plans so that paramedics have timely access to these care plans before they arrive with the patient.
- Ambulance service involvement with the development of end of life registers, potentially ambulance services can host these registers.
- Direct access to specialist palliative advice/services 24/7 for ambulance clinicians.
- Commissioning of bespoke transport and booking processes to ensure rapid discharge or transfer for patients who are at the end of life.
- Investment in regular education and training in end of life care for ambulance clinicians.
- Develop procedures around how paramedics can administer appropriate end of life medications to support patients who have accessed the ambulance service.
- Commissioning of integrated information systems, education programmes and appropriate arrangements for urgent 24/7 care provision.

As already stated, paramedics can find themselves in attendance at a patient who is near the end of their life which can occur as a result of numerous reasons. Conversations with the patient themselves or family members who might be in attendance can be very difficult, which sometimes result in becoming very clinically focused. It is important to remember that although there are some immediate decisions and assessments to be made, how this is handled will have a lasting effect on everyone involved (see Case study 15.1).

Case study 15.1

Joan is an 80-year-old lady with chronic obstructive pulmonary disease (COPD), she has been prescribed antibiotics by her GP for a recent chest infection. Joan is on the palliative care register as she is entering the end phase of her life, she has an advance care plan which states that wants to stay at home and also has a DNACPR. However, she is breathless and confused and incoherent so her anxious family has called an ambulance.

Consider how you might approach this situation, how might you interact with Joan and her family to ensure her needs and wishes are met and that, despite Joan's confusion, she is treated as a person and can remain at home?

Some key practical tips to help in end of life care situations

- *Consider the person* – try to establish something about the person that recognises them as a unique individual. People often try to cope with their illness by maintaining a sense of normality. Talking to the person or family about them while undertaking vital assessments helps them to feel more like a person than a patient. Sometimes there are clues in a person's home which help, photographs, trophies, pets, anything to help try to make a connection.
- *Recognise their importance* – remember that the person you are treating is so significant and important to members of their family. This is why care needs to be compassionate and communication needs to be honest and clear.
- *Personhood* – life-threatening illness can erode a person's sense of identity; they can suffer a variety of losses and changes. Illness affects how they look physically and how they are able to fulfil their roles in their family and society. All the interactions by healthcare professionals can have an impact on their self-esteem and feelings of self-worth, so all aspects of communication need to be person-centred.

BREAKING BAD/SIGNIFICANT NEWS

There are several models that can help guide difficult conversations, one example is the SPIKES model (Baile et al. 2000). This focuses on the delivery of significant news and the factors that influence how this news is given. It guides the information giver to consider the setting where the news is given, what is already understood, and encourages information to be given in small chunks so that understanding can be assessed. It is important to consider how news might be received and the emotional responses people may have, such as denial, anger and distress, all of which should be respected and supported. Finally, the model encourages the discussion of the next steps, ensuring no one is left uncertain of what will happen. For example, the attendance of the police officer, funeral director, or admission into hospital.

Chapter 1 for other models of communication that may be useful and **Chapter 2** for the power of reflection in such difficult situations.

 Reflection: points to consider

Reflect on an occasion where you had to give some difficult or significant news to a patient or relative. What went well? What would you do differently and how did you feel?

CONCLUSION

In conclusion, this chapter has introduced you to the policies and frameworks underpinning end of life care. The delivery of high quality end of life care can be a challenging part of your role as a paramedic or ambulance clinician. It requires multidisciplinary working and the successful implementation of the identified policies and initiatives to meet the needs of patients at the end of life. The GSF factsheet for paramedics suggests the following points for consideration before transporting a patient:

- Is there an advance care plan which may include information for DNACPR or where the patient wants to be cared for?
- Is there a decision to refuse treatment?
- Can you access the information you need?
- Can you use other options to avoid unnecessary admission?
- Is admission appropriate or could other services help?
- Can you avoid transporting a patient who is in the last weeks/days of their life when they wish to die in their home or care home?

Chapter key points:

- An understanding of the policies and frameworks underpinning end of life care will inform your practice.
- Multidisciplinary working is key to ensuring patients' needs are met.
- Too few people die at home or in their preferred place of choice.
- Initiating discussions about preferences for end of life care is essential.
- Everyone is involved in end of life care.

REFERENCES AND SUGGESTED READING

Baile, W., Buckman, R., Lenato, R., Glober, G., Beale, E.A. and Kudelka, A.J. (2000) SPIKES: A six step protocol for delivering bad news: Application to the patient with cancer. *The Oncologist*, 5(4): 302–11.

Brady, M. (2014) Challenges UK paramedics currently face in providing fully effective end-of-life care. *International Journal of Palliative Nursing*, 20(1).

Brown, S.N., Kumar, D. and Millins, M. (eds for JRCALC and AACE) (2016) *UK Ambulance Service Clinical Practice Guidelines*. Bridgwater: Class Professional Publishing.

Clark, D., Small, N., Wright, M., Winslow, M. and Hughes, N. (2005) *A Bit of Heaven for the Few? An Oral History of the Modern Hospice Movement in the United Kingdom*. Lancaster: Observatory Publications.

DH (Department of Health) (2005a) *Mental Capacity Act*. London: HMSO.

DH (Department of Health) (2005b) *Mental Capacity Act Code of Practice*. Available at: www.dca.gov.uk/legal-policy/mentalcapacity/mca-cp.pdf (accessed 11 February 2017).

DH (Department of Health) (2007) *Promoting Innovative End of Life Care Practice within Ambulance Trusts*. London: DH.

DH (Department of Health) (2008a) *High Quality Care for All: NHS Next Stage Review*. London: DH.

DH (2008b) *End of Life Care Strategy: Promoting High Quality Care for All Adults at the End of Life*. London: DH.

DH (Department of Health) (2010a) *End of Life Care Strategy: Promoting High Quality Care for All Adults at the End of Life*. London: DH.

DH (Department of Health) (2010b) *End of Life Care Strategy: Second Annual Report*. London: DH.

DH (Department of Health) (2013a) *More Care, Less Pathway. A Review of the Liverpool Care Pathway*. London: DH.

DH (Department of Health) (2013b) *Advance Decisions to Refuse Treatment: A Guide for Health and Social Care Staff*. London: DH.

DH (Department of Health) (2015) *Long-Term Health Conditions*. London: DH.

Dying Matters (2015) http://www.dyingmatters.org/

Gold Standards Framework (GSF) (2009) *Factsheet 6: Paramedics,* May 2009. Available at: http://www.goldstandardsframework.org.uk/ (accessed 11 August 2017).

House of Commons (2004) *House of Commons Health Committee: Palliative Care. Fourth Report of Session 2003–2004*. London: The Stationery Office.

National Ambulance Service Medical Directors (NASMeD) (2014) *Future National Clinical Priorities for Ambulance Services in England*. Available at: http://aace.org.uk/wp-content/uploads/2014/05/Future-national-clinical-priorities-for-ambulance-services-in-England-FINAL-2.pdf (accessed 1 August 2017).

National Council for Palliative Care (2010) *End of Life Care Manifesto*. London: NCPC.

National Council for Pallative Care (2015) *Every Moment Counts: A New Vision for Co-ordinated Care for People Near the End of Life Calls for Brave Conversations*. London: NCPC.

National End of Life Care Intelligence Network (NELCIN) (2014) http://www.endoflifecare-intelligence.org.uk/home (accessed 1 August 2017).

National End of Life Care Programme (2007) *Promoting Innovative End of Life Care Practice Within Ambulance Trusts*. London: DH.

National End of Life Care Programme (2008) *Advance Care Planning: A Guide for Health and Social Care Staff*. London: DH.

National End of Life Care Programme (2013) *The Route to Success in End of Life Care: Achieving Quality for Ambulance Services*. London: DH.

National Palliative and End of Life Care Partnership (2015) Ambitions for palliative and end of life care: a national framework for local action 2015–2020. www.endoflifecareambitions.org.uk

NHS England (2014) *Actions for End of Life Care: 2014–16*. London: NHS England

NICE (2011) NICE Quality Standards for End of Life Care. Available at: https://www.nice.org.uk/guidance/qs13

Northern England Clinical Network (2014) Deciding Right. Available at: http:/www.necn.nhs.uk/common-themes/deciding-right/

Resuscitation Council UK (2016) *Decisions Relating to Cardiopulmonary Resuscitation. Guidance from the British Medical Association, the Resuscitation Council and the Royal College of Nursing*. 3rd edn. London: NHS Improving Quality.

Rosenberg, M., Lamba, S. and Misra, S. (2013) Palliative medicine and geriatric emergency care: challenges, opportunities, and basic principles. *Journal of Clinical Geriatric Medicine*, 29(1): 1–29.

Saunders, C. (2005) *Watch with Me*. Lancaster: Observatory Publications.

Stone, S., Abbott, J., McClung, C.D. et al. (2009) Paramedic knowledge, attitudes and training in end of life care. *Prehospital and Disaster Medicine*, 24(6): 529–34.

Storey, L., Pemberton, C., Howard, A. and O'Donnell, L. (2003) Place of death: Hobson's choice or patient choice? *Cancer Nursing Practice*, 3: 33–8.

Thomas, C., Morris, S.M. and Clark, D. (2004) Place of death: preferences among cancer patients and their carers. *Social Science and Medicine*, 58: 2431–44.

WHO (World Health Organisation) (2010) Available at: http://www.who.int/cancer/palliative/definition/en/ (accessed 15 August 2017).

Leadership styles and the impact on practice

Alison Cork and Kath Jennings

In this chapter:

- Introduction
- Why is this relevant?
- Paramedic leadership within a multi-professional context
- Leadership styles and the impact on practice
- Conclusion
- Chapter key points
- References and suggested reading

INTRODUCTION

This chapter discusses the variety of leadership styles and the work of several eminent theorists in this field. The subject of leadership is discussed in relation to the pre-hospital environment and the unique work of paramedics, where applicable and appropriate. Chapter 17 looks at the theory which lies behind the decision-making process.

WHY IS THIS RELEVANT?

Paramedics make leadership decisions on a daily basis. Some involve life and death decisions; others are less urgent but may still impact on the outcome for many patients and their families. It is hoped that the content of this chapter may impact on your future patient care.

PARAMEDIC LEADERSHIP WITHIN A MULTI-PROFESSIONAL CONTEXT

There are a number of key sources of evidence with which students of paramedic leadership should become familiar. These include documents on the required Standards of Proficiency at the point of registration from the paramedics' regulatory body, the Health and Care Professions Council (HCPC); advisory documents from paramedics' professional body, the College of Paramedics (CoP); commentary documents from renowned and respected organisations such as the King's Fund, and quality benchmark statements from the government agency on paramedic education, the Quality Assurance Agency

(QAA). In addition to these, there is a small but growing body of research in the field of pre-hospital, out-of-hospital, paramedic, and ambulance service leadership.

The HCPC specifically identify that registered paramedics should 'understand the concept of leadership and its application to practice' (HCPC 2014: 12). The Subject Benchmark Statements for paramedics (QAA 2016) number one key change from their previous publication in 2004 is the development of clinical leadership for paramedics and specifically that 'graduate paramedics should be able to articulate and rationalise clinical leadership, problem-solving and decision-making processes associated with paramedic practice as a registered healthcare professional' (QAA 2016: 18).

Team working is implicit in the Standards of Conduct, Performance and Ethics (HCPC 2016), and the QAA include knowledge of leadership and teamwork theories as knowledge applicable to safe and competent practice as a paramedic. Delegation is explicitly identified in the Standards of Proficiency for Paramedics (HCPC 2014), Standards of Conduct, Performance and Ethics (HCPC 2016a) for registrants as well as the Guidance on Conduct and Ethics for Students (HCPC 2016b). The standards and statements demonstrate the attributes desirable for every graduating paramedic and emphasise the link between leadership, team working and delegation.

Since the Bradley Report (DH 2005), there have been a number of leadership strategies and frameworks introduced by the NHS. These can be confusing to navigate through since they all have similar-sounding titles and superficially focus on the same thing. However, there are differences which reflect the paradigm shift from the individual to teams. The early frameworks focused initially upon doctors (Medical Leadership Competency Framework, NHS Institute for Innovation and Improvement 2009), then were widened to all clinical staff (Clinical Leadership Competency Framework, NHS Leadership Academy 2011) via the newly established NHS Leadership Academy.

Link to **Chapter 8** in *Clinical Leadership for Paramedics*, edited by Blaber and Harris (2014).

The domains identified in the Clinical Leadership Competency Framework have titles suggestive of a focus on management, yet they can be applied to all paramedics at every level of their development. They are setting direction, improving services, managing services, with personal development domains identified as demonstrating personal qualities and working with others. The Leadership Framework (NHS Leadership Academy 2011) mirrored these domains and sought to develop leadership behaviours among wider groups of individuals within large organisations rather than leave leadership matters to nominated and named persons. In paramedic practice, these domains relate to a range of behaviours, such as developing networks and building relationships, and are demonstrated in multi-professional working, sharing responsibilities, team working

Case study 16.1

Peter is a 59-year-old cardiac patient experiencing abdominal discomfort. After calling 999 for help, he is assessed by a paramedic who discovers that Peter is prescribed more than five different types of medication in tablet form to be taken per day. Peter collects his prescription boxes every two weeks from the pharmacy, returns home and then transfers all the tablets into one large old vitamin bottle. Each day he shakes a few out into the palm of his hand and swallows them with water. The paramedic ascertains that while Peter is able-bodied and self-caring, he has no idea what quantity of any drug he is taking each day but that he believes he is compliant with his medication regime. Peter agrees to be seen by a doctor that day but also requires better medicine management.

En route to hospital the ambulance stops at Peter's local pharmacy and, with Peter's consent, the paramedic requests a blister pack for future dispensation of medications. The paramedic then communicates this decision to Peter's GP by telephone, while on the way to the hospital.

and crew resource management. They are evident when a crew plan the best course of action in the best interests of a patient, no matter how small the intervention appears.

The Healthcare Leadership Model (NHS Leadership Academy 2013) now surpasses previous frameworks. While maintaining a focus on behaviours, it relates easily to those who identify themselves as working in teams and explicitly links leadership development with positive outcomes for both staff and for patients.

In Case study 16.1 the paramedic has demonstrated leadership by using joint decision-making to seek a more effective use of the existing services provided to the patient. He has used problem solving, decision-making and communication skills, and has cooperated with the patient and other stakeholders to improve quality of care.

It is now common for paramedics to make decisions together with service users which result in the utilisation of a pathway or referral process and that does not result in a trip to the emergency department. Collaboration with other healthcare professionals involved in patient care can influence decision-making and highlights a need for collective leadership to extend beyond the small team.

In Case study 16.2 the paramedic not only assesses and manages the presenting medical emergency but goes on to demonstrate leadership within a multi-professional context through her liaison with other stakeholders involved in the care of the patient. A shared decision is reached between the paramedic and the patient which empowers the patient. Key players in the successful patient interaction are the GP, the respiratory nurse and the pharmacist. There is recognition on the paramedic's part that

Case study 16.2

Anne is a 65-year-old patient experiencing an acute episode of COPD. She is tachyp-noeic with shortness of breath and a wheeze on auscultation. Anne usually manages her condition well and has an emergency pack for such episodes but has not had it replaced since her last attack 6 months ago. Anne is reluctant to attend hospital.

The paramedic conducts a full assessment and begins to reverse the acute episode with medication. She then contacts Anne's respiratory nurse to discuss the episode and together with Anne they make a plan. The paramedic contacts Anne's GP to report the episode, share the plan and to arrange a replacement emergency pack, which is available for collection at the local pharmacy. Anne's respiratory nurse calls back and brings forward her next home assessment.

appropriate, compassionate and patient-centred care cannot be met by intervention by just one profession (Richardson 2014).

 Link to **Chapter 6** in *Clinical Leadership for Paramedics*, edited by Blaber and Harris (2014).

LEADERSHIP STYLES AND THEIR IMPACT ON PRACTICE

Leadership is a complex process by which a person influences others to accomplish a mission, task or objective and it is a role which is implicit in paramedic practice. From leading the coordinated approach to a multiple casualty situation, to working with a colleague and assuming control of the situation, the philosophy of leadership is similar. By examining different models this section of the chapter will then concentrate on the characteristics of a good leader. Finally, it will look at the requirements of a good follower, which is essential if the process is to succeed.

What constitutes a leader?

Good leaders develop through a continuous process of reflection, education and experience. However, in order to provide good leadership, you must commence with the conclusion in mind in order to have a clear understanding of your destination. Leadership is a multifac-eted process by which a person influences others to achieve a mission, task or objective and directs the organisation in a way that makes it more unified and consistent. North-ouse (2015) argues that some people are leaders because of their formal position within an organisation whereas others are leaders because of the way other group members respond to them. He describes these two types of leadership as 'assigned' and 'emer-gent' respectively. The assigned leader would be the boss. The emergent leader would be the person within the group who has the most influence, regardless of their title.

Emergent leadership is acquired through other people in the organisation who support and accept the person's behaviour and it is always salutary to remember that being the boss does not make you the leader; it merely gives you the power.

The work of John Adair

John Adair, a military tutor by background, developed his 'Action-centred Leadership model' while lecturing at Sandhurst Royal Military Academy. He helped change the accepted perception of management to encompass leadership and has written over 25 books on the subject. Adair (2009) asserts that there are core functions of leadership which can be applied in any situation:

- *Planning* – seeking information, setting aims, defining tasks.
- *Initiating* – briefing, task allocation, setting standards.
- *Controlling* – maintaining standards, ensuring progress, ongoing decision-making.
- *Supporting* – monitoring and rewarding individuals' contributions, encouraging team spirit, morale boosting, reconciling.
- *Informing* – clarifying tasks and plans, updating, receiving feedback and interpreting.
- *Evaluating* – feasibility of ideas, performance, enabling self-assessment.

Action-centred leadership

The action-centred leadership model is a simple model which is easy to remember and straightforward to apply in clinical practice in relation to both leadership and management. Adair (2009) recognises there are three elements to effective leadership that require attention from individuals in a leadership position:

- Task
- Team
- Individual

It is part of an integrated approach and although the three elements are collectively dependent, they are also independently crucial. In his model Adair represents the three areas as circles and the point where all three circles overlap (see Figure 16.1) he considers to be where effective leadership is occurring and all three elements are in perfect balance.

Adair maintains that good leaders should have full control of the three main areas and that being able to do all these things and keep the balance right gets results by developing the team and productivity, building morale and enhancing quality, and this is the mark of a successful manager and leader.

Within each domain there are certain elements for the leader to consider and achieve (see Box 16.1).

Within the clinical field, all the above factors happen simultaneously and are rarely analysed in any great depth. For example, when managing a multiple casualty situation,

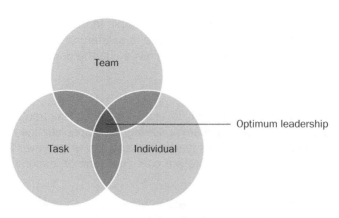

Figure 16.1 Example of overlapping circles

Box 16.1 Elements which require completion

The task	The team	The individual
Define the task	Resolve conflict	Assist and support individuals
Identify resources	Develop team working	Agree individual responsibilities
Create the plan	Encourage the team to achieve the task	Give recognition and praise
Establish the responsibilities	Give feedback to the group	Develop individual freedom and autonomy
Set the standards	Understand the team members	
Control and maintain the activities		
Monitor overall performance		
Review, reassess, adjust plan		
Establish standards of performance and behaviour		
Monitor and maintain discipline and integrity		

---

the focus will be on the task, i.e. the prioritisation of care and safe transfer to definitive facilities. One of the leader's aims is to identify the resources available, i.e. the people and equipment required and available to manage the situation. Responsibilities should be established and all team members should be aware of their role and that of their colleagues in order to achieve the task. Activities should be controlled and maintained by the leaders and regular reports on progress should be imparted to the team.

The team are established in that they are the available people to manage the situation. The responsibilities of the leader are to focus the group on their objectives and encourage them to achieve their aims. Effective communications should be established both within the team and with external agencies in order that feedback on overall progress and achievement may be attained.

The leader should recognise the individual variants in terms of personality, skills, strengths and needs. The team members should be given recognition for their achievements and support when they need guidance or tuition. This should be embedded in all teams in order for them to function at a productive level; however, the leader should recognise extraordinary contributions to the team and reward these appropriately.

Leadership is the style and manner in which a situation is approached. There are normally three styles and the emphasis of power is different for each one (Box 16.2):

- *Authoritarian*: With an authoritarian style the dominant power base lies with the boss and employees hold a non-dominant power base.
- *Participative*: Both the boss and employees hold a dominant power base with this style of leadership.
- *Delegative*: The power base of dominance lies with employees and the non-dominant power base is held by the boss.

While it is inevitable that one style will dominate behaviour, a good leader will use all three approaches and be able to alter this in any given situation. However, there are certain factors which will determine the style to be used and these are:

- Resources available, i.e. time, financial, equipment.
- Basis of relationships, i.e. trust, distrust.
- Who holds the information: you, the employees, both?
- Knowledge and skills of you and your employees.
- Internal dynamics of the team.
- Positive and negative stress levels.

Box 16.2 Emphasis of power with different approaches

Power style	Dominant power base	Non-dominant power base
Authoritarian	Boss	Employees
Participative	Boss and employees	
Delegative	Employees	Boss

Adapted from Adair (2009)

Reflection: points to consider

What style of leadership do you think best describes you? Is this how others see you?

Authoritarian

This is a style which does not look for the advice of followers; rather it is used when the leader tells the employees what they want done and how they want it done. This is most commonly used when all the information to solve the problem is available, employees are well motivated and time is of the essence. There is no room for negotiation within the decision. This could be an approach to be used in resuscitation. In this situation the leader is very much in command. From the didactic approach of resuscitation courses, all members of the team will know their roles. The leader has to assess the problem quickly, work out a management plan and then give clear orders to the rest of the team. Although the leader will listen to suggestions from the members of the team, most of the direction and orders will come from the leader. Here the needs of the individual staff members are of a low priority while the key objective of saving the patient's life is paramount.

Although one can understand the reasons why this style is adopted in this situation, the good leader will recognise that the casualty of this style of leadership is the follower. This style can be used when working with a non-registered practitioner who is new to the job and needs direction and firm guidance. However, it must be noted that taking such an inflexible approach does not allow the followers to develop problem-solving skills for themselves and limits individual growth; this is acceptable if, in the whole scheme of the work scenario, it is tempered with periods of participative styles of leadership.

Participative

This style of leadership involves employee participation in the decision-making process. Within this style one or more followers are involved in the decision-making process. However, the leader maintains the final decision-making authority. This is a sign of strength that employees will respect and is normally used when you have part of the information and your employees have other parts. It is inclusive and acknowledges that employees have a valuable contribution to make when shaping the service within which they work. This style sends the message that the leader cannot be expected to know everything and this is why you employ skilful and knowledgeable employees. This style may be adopted when working with an experienced crew who know their job. The leader knows the problem and the workers know their job and can offer advice on how to solve it.

Delegative (free rein)

In this style the decision is made solely by the employees, but the leader still carries the responsibility. This is used when the followers are able to analyse the situation and determine what needs to be done and how to do it. This style is to be used when you have full trust and confidence in the people around you as you cannot blame others when things go wrong. This would be used with a crew who knew more about the job than you did. Although you may be first on scene and assume overall command of the situation, if a crew arrived to assist who had been in the same situation before, then you would delegate the role of leadership to them.

The example in Case study 16.3 demonstrates paramedic leadership, team working, communication, and delegation skills in the provision of advanced life support to a patient experiencing an out-of-hospital cardiac arrest. The authors of the Research Council United Kingdom's (RCUK) guidelines on the management of pre-hospital resuscitation are clear in their emphasis on the team approach and the establishment of both clearly identified roles and a system for managing the emergency (Deakin et al. 2015). The systematic management of out-of-hospital cardiac arrest led to this historically been interpreted as an example of authoritarian leadership by paramedics. However, in step with the evolution of theory and practice, the skills demonstrated in the example above are more demonstrative of situational or relational leadership.

Transformational leadership

Although in contemporary practice an authoritarian and task-led approach to leadership is sometimes used, there are other models that incorporate the softer side of leadership which can be equally successful. The transformational approach to leadership challenges the autocratic unilateral leadership style of former years. It strives to elevate the needs of followers that are harmonious with their own goals and objectives and it achieves this through charisma, intellectual ability and individual consideration. The transformational leader is characterised as a visionary or catalyst for change who can

---

Case study 16.3

A paramedic crew respond to a 56-year-old male in cardiac arrest. After initiating basic life support they are assisted by a second ambulance crew. Immediately on their arrival the crews exchange names and roles, and a handover is given without interruption to chest compressions. The lead paramedic delegates tasks and responsibilities associated with advanced life support checking for understanding and confirming actions. Upon return of spontaneous circulation, a reversible cause is established and the crew work together under the leadership and delegation of the lead paramedic to haemodynamically stabilise the patient, before preparing him for transfer to an appropriate receiving facility.

motivate and energise staff to pursue mutual goals, share vision and create an empowering culture. With transformational leadership, both the leader and the follower have the same purpose and they raise one another to higher levels of performance. It also relies on mutuality, cooperation rather than competition, networking rather than hierarchy and empowerment of all employees. It recognises individuals' potential and will go further to satisfy higher-level needs such as self-esteem and achieving their full potential (Giltinane 2013). The results of such an approach are that of increased work satisfaction and a low staff turnover. Workers are more likely to stick with an organisation that values their ideas and thoughts and which creates an empowering culture.

When examining the concept of recognising the value of workers through thoughts and ideas, the ideology of emotional intelligence is worthy of note. Taylor and Armitage (2012) cogently argue that leadership as a concept is fundamentally human. It is widely accepted that not all communication is verbal, and recognising and understanding the non-verbal cues that co-workers emit is paramount in managing expectations. 'Emotional intelligence' can be described as the ability to recognise and interpret their own and others' emotions in a situation, using this as a guide in leadership situations. Giltinane (2013) cites Goleman (1998), who states that the most effective leaders possess emotional intelligence. Furthermore he asserts that regardless of all other variables in leadership abilities, a leader will never be great without emotional intelligence. However, this is an alternative view of leadership for paramedics to consider. Delmatoff (2014) claims that for many leaders maintaining the status quo is not an ideal, and recommends that by adopting an emotionally and behaviourally intelligent style of leadership, staff will feel a greater sense of empowerment. He explains this by considering that emotional intelligence starts with self-awareness. Having the ability to objectively understand one's own emotional and behavioural reactions helps to recognise the effect those reactions have on others, thus mitigating undesired effects. Emotional awareness then goes one step further in that it is the ability to pick up on others' reactions and analyse why such reactions may be given. This can be used in a clinical situation, Johnson et al. (2013) argue that leadership is a core function of the paramedic, whether in clinical or management roles. Standards of leadership affect relationships with patients, colleagues, multi-agency partners and within organisational frameworks. For some paramedics, the concept of emotional leadership may be deemed as soft and too 'squishy' to give any practical value. Delmatoff (2014) insists that enlightened leaders in the military, industry and business are finding real value in understanding the concept of emotional leadership and incorporating it into their style of leadership.

 Reflection: points to consider

Have you been in a situation where emotional leadership has been used? How can you ensure that you incorporate it into your leadership style?

Although there are more than three hundred definitions of leadership currently available, Cullen (2007) urges caution and suggests that effective leaders operate in a multi-dimensional framework that combines a multitude of skills, styles, attributes and abilities. He cites numerous leaders in history and argues that it is only the effective parts of their leadership that are concentrated upon, with the narrative largely ignoring the less helpful aspects.

Chapter 1 for more in-depth information about communication theory: **Chapter 2** to explore the potential value of reflective practice and **Chapter 6** for detail on human factors.

Along with the emerging styles of leadership, there is an acknowledgement that the topic of followers is also worthy of further study. Barr and Dowding (2015) stipulate that without followers, there cannot be leaders and vice versa.

Followers will go along with the leaders for a number of different reasons, some personal, others more objective. Some examples might be if the followers respect both the leader and the solution, if they trust the leader not to lead them into disarray, or if they like the personal characteristics of the leader. Northouse (2015) claims that the degree to which followers have the competence and commitment necessary to accomplish a given task or activity is their developmental level. This is supported by Hughes et al. (2011), who state that junior followers will need almost constant guidance, coaching and comment whereas senior ones only need general guidance and periodic feedback in order to maintain high levels of performance. Moreover, they assert that the inexperienced refer to the experienced for guidance and advice on how to improve their performance. Within the framework of work-based learning for the student paramedic and support worker, the student would look to the senior for guidance and feedback on performance. This model also helps to create new leaders as good leaders create good followers who then become good leaders, and so on. However, it has to be acknowledged that in order for the follower to develop the leadership skills required, they must be empowered to do so. Rolfe (2011) maintains that empowered followers possess higher core qualities, such as loyalty to the organisation, motivation to succeed and job satisfaction. Furthermore, this in turn leads to decreased levels of sickness and promotes a positive work environment.

This shows that success or failure is not dependent on the leader but the followers have a role to play and this must be recognised.

Reflection: points to consider

Think of examples where you have been a follower or a leader. Which skills are required for each?

CONCLUSION

Many emerging leaders are rather confused about their leadership style and the approach that they wish to adopt with their team. It must be recognised that leadership starts at the point of qualification and the role develops alongside the individual. The role of followers in the leadership strategies must be examined, as this will enable the true leader to understand the levels of support that they are given. Paramedics are leaders of care, teams and themselves on a daily basis. In order for this leadership role to develop, there needs to be investment and education at an early stage in order that paramedics can critically analyse their leadership style and develop accordingly.

Chapter key points:

- Being the boss does not make you the leader; it merely gives you the power.
- Leadership does not have to be on a large scale; rather it can be on a 'job-to-job' basis.

REFERENCES AND SUGGESTED READING

Adair, J. (2009) *Effective Leadership*. London: Pan.

Barr, J. and Dowding, L. (2015) *Leadership in Health Care*, 3rd edn. London: Sage.

Cullen, J. (2007) Front line leadership: a challenge to the continual search for the holy grail of an all-encompassing leadership model. *Leadership in Public Services*, 3(1): 4–16.

Deakin, C., Brown, S., Jewkes, F., Lockey, D., et al. (2015) *Prehospital Resuscitation*. Resuscitation Council (UK). Available at: https://www.resus.org.uk/resuscitation-guidelines/prehospital-resuscitation/

Delmatoff, J. (2014) The most effective leadership style for the new landscape of healthcare. *Journal of Healthcare Management*, 59(4): 245–9.

DH (Department of Health) (2005) *Taking Healthcare to the Patient: Transforming NHS Ambulance Services*. London: Department of Health.

Giltinane, C.L. (2013) Leadership styles and theories. *Nursing Standard*, 270(41): 35–9.

Goleman, D. (1998) The emotionally competent leader. *The Healthcare Forum Journal*, 41(2): 36–43.

Grohar-Murray, M. and DiCroce, H. (2010) *Leadership and Management in Nursing*, 4th edn. London: Prentice-Hall.

Health and Care Professions Council (2014) *Standards of Proficiency: Paramedics*. London: Health and Care Professions Council.

HCPC (Health and Care Professions Council (2016a) *Standards of Conduct, Performance and Ethics*. London: Health and Care Professions Council.

Health and Care Professions Council (2016b) *Guidance on Conduct and Ethics for Students*. London: Health and Care Professions Council.

Hughes, R., Ginnett, R. and Curphy, G. (2011) *Leadership: Enhancing the Lessons of Experience*, 7th edn. London: McGraw-Hill.

Johnson, D., Bainbridge, P. and Hazard, W. (2013) Understanding a new model of leadership. *Journal of Paramedic Practice*, 5(12): 686–90.

McCormick, S. and Wardrope, J. (2003) Major incidents, leadership, and series summary review. *Emergency Medicine Journal*, 20: 70–4.

Murphy, L. (2005) Transformational leadership: a cascading chain reaction. *Journal of Nursing Management*, 12: 128–36.

NHS Institute for Innovation and Improvement (2009) *Medical Leadership Competency Framework*, 2nd edn. London: Royal Medical Colleges.

NHS Leadership Academy (2011) *Leadership Framework*. Coventry: NHS Institute for Innovation and Improvement.

NHS Leadership Academy (2013) *Healthcare Leadership Model: The Nine Dimensions of Leadership Behaviour*. Version 1. Available at: https://www.leadershipacademy.nhs.uk/wp-content/uploads/2014/10/NHSLeadership-LeadershipModel-colour.pdf (accessed 30 August 2017).

Northouse, P. (2015) *Leadership Theory and Practice*, 7th edn. London: Sage.

Quality Assurance Agency (2016) *Subject Benchmark Statements. Paramedics*. Gloucester: The Quality Assurance Agency for Higher Education.

Richardson, M. (2014) Working as a team: understanding group dynamics. In A.Y. Blaber and G. Harris (eds) *Clinical Leadership for Paramedics*. Maidenhead: Open University Press.

Rolfe, P. (2011) Transformational Leadership Theory: what every leader needs to know. *Nurse Leader*, 9(2): 54–7.

Taylor, J. and Armitage, E. (2012) Leadership with the ambulance service: rhetoric or reality? *Journal of Paramedic Practice*, 4(10): 546–68.

The King's Fund (2015). *Leadership and Leadership Development in Health Care: The Evidence Base*. London: The King's Fund.

Theories of decision-making
Alison Cork and Mike Brady

In this chapter:

- Introduction
- Why is this relevant?
- What is decision-making?
- Critical thinking
- Models of decision-making
- Remote clinical decision-making
- Conclusion
- Chapter key points
- References and suggested reading

INTRODUCTION

Paramedics make decisions every day while planning and delivering care within their scope of practice. Successful and reliable decision-making requires the gathering and use of relevant data as well as higher-order thinking skills such as decision-making and critical thinking. This chapter will explore theories of decision-making, its various influences and relate it to the paramedic's practice.

WHY IS THIS RELEVANT?

Simpson et al. (2017) propose that traditionally the role of the paramedic has been a largely protocol-driven vocation with minimal autonomy and limited clinical responsibility. However, they argue that this is changing and the role now encompasses a much broader scope of practice which demands higher levels of clinical decision-making, professional judgement and accountability than ever before. Given the current demands of the service, this can only be anticipated to increase.

In order for paramedics to meet the current and future demands of clinical practice, it is fundamental that they must reflect upon and analyse decisions made. In order to achieve this, it is beneficial to use a model which deconstructs the decision-making process into its component parts. This allows the practitioner to learn from their experiences and formulate action plans for the future in order to improve practice and ultimately patient care. However, decision-making is not linear or exempt from outside influences, but by increasing awareness of external influences, the paramedic can view decision-making in a more effective manner.

WHAT IS DECISION-MAKING?

Effective decision-making is a pivotal role in the delivery of quality care and the advancement of clinical services at both an organisational and an individual level. It is a process which happens with every episode of patient contact, although the progression or external influence of the decision is rarely analysed in any depth. Muoni (2012) suggests that a competent decision-maker should develop the skills to be able to analyse multi-faceted problems and outcomes concurrently. Although reflection is embedded in practice for all, this often only happens when the outcome of a decision is adverse. Rarely are decisions analysed in any depth when a positive outcome is gained. This then denies the learning process that could accompany it.

 Chapter 2 for examples of models of reflection.

Following a decision-making model enables the component parts of any action to be analysed and the weakness or strength of the decision-making process to be recognised. However, decisions in clinical practice rarely follow a linear logical pattern; theories are printed in black and white and much of paramedic practice occurs in the grey area.

Intertwined with clinical decision-making is that of problem-solving and these two concepts are often used interchangeably, though there are subtle differences. Decision-making is where alternative courses of action are judged on their merits and only one of these is ultimately selected, whereas problem-solving is a process in which a dilemma, once analysed, is identified and the cause then corrected. It encompasses the decision-making process, which is said to be synonymous with management and is one of the criteria on which management expertise is judged. Problem-solving is a systematic process that focuses on analysing a difficult situation; considerable time and energy are spent on identifying the real problem and it can be described as the precursor to decision-making. In practice, however, it is sometimes difficult to separate the two, for example, the paramedic dealing with a violent patient might choose not to solve the root cause of the violent conduct, such as personality trait, alcohol or drug intoxication or dependence. As an alternative, he may choose to use only decision-making skills to call for police assistance to facilitate removal of the patient to police custody. The paramedic has, therefore, made the decision to remove the problem, i.e. the violent patient, rather than examine the cause of the patient's behaviour and address that. This is not opting out of the situation; rather it is identifying the resources available and using them to best advantage. Muoni (2012) advocates that prior to making any decision, there should be recognition that all available information about the problem is available. This ensures that informed decision-making becomes the norm.

What can help us make decisions?

Decision-making exists within a framework of classifications. Routine decisions are those that are made when the problem is well defined and commonplace in practice. There are usually established policies and procedures which can be used to guide decision-makers as the problem has been examined and solved by previous practitioners before them. The JRCALC Clinical Practice Guidelines (Brown, Kumar and Millins 2016) are a good example of this as they guide the practitioner through a range of situations which lead to the obvious treatment plans. In contrast, adaptive decisions are where problems and alternative solutions are somewhat unusual and only partially understood. There may be a policy to support the decision-making process but as the problem and solution are ill defined, creative thought may be necessary. The last area is that of innovative decisions. This is when the problem is unusual and unclear and in order to make a decision, creative thinking and innovative solutions are necessary (Sullivan and Garland 2013). An example of this would be referring a patient with a mental health problem directly to her community psychiatric nurse rather than her general practitioner because of the patient's preference. This decision would circumnavigate the accepted practice of contacting the general practitioner but would be more individualised for the patient. The chance to discuss these decisions with colleagues is invaluable and individual ambulance services have implemented strategies of clinical telephone advice desks. These enable practitioners to talk through complex patients who may require treatment which is beyond current protocol. The paramedic who provides the telephone advice has access to a range of software, literature and medical advice to help guide the practitioner in the decisions that they make. Within emergency work there are routine decisions that fall within policy and procedures, but there may be the need for innovative decisions if the patient's situation warrants it. It is then that an understanding of the decision-making process will be invaluable to guide the paramedic to the best course of action. Jenson et al. (2009) feel that there is a paucity of research within the paramedic population in relation to decision-making. Moreover, they add that it is most likely that weak abilities in the clinical decision-making process may lead to clinical errors.

 Reflection: points to consider

What enables you to make decisions? Think of an example where you may not have agreed with policy and procedures. What difference might it have made to a patient outcome?

Decision-making is a complex cognitive process that is often described as *choosing a particular course of action*, implying that there are several courses of action that could be taken and that a considered judgement is required to decide which route to follow. Inherent within decision-making is the concept of 'critical thinking'. This is purposeful, goal-oriented thinking that is based on a body of knowledge which is derived from research and other sources of authenticated evidence (Ignatavicius 2001). It is more complex than problem-solving and decision-making because it involves a higher level of reasoning and deductive thinking.

CRITICAL THINKING

Decision-making relies heavily on critical thinking skills and those who are successful will possess some or all of the skills required. Heidari and Shahbazi (2016) maintain that in order to make competent decisions and maintain professional competence, possessing the competence of critical thinking is essential.

Furthermore, they develop this concept and recommend that the best setting for teaching these higher-order skills is the clinical setting, so being able to combine authenticity and patient centredness. They support this by arguing that case-based lectures do not allow the learner to develop these skills due to the physical separation between student and teacher and the passive nature of learning in these settings.

Sullivan and Garland (2013) quantify the concept and describe it as the process of probing underlying assumptions, interpreting and evaluating arguments, imagining and exploring alternatives and developing a sense of reflective criticism. This supports Marquis and Huston (2012), who affirm that critical thinking is related to evaluation, which in itself is broader than decision-making and requires the skills of conceptualisation, analysis, synthesis and evaluation of information. These are all integral to effective practice and are described in Box 17.1.

There are certain qualities that successful decision-makers will possess. They have to have the willingness to take a risk, the sensitivity to react to both the situation and the other members involved in the decision-making process, the energy to make things happen, and the creativity to develop new ways to solve problems. Such people have a

---

Box 17.1 Critical thinking skills

- Interpretation – clarifying, examining data
- Analysis – understanding data
- Evaluation – determining the desired outcome
- Inference – coming to your conclusions
- Explanation – justifying actions taken based on data collected
- Self-regulation – examining your own practice.

Adapted from Ignatavicius (2001)

lot of 'balls to juggle', but they do possess a repertoire of skills that they can call on to assist them in the decision-making process. They are:

- open to new ideas;
- intuitive;
- having plenty of energy;
- the ability to analyse;
- good communicators;
- assertive;
- adaptable in their thinking;
- resourceful;
- willing to change;
- flexible;
- focused on outcomes;
- insightful;
- creative.

Paramedics regularly work in stressful conditions, managing complex and dynamic cases in a time-critical manner. Moilanen (2014) proposes that in order to meet this challenge, they require highly developed critical thinking skills in order to operate in the midst of chaos and make informed decisions immediately.

 Reflection: points to consider

Do you possess any of the traits of a critical thinker? How might your personality traits make your working life more frustrating, if you feel constrained by your organi-sation's policies/procedures?

External influences on decision-making

With any decision there are individual variations which may affect the outcomes. Any choices generated and made are affected by personal values and bias. These are moral and ethical codes socialised within us as part of our culture, exposure and experience. These could be those that have been instilled in us as children or those values that we have acquired through our workplace culture and customs.

When reviewing any decision, it is important not only to examine the component parts of the decision but also to look at the external factors that have influenced it. The impact of factors such as evidence-based practice, working culture and bias on decision-making cannot be underestimated.

Evidence-based practice (EBP) should be the cornerstone of contemporary clinical prac-tice. We no longer do things because we have always done it that way but because the evidence has demonstrated that the approach recommended works and has proven to be beneficial through rigorous scientific testing and research, however, this is not always the case. Chew (2014) explored the factors influencing the development and implementation of evidence-based healthcare practice in the emergency care setting. He concluded that there is a tardy integration of EBP into contemporary practice despite there being valid and legitimate reasons for doing so. Some of the organisational factors that Chew (2014) offered for this were time, support and culture.

One of the reasons for this reluctance may lie in the theory of change management. Cork (2012) cogently argues that change is inevitable in any organisation, especially those following an EBP agenda. Practitioners who understand change are more likely to embrace, influence and accept it. However, in order to embrace change, we have to accept that what we are doing can be improved, i.e. it is not the best that we can do; this is an uncomfortable position for any paramedic. Nevertheless, it is unavoidable and in order to make decisions which are based on contemporary evidence, we need to ensure that the culture within which we work is conducive to change (Cork 2012).

The Oxford English Dictionary (2017) defines culture as 'the ideas, customs and social behaviour of a particular people or society'. The Ambulance Service in itself is a society with leaders, followers, rules and regulations, based on legal frameworks, evidence-based practice, tradition, cultural norms and social influences.

 Chapter 9 for more on sociological theory.

Schobel et al. (2016) conducted a study to explore social influences in sequential decision-making. They claim that individuals will often follow the behaviour of others and ignore their own opinions, even if the behaviour of others is misinformed.

Parallels can be drawn to this in the paramedic world. As team members and working closely alongside colleagues, individual practitioners are exposed to external opinions and pressures to conform to what is seen as the cultural norm. To step outside of this can sometimes place the individual in an uncomfortable situation, however, in order to ensure that decisions reflect current clinical excellence, it is sometimes necessary.

An example of this could be the use of gloves in clinical practice. Although a relatively low priority area in relation to the wealth of decisions made on a daily basis, the use of gloves has direct consequences on patient care, interpretation of clinical data, and ultimately financial resources. In university, the use of Personal Protective Equipment (PPE) is high on the teaching agenda and students are taught, according to the latest evidence, to assess their likely exposure to bodily fluids and then make an informed decision if gloves are required (WHO 2014). From working with and teaching various groups of paramedics and student paramedics, it has become apparent that gloves are sometimes donned by practitioners prior to entering the patient's environment. This may limit their ability to assess the patient using the sense of touch and may also impede the development of a therapeutic relationship with the patient due to negative perceptions of the use of gloves. Although the individual practitioner is aware of the evidence surrounding the use of PPE, this practice becomes embedded into the culture and perpetuated for the future, thus dictating decisions from a cultural norm rather than an evidence base. Furthermore, they describe what they call the 'authority influence hypothesis' (Schobel et al. 2016: 5). This predicts that hierarchy and the individual's position in the organisation will influence people's behaviour. Schobel et al. (2016) state that the individual will often ignore their own opinions, and favour the opinions of seniors even when they provide inaccurate information.

Finally, individual biases have to be acknowledged to ensure that decision-making is based on altruistic principles. Biases are a product of each individual's experiences, learned either explicitly or implicitly within cultural contexts. These are often unconscious and not immediately apparent to us. Sporek (2015) advises that although we may feel our decisions are based on facts, they are frequently influenced by hidden feelings and thoughts that we are not even aware of. This is supported by Marquis and Huston (2012), who maintain that value judgements will always be encompassed within a decision, no matter how objective the criteria. Furthermore, they apply this and propose that the alternatives generated and the final choices are limited by each person's value system. Stone and Moskowitz (2011) propose that in order to reduce the unintentional acts of discrimination, training should be in place in all healthcare programmes.

The consequences of decision-making in line with cultural norms rather than the evidence which supports it are immense. As a registrant, the HCPC requires you to use your judgement so that you make informed and reasonable decisions and meet the standards. In addition, they mandate that you must always be prepared to justify your decisions and actions (HCPC 2016). You are also accountable first and foremost to your patients and they have the right to pursue this through the civil and criminal courts. Any practitioner must be prepared to justify the decisions made to an expert audience.

 Reflection: points to consider

Have you ever been in a situation where you have felt pressured to conform to cultural norms? What could you do in future to manage this situation?

 Chapter 6 to read about human factors affecting paramedic practice.

The value of experience

Within the process of decision-making, we use our life experiences to guide the way in which we act. Although dated, Cioffi (1997) remains the forerunner of this concept and defines this as intuitive knowing associated with past personal experiences, which she refers to as heuristics in her literature. The more mature a person, the greater range of alternatives he may identify. This may not be maturity in the traditional meaning of age but of time spent in his chosen career. Past experiences and outcomes all guide us to make certain decisions as we draw on these to guide our thinking. This is supported by Lyneham et al. (2008), who debate the concept of intuition in their work. Furthermore, they claim that the expert will make decisions faster and with greater accuracy than at any other stage of professional development. This could be attributed to the tacit knowledge that we all carry, however, it is rarely acknowledged. Banning (2008) cites Benner (1984) when describing how the inexperienced practitioner will use procedures and guidelines to make decisions, but as they become more experienced, decision-making becomes intuitive, drawing on past experiences to inform future actions. Marquis and Huston (2012) support this and maintain gut-level feelings have a part to play when experienced practitioners take strategic action that positively impact upon patient outcomes.

This could be explained by Muoni (2012) who agrees and adds that the advantage of heuristics is speed, allowing practitioners to process data faster than if using analytical methods. However, she urges caution as this can lead to errors. She defends this by adding that not all information is given equal status due to its enormity and complexity. The process of reflection then becomes paramount.

There are those, however, who do not re-examine decisions that they have made and therefore do not learn from their experiences. It is always advisable to remember that we

---

Box 17.2 Heuristic decision-making

- *Pattern recognition* – in responses presented by patients you have previously treated, i.e. we recognise answers to questions (from previous patients) we have asked our patient and should sometimes delve further rather than assuming the same as with other patients.
- *Similarity recognition* – comparison of similar and dissimilar characteristics of past patients who have had similar conditions.
- *Common-sense understanding* – understanding diversity from a selection of information, i.e. vital signs that give subtle trends/indications about a patient.
- *Skilled knowhow* – that considers possibilities for each patient.
- *Sense of salience* – perceptions about a patient that stand out as more important.
- *Deliberative rationality* – selective attention to certain aspects/events.

Adapted from Cioffi (1997: 205)

...arn by doing, rather we learn by doing and then reviewing. Cioffi (1997) states that intuitive, heuristic judgements are qualitative, critical, discriminating and associated with past experiences and she identifies six key aspects of heuristic decision-making, maintaining that they can be used in complex decision-making situations (see Box 17.2).

MODELS OF DECISION-MAKING

In order to support the decision-making process, various models are available and within the process there are critical elements that determine outcome. These are as follows:

- determine the goal;
- gather data carefully;
- generate many alternatives;
- think logically;
- choose and act decisively.

Marquis and Huston (2012) describe a traditional problem-solving model that is commonly applied to healthcare situations. The model consists of seven steps:

1 Problem identification.
2 Data gathering of causes and consequences which are analysed.
3 Possible alternatives are explored.
4 Alternatives are then evaluated.
5 The solution is then chosen to suit the situation (steps).
6 This is then implemented.
7 The results are then evaluated and reflection occurs.

Marquis and Huston (2012) recognise that the decision-making process does not take place until step 5. Although this could be construed as a weakness, it is important not to minimise the importance of examining the problem in full in order to collect the maximum data to enable informed decision-making. Furthermore, it could be said that the amount of time needed for proper implementation and the lack of initial objective setting do not lend themselves to use in a real-time situation.

A model of decision-making supported by Ryan and Halliwell (2012) is the hypothetico-deductive model. This involves the paramedic assessing the impact of the data collected on the situation and then ruling in or ruling out data required in order to make informed decisions. An example of this is the ABCDE model of assessment where clinical findings are ruled in and out of the decision-making process depending on the significance and severity of their consequences.

They assert that in order to make informed decisions there are three important areas of reasoning:

1 The paramedic will make a *conscious* decision to rule in or out data involving actively considering the significance of findings.

2 The paramedic will understand the *evidence* which supports the decision and so follow best practice.

3 The paramedic will understand that their practice has to *withhold scrutiny* from relevant stakeholders, patients, peers, and the HCPC.

They recognise the many attributes of intuitive decision-making and the hypothetico-deductive model, however, when they conducted a comparison of those who followed an Institute of Health Care Development (IHCD) route and those who followed a university route, they found significant differences. They reported that those who followed the IHCD route were very confident in using intuitive mechanisms, whereas the graduates had more confidence in following the template, due to their lack of experience and confidence.

In order to overcome this, they recommend the combined approach. By using a model of decision-making and incorporating observational experience, the paramedic can ensure that they are using all the available resources to them.

In the climate in which the paramedic currently practises, there are numerous opportunities for barriers to effective decision-making to exist. These reflect closely the barriers that are discussed in relation to change management.

Barriers to decision-making

Barriers may exist at both an operational and an organisational level. At an organisational level there can be a lack of managers who have been adequately prepared to take on the role of decision-makers (Finkelman 2006). They may lack the skills to communicate effectively with their teams in order to promote the message of the decision that has been made. A lack of staff participation will effectively immobilise the decision as it should include all stakeholders, a huge although not unachievable task, when examining the ambulance clinician provision within the United Kingdom. The lack of staff participation can be attributed to many factors, but it has to be acknowledged that the most common are the exclusion of team members by the decision-maker and the lack of impetus to participate by staff due to low morale.

At a more local operational level, one of the main barriers is that of taking short cuts within the process (Sullivan and Garland 2013). This can limit the amount of data collection and the quantity and quality of the alternatives that are generated and then considered. This may be due to the decision-maker relying on past experience and not being willing to acknowledge that there may be other alternatives to bring about a solution.

 Chapter 1 to explore the value of communication and barriers to effective communication, and **Chapter 6** for further explanation of the human factors affecting paramedic practice.

A barrier which straddles both organisational and operational levels is that of rigid ideas and points of view. If the stakeholders do not want to embrace the decision because of preconceived ideas or past experiences, the decision-maker will have to ensure that these views are discussed and new ways forward negotiated. This will be demonstrated in the clinical setting with phrases such as 'We have always done it this way; it did not work when we tried to change it before; it is easier to keep it as it is.' It must be recognised by the decision-maker that the opposition is ignored at the peril of the decision failing.

At a more individual level, the personality trait of the decision-maker can act as a barrier. One's personality can and does affect the decision-making process. The decision-making could be based on approval-seeking if the manager is inexperienced and seeking acceptance from the workers. Rather than face rejection, when a truly difficult decision arises, the manager will make a decision which is based on the fact that it will placate people, thus increasing the manager's popularity. Although at first this may seem like a successful model of leadership, it puts the need of the team above the needs of the task, which will have detrimental consequences for the decision. Alternatively, a manager may make a decision based on her own personality traits, rather than that of her workers. The 'workaholic' boss may deem it acceptable to ask the staff to work overtime without payment if this is what she herself would do. This can lead to resentment and a feeling among staff that the decision-maker has not looked at the consequences of the problem. This is a common pitfall of managers and they must work hard to embrace all personality types into the team and not judge others by their own standards if these are not the norm.

Reflection: points to consider

Do any of the above comments apply to you?

REMOTE CLINICAL DECISION-MAKING

The term remote clinical decision-making (RCDM), within the context of this chapter, refers to a clinician's role and responsibility in assessing, triaging, and/or making any decision about the outcome and/or onward referral of a patient in the absence of a face-to-face patient–clinician interaction (Brady 2016). RCDM is also commonly known in the UK as telephone triage or 'hear and treat', and is an established strategy used within emergency and primary care to manage an increasing patient demand. While there remain differing views surrounding the best definition of RCDM (Brady and Northstone 2017), various studies have demonstrated high degrees of patient safety associated with its use (Meer et al. 2010; Huibers et al. 2011); and of the 10.68 million 999 calls received by NHS ambulance services in the year 2015/16, 10.2 per cent were treated remotely (AACE 2016).

Many professionals undertake RCDM, such as nurses, paramedics, midwives, doctors, and psychiatrists. The goal of RCDM differs depending on the context of its use, but from an out-of-hospital perspective RCDM predominantly involves the enhanced triage of patients calling 999/911/112. Most ambulance services internationally use a computer or card-based triage sieve system to rapidly assign a priority level and dispatch code to those calling. This role is usually carried out by non-medically trained call handlers who use strictly scripted protocols for each presenting complaint. While this sieve-based method is highly sensitive in detecting critically ill patients, it can 'over-triage' conditions and result in patients being attended by paramedics who do not require emergency treatment and transportation. In contrast to this, however, many people calling 999/911/112 do so in panic or misunderstanding and the triage sieve method can also determine patients who do not require emergency treatment and transportation, but who may benefit from a more in-depth assessment by a RCDM clinician. It is the role of nurses and paramedics within emergency clinical hubs to intercept cases of 'over-triage' and 'under-triage' and carry out a clinical assessment to establish the level of urgency of patient need, rather than to diagnose. Equally so, nurses and paramedics carry out routine clinical assessments of those patients identified as having a non-emergency complaint, to again establish the level of urgency of patient need. These consultations often involve giving patients self-care advice or advising an onward referral. This model is similar in urgent care settings such as NHS Direct, NHS 24, and NHS 111. RCDM, however, can mean much more than undertaking a clinical assessment, and can involve providing remote senior clinical support to face-to-face colleagues, advising dispatch staff, providing support to non-medically trained call handlers, and monitoring call/response queues. These responsibilities involve making decisions about the outcome and/or onward referral of patients in the absence of a face-to-face patient–clinician interaction. Again, the goal of RCDM differs depending on the context of its use, and some remote interactions do not involve vehicular responses, such as midwifery advice lines. Such advice lines involve registered midwives assessing expectant mothers, and providing remote support to non-midwifery trained staff. General practitioners also often work remotely as many of their patients do not require face-to-face appointments or assessments, and so can be assisted more economically and efficiently. With such diversity in what is considered RCDM, it is important to consider the type of clinician who might undertake such a role.

Who should undertake RCDM?

Holmström (2007) describes remote decision-making as a highly complex process, which is neither mechanical nor linear in nature, but rather a highly skilled knowledge-intensive specialty. For many years, greater emphasis has been placed upon the knowledge derived from systematic, scientific, and empirical data to inform clinical decisions. Working remotely from a patient, however, often means that such systematic and scientific data is not available to the clinician; and that skills derived from face-to-face clinical practice have to be transferred to working in this alternative way. Other forms of knowledge have been widely recognised as having an impact on how decisions are made in clinical practice (Chinn and Kramer 2011), such as tacit or intuitive knowledge. Polanyi (1967) defined tacit knowledge as occurring when something is known only by relying on an awareness of it for attending to a secondary activity (proximal and distal knowledge). Marsden (1999; 2000) posits that tacit knowing and intuitive knowing are accepted by most authors as being an integral part of expert decision-making – including RCDM, where systematic, scientific, and empirical data is often unavailable. Thus, it is reasonable to assert that unless one has a developed tacit knowing of their clinical area, then they are unable to be considered an expert. Therefore, considering that tacit knowing is integral to areas such as RCDM, it is reasonable to assert that only experts should be able to undertake this highly complex process; although it is also recognised that one can develop an expertise in RCDM.

McHugh and Lake (2010) describe clinical experts as being distinguished from their colleagues by their often-intuitive ability to efficiently make critical clinical decisions while grasping the whole nature of a situation. Such knowledge is acquired during experiences in special domains and is linked closely with experience-guided working (Herbig et al. 2001). There is evidence to indicate that length of clinical experience has an impact on RCDM in emergency and out-of-hour care settings (Varley et al. 2016). A study of 60,794 calls managed by 296 NHS Direct nurses, for example, reported a positive relationship with years of nursing experience and call disposal patterns. Nurses of less than 10 years' clinical experience were less likely to arrive at self-care dispositions than nurses with more than 20 years' experience (O'Cathain et al. 2004). Thus, it is also reasonable to assert that only experienced clinicians should be able to undertake RCDM.

The assertion that only expert and experienced clinicians should undertake RCDM is complicated by the viewpoint that experience is a necessary but not sufficient condition for expertise; and that not all experienced clinicians are themselves experts. Indeed, while expertise and experience are related, they are overtly different concepts (McHugh and Lake 2010). Experience is defined by Benner (1984) as both time in practice and self-reflection that allows preconceived notions and expectations to be confirmed, refined, or disconfirmed in real circumstances. Benner (1984) continues to posit that merely encountering patient conditions and situations is not experience; rather, experience involves clinicians reflecting on encountered circumstances to refine their moment-to-moment decision-making at an unconscious level.

There is a lack of consensus within the literature pertaining to the best attributes of an RCDM clinician. What is clear, however, is that an RCDM clinician requires experience in real terms of their clinical area, which is developed through learning from errors, reflecting, and critical thinking. In turn, this experience should influence the expert tacit knowledge that RCDM clinicians should have, which contributes to decision-making. Working remotely is so inherently different from working face-to-face that often despite experience and expertise being used, clinical decisions often require further support.

 Chapter 2 for more theory on reflection.

Supporting remote clinical decision-making

Unlike working in face-to-face clinical practice, RCDM involves working with limited senses – effectively blindfolded. Clinicians normally rely both explicitly and implicitly on what is performed non-verbally and what they physically see during a consultation. Working remotely involves being unable to see the home environment, the patient's colour or condition, and being unable to palpate the patient's anatomy and provide the therapeutic physical contact normally provided to emotionally upset patients and family. Equally so, clinicians are unable to smell any overt urinary infection, the odour of diabetic ketoacidosis, or the alcohol on a patient's breath. Subsequently RDCM clinicians have to find methods of gathering information that would otherwise be readily accessible to them and find methods of transferring face-to-face skills, built up through many years of practice, to working remotely. Pettinari and Jessopp (2001) describe the process of picture building or visualisation of the patient and the situation as a recognised strategy in RCDM. They explain that clinicians develop skills to manage the interaction with callers in order to compensate for the absence of visibility. Such skills involve the use of non-bias, non-leading, open and closed questioning, which describes various aspects of the patient's condition. This process of picture building and information gathering is often facilitated and aided by clinical decision support software (CDSS).

Remote clinicians often use clinical decision support software to help guide, structure, and record their assessments, providing clinical assessment and advice in an auditable, evidence-based way. CDSS allows remote clinicians to ask questions to which the answers would be obvious if they were working in face-to-face clinical practice, and thus, might be forgotten. Remote clinicians should, however, not rely on CDSS, as such software cannot assess and plan for every clinical eventuality and cannot replace the nuances of extensive clinical experience. Remote clinicians are more likely to override CDSS recommendations, in either direction, if they have detailed knowledge of the health problem under consideration, and rely more heavily on CDSS for conditions about which they have limited clinical knowledge (O'Cathain et al. 2004). While Sahota et al.'s (2011) systematic review of the literature found that the majority of CDSSs demonstrated improvements in process of patient care, there remains a lack of evidence showing definitely that the use of CDSS leads to positive patient outcomes; with Randell et al. (2007) calling for more research into these complex systems. For those clinicians who do not use CDSS, other consultation models can be used. Such models record and provide structure, consistency, and auditability to remote clinical practice, and further aid the picture building and patient visualisation.

Warner (2008) explains that if remote clinicians err slavishly on the side of caution, they effectively become a receptionist and not a clinician. If they stick rigidly to established algorithms, they could spend a quarter of an hour consulting with a patient who has a pimple on his chin, while a potential heart attack or stroke case might still be in the queue.

If they skim over a triage encounter, lose concentration, get interrupted, or forget to ask a vital question, patients could ultimately die. Warner's (2008) narrative is an apt description of the complexity of RCDM and outlines how challenging working without senses can be in clinical practice.

As the modern healthcare system struggles to cope with the rising patient demand effectively, and economically, RCDM will play a much larger role in the emergency, urgent, and primary care setting. More clinicians will inevitably be called upon to work in this way to efficiently and safely manage the needs of the population. Being a clinically experienced expert, as well as being well-armed with a factual evidence base, while also being supported by CDSS or a consultation model, can help clinicians transfer their face-to-face skills to working remotely. As technology advances, so will the use of RCDM. Mobile heart rate monitors are already being integrated into wrist watches, and home blood pressure, oxygen, and blood glucose monitoring continues to be introduced within the community and relayed digitally and telephonically to remote clinical hubs. Internet and mobile-phone video call facilities will allow remote clinicians to be able to view their patients and assess their needs in a way that has until now been impossible.

This chapter has demonstrated that with any decision made in practice, there should be a process of reflection afterwards. Decisions are made all the time but are rarely reflected upon unless something untoward happens. It is important to be aware of the barriers to effective decision-making in order to reduce these, or at least acknowledge that they exist and can affect the outcome. In order to ensure that decisions made are effective, the process of following a model will enable logical analysis to be applied.

CONCLUSION

Overall this chapter has demonstrated that decision-making skills are not in addition to, but part of, the clinical repertoire that enables effective skilled care to be delivered to the patient. Although not obvious at the point of care delivery, an understanding of the ways in which decision-making is approached and the importance of experience will develop an understanding of the wider issues of working within the organisation.

Chapter key points:

- Understanding the component parts of the decision-making process enables a higher level of reflection.
- All decisions, whether on an organisational, local or personal basis, have consequences which should be explored prior to the decision being taken.

REFERENCES AND SUGGESTED READING

Association of Ambulance Chief Executives (2016) *Annual Report 2015/2016*. London: Association of Ambulance Chief Executives.

Banning, M. (2008) A review of clinical decision making: models and current research. *Journal of Clinical Nursing*, 17: 187–95.

Benner, P. (1984) *From Novice to Expert: Excellence and Power in Clinical Nursing Practice*. Menlo Park, CA: Addison-Wesley.

Bickley, L. (2008) *Bates' Guide to Physical Examination and History Taking*. Philadelphia, PA: Lippincott Williams and Wilkins.

Brady, M. (2016) Remote clinical decision making: transition to higher education. *Journal of Paramedic Practice*, 8(3): 115–17.

Brady, M. and Northstone, K. (2017) Remote Clinical Decision Making: a clinician's definition: short report. *Emergency Nurse Journal*, 25(2): 24–8.

Brown, S.N., Kumar, D. and Millins, M. (eds for JRCALC and AACE) (2016) *UK Ambulance Service Clinical Practice Guidelines*. Bridgwater: Class Professional Publishing.

Chew, B. (2014) Exploring factors influencing the development and implementation of evidence-based healthcare practice in emergency care setting. *Singapore Nursing Journal*, 41(2): 29–34.

Chinn, P. and Kramer, M. (2011) *Integrated Theory and Knowledge Development in Nursing*. 8th edn. London: Mosby Elsevier.

Cioffi, J. (1997) Heuristics, servants to intuition, in clinical decision-making. *Journal of Advanced Nursing*, 26(1): 203–8.

Cork, A. (2012) Change management theory and its usefulness to practice. In A.Y. Blaber (ed.) *Foundations for Paramedic Practice*, 2nd edn. Maidenhead: Open University Press.

Curtis, S. and Scott, C. (n.d.) CLEAR Telephone Consultation Model. Unpublished.

Finkelman, A. (2006) *Leadership and Management in Nursing*. London: Prentice-Hall.

Health and Care Professions Council (2016) *Standards of Conduct, Performance and Ethics*. London: HCPC.

Heidari, M. and Shahbazi, S. (2016) Effect of training problem-solving skill on decision-making and critical thinking of personnel at medical emergencies. *International Journal of Critical Illness and Injury Science*, 6: 182–7.

Herbig, B. et al. (2001) The role of tacit knowledge in the work context of nursing. *Journal of Advanced Nursing*, 34(5), 687–95.

Holmström, I. (2007) Decision aid software programs in telenursing: not used as intended? Experiences of Swedish telenurses. *Nursing and Health Sciences,* 9: 23–8.

Huang, G., Lindell, D., Jaffe, L. and Sullivan, A. (2016) A multi-site study of strategies to teach critical thinking: 'why do you think that?' *Medical Education*, 50: 236–49.

Huibers, L., Smits, M., Renaud, V. et al. (2011) Safety of telephone triage in out-of-hours care: a systematic review. *Scandinavian Journal of Primary Health Care*, 29(4): 198–209.

Ignatavicius, D. (2001) Critical thinking skills for the bedside nurse. *Nursing Management,* 32(1): 37–9.

Jenson, J., Croskerry, P. and Travers, A. (2009) Paramedic clinical decision making during high acuity emergency calls: design and methodology of a Delphi study. *BMC Emergency Medicine*, 9(17): 1–40.

Lyneham, J., Parkinson, C. and Denholm, C. (2008) Explicating Benner's concept of expert practice: intuition in emergency nursing. *Journal of Advanced Nursing*, 64(4): 380–7.

Marquis, B. and Huston, C. (2012) *Leadership Roles and Management Tools for the New Nurse*, 7th edn. Philadelphia, PA: Lippincott Williams and Wilkins.

Marsden, J. (1999) Expert nurse decision-making: telephone triage in an ophthalmic accident and emergency department. *Nursing Times Research*, 4(1): 44–52.

Marsden, J. (2000) *Telephone Triage in Ophthalmic A&E Department*. London: Whurr Publishers.

McHugh, M. and Lake, E. (2010) Understanding clinical expertise: nurse education, experience, and the hospital context. *Research in Nursing & Health,* 33: 276–87.

Meer, A., Gwerder, T., Duembgen, L. et al. (2010) Is computer-assisted telephone triage safe? A prospective surveillance study in walk-in patients with non-life-threatening medical conditions. *Emergency Medicine Journal*, 29(2): 124–8.

Moilanen, J. (2014) The wisdom of tacit knowing-in-action and mission command. In C.J. Boden-McGill and K.P. King (eds) *Developing and Sustaining Adult Learners*. New York: IAP Information Age Publishing, pp. 283–304.

Muoni, T. (2012) Decision-making, intuition, and the midwife: understanding heuristics. *British Journal of Midwifery*, 20(1): 52–6.

O'Cathain, A. et al. (2004) Do different types of nurses give different triage decisions in NHS Direct? A mixed methods study. *Journal of Health Services Research & Policy*, 9(4): 226–33.

Oxford English Dictionary (2017) Culture. Oxford: Oxford University Press.

Pettinari, C. and Jessop, L. (2001) 'Your ears become your eyes': managing the absence of visibility in NHS Direct. *Journal of Advanced Nursing*, 36(5): 668–75.

Polanyi, M. (1967) *The Tacit Dimension*. London: Routledge & Kegan Paul.

Randell, R. et al. (2007) Effects of computerized decision support systems on nursing performance and patient outcomes: a systematic review. *Journal of Health Services Research & Policy*, 12(4): 242–9.

Ryan, L. and Halliwell, D. (2012) Paramedic decision making – how is it done? *Journal of Paramedic Practice*, 4(6): 343–51.

Sahota, N. et al. (2011) Computerized clinical decision support systems for acute care management: a decision-maker–researcher partnership systematic review of effects on process of care and patient outcomes. *Implementation Science*, 6: 91.

Schobel, M., Rieskamp, J. and Huber, R. (2016) Social influences in sequential decision making. *PLoS ONE*, 11(1): e0146536.

Simpson, P., Thomas, R., Bendall, J., Lord, B., Lord, S. and Close, J. (2017) 'Popping nana back into bed' – a qualitative exploration of paramedic decision making when caring for older people who have fallen. *BMC Health Services Research*, 17: 299.

Sporek, P. (2015) Unconscious bias. *British Journal of Midwifery*, 23(12): 910.

Stone, J. and Moskowitz, G. (2011) Non-conscious bias in medical decision making: what can be done to reduce it? *Medical Education*, 45: 768–76.

Sullivan, E. and Garland, G. (2013) *Practical Leadership and Management in Healthcare*. London: Pearson.

Varley, A. et al. (2016) The effect of nurses' preparedness and nurse practitioner status on triage call management in primary care: a secondary analysis of cross-sectional data from the ESTEEM trial. *International Journal of Nursing Studies*, 58: 12–20.

Warner, J. (2008) Telephone triage requires high-quality nursing skills. *Nursing Times Online*. Available at: https://www.nursingtimes.net/telephone-triage-requires-high-quality-nursing-skills/1847744. article (accessed August 2017).

WHO (2014) *WHO Surgical Site Infection Prevention Guidelines. Web Appendix 21. Summary of a Systematic Review on the Use of Surgical Gloves*. Geneva: WHO. Available at: http://www.who.int/gpsc/appendix21.pdf (accessed 13 June 2018).

Continuing professional development (CPD) pre-and post-registration

Graham Harris and Bob Fellows

In this chapter:

- Introduction
- Why is this relevant?
- Pre-registration and the role of the HCPC
- Post-registration and the role of the HCPC
- What is continuing professional development (CPD)?
- Standards for CPD
- The HCPC audit
- Examples of types of CPD activity
- The purpose of each part of the profile
- What happens to your completed CPD profile?
- Conclusion
- Chapter key points
- References
- Useful websites

INTRODUCTION

This chapter incorporates the appropriate and updated information from the previous edition of the text. It now includes and differentiates between CPD for the pre-registered student and the registered paramedic. From the Health and Care Professions Council (HCPC) perspective, there are differing requirements for a pre-registered student and the registered paramedic who needs to maintain registration to be employed as a paramedic and continue to practise.

WHY IS THIS RELEVANT?

Whether you are a student on a HCPC approved programme of education leading to eligibility to apply to the register, or an existing qualified and registered paramedic with the HCPC, we all as health professionals need to demonstrate and maintain a record of what we do for our CPD.

PRE-REGISTRATION AND THE ROLE OF THE HCPC

To use the protected title of *paramedic*, the student paramedic needs to successfully complete a pre-registration programme of education and training that meets the requirements of the registrant body, currently the Health and Care Professions Council. A programme which meets the HCPC standards of education and training (SETs) allows a student who successfully completes that programme to meet the relevant standards of proficiency. They are then eligible to apply to the HCPC for registration. To enable an education provider or a higher education institute (HEI) university to deliver such a programme, they must apply to the HCPC for the programme to be approved. The curriculum would be mapped against and meet the following standards:

- College of Paramedics (2017) *Paramedic Curriculum Guidance*, 4th edition;
- Quality Assurance Agency (QAA) (2016) *Subject Benchmark Statement – Paramedics*;
- Health and Care Professions Council (2014) *Standards of Proficiency – Paramedics*;
- Health and Care Professions Council (2017a) *Standards of Education and Training*.

As a student on such a programme you will be expected to adhere to the HCPC *Guidance on Conduct and Ethics for Students* (2016a), and aspire to the HCPC *Standards of Conduct, Performance and Ethics* (2016b). Throughout the duration of education and training you will need to compile a 'portfolio of evidence', which provides confirmation of your continuing professional development throughout the period of education and training to enable you to demonstrate your achievement. Successful completion of such a programme entitles the individual to be eligible to apply for registration with the HCPC as a paramedic. Once registered as a paramedic, CPD continues throughout the individual's career.

POST-REGISTRATION AND THE ROLE OF THE HCPC

The regulatory body requires all registrants to meet their standards for continuing professional development (HCPC 2017b). The HCPC carries out an audit each time a professional renews their registration – every two years – to make sure that their standards are being met. This requires the paramedic to sign a 'professional declaration' once every two years in order to remain registered (HCPC 2017c). Signing the declaration confirms that the paramedic has:

- continued to practise their profession since the last registration; or
- not practised their profession since the last registration, but has met the (HCPC 2017d) *Returning to practice* requirements.

They are also confirming that:

- they continue to meet the HCPC's Standards of Proficiency – Paramedics;

- since the last registration there has been no change relating to their good character (this includes any conviction or caution, if any, that they are required to disclose), or any change to their health that may affect their ability to practise safely and effectively;
- they continue to meet the HCPC's standards for professional development; and,
- they either have a professional indemnity arrangement in place which provides appropriate cover, or they are not practising at the time of their renewal, but understand the requirement to have a professional indemnity in place which provides appropriate cover, and will have this in place when they practise.

To stay registered you will need to ensure that you continue to meet all the above standards and can sign the professional declaration on your renewal form. Bear in mind that if you come off the register, you will not be able to use the title 'Paramedic' to refer to yourself or to your work. You should also consider that you may need to update your skills to come back onto the register at a future date.

For the purpose of registration renewal, the HCPC defines 'practising your profession' as using and drawing upon your professional skills and knowledge in the course of your work. Therefore, if you work in education, leadership and management or research, the HCPC regards this as practising your profession. If you have moved to a non-clinical area of work but wish to stay on the register, you need to ensure that you keep up to date with your profession and that you stay within your scope of practice. If you return to clinical work or change your scope of practice, then you may need to update your skills.

When you are planning or undertaking your CPD, you will need to make sure that it is relevant to your work. Similarly, to stay registered, you need to make sure you keep within the 'scope of your practice'. This refers to the particular area in which you are trained to practise, lawfully, safely and effectively in a way that meets the HCPC standards and does not present any risk to the patients, the public or to yourself. Scope of practice may vary between paramedics and will relate to job role, experience and training. For example, two paramedics will both meet the HCPC's (2014) *Standards of Proficiency: Paramedics*, but may then have gone on to develop in different areas. If they were then to perform each other's roles without training, they may be practising outside their scope of practice, as their lack of experience in the different area may lead to unsafe practice, or pose a risk to a patient or to themselves.

The *Standards of Proficiency: Paramedics* are the standards which every registrant must meet in order to be registered and must continue to meet in order to stay on the register. They set out the required knowledge, understanding and skills for the practice of paramedics. Registrants must also read and agree to abide by the HCPC *Standards of Conduct, Performance and Ethics* (HCPC 2016b), and adhere to the *Confidentiality – Guidance for Registrants* (HCPC 2017e).

If someone is no longer fit to practise their profession and does not remove themselves voluntarily, the HCPC can take action using the fitness to practise process. If you feel that for any reason you no longer meet the HCPC standards, then you should come off the register. This is known as professional self-regulation, which means that you (the registrant) are in the best position to judge your ability to practise safely and lawfully. It is your responsibility to stay on the register, or to decide if you need to come off for any reason. Likewise, you need to inform the HCPC of any changes in your circumstances which may affect your ability to practise safely. It is felt that as an accountable registered professional, you are in the best position to make professional judgements of this nature and the HCPC trusts you to do so.

WHAT IS CONTINUING PROFESSIONAL DEVELOPMENT (CPD)?

The HCPC defines CPD as 'the way in which registrants continue to learn and develop throughout their careers so they keep their skills and knowledge up to date and are able to practise safely and effectively' (HCPC 2017c: 5). Quite simply, CPD is not only about undertaking formal courses but any activity from which you learn and develop.

Why do I need to record my CPD?

In addition to being linked to your HCPC registration, CPD is an essential part of your development as a professional. Recording your CPD is as valuable as doing your CPD in the first place. However, without the evidence of the value of your CPD, how will you be able to show it really was worthwhile to your service? If you do not have an up-to-date record of your CPD, in essence, you cannot demonstrate that you have developed professionally. The College of Paramedics provides support with CPD activities including arranging regional CPD events, and e-learning CPD, details of which can be found on the College website: www.collegeofparamedics.co.uk

STANDARDS FOR CPD

Registrants must do the following (HCPC 2017c: 5):

1   maintain a continuous, up-to-date and accurate record of their CPD activities;
2   demonstrate that their CPD activities are a mixture of learning activities relevant to current or future practice;
3   seek to ensure that their CPD has contributed to the quality of their practice and service delivery;
4   seek to ensure that their CPD benefits the service user; and,
5   upon request, present a written profile (which must be their own work and supported by evidence) explaining how they have met the Standards for CPD.

THE HCPC AUDIT

2016 saw the publication of the 2013–15 *Continuing Professional Development Audit Report* (HCPC 2016c). Some 2.5 per cent of registrants were selected for audit which equated to 487 paramedics of which 430 (88.3 per cent) were accepted, 32 deferred and 17 voluntarily deregistered, while a further 8 were deregistered due to their registration lapsing, and none were removed from the register. If you are audited, the HCPC will ask you to fill in a form (the CPD profile). This is a form that you will be given. In it you must write a statement which tells them how your CPD has met the standards. When you send this in, you must also send in supporting evidence from your personal CPD record. You need to complete your CPD profile honestly and accurately. If you provide false or misleading information in your CPD profile, the HCPC will evoke their fitness to practise procedure. This could lead to you being struck off the register so that you can no longer practise.

EXAMPLES OF TYPES OF CPD ACTIVITY

The following are activities that the HCPC suggests might make up your CPD profile (HCPC 2017b, Appendix 1):

Work-based learning

- learning by doing;
- case studies;
- reflective practice;
- coaching from others;
- audit of service users;
- peer review;
- discussions with colleagues;
- gaining and learning from experience;
- involvement in the wider, profession-related work of your employer (e.g. member of a committee);
- job rotation;
- journal club;
- in-service training;
- expanding your role;
- project work or project management;
- secondments;
- supervising staff or students (Practice Educator);
- filling in self-assessment questionnaires;
- significant analysis of events;
- work shadowing.

Professional activity

- being a national assessor;
- being a tutor;
- being an external examiner;
- being an expert witness;
- organising journal clubs or other specialist groups;

- giving presentations at conferences;
- involvement in your professional body (special interest group, or other groups);
- lecturing or teaching;
- maintaining or developing specialist skills (for example, musical skills);
- mentoring or coaching new staff (Preceptor – Practice Educator);
- organising accredited courses;
- supervising research or students.

Formal/educational

- attending conferences (College of Paramedics National Conference, Life Connections, Trauma Care, Sepsis, Emergency Services Show, etc.);
- courses accredited by your professional body (College of Paramedics);
- distance or online learning;
- further education;
- going to seminars;
- planning or running a course;
- research and audit;
- writing or editing a chapter in a book;
- writing articles or papers.

Self-directed learning

- keeping a file of your progress;
- reading journals/articles (*British Paramedic Journal*; *Emergency Medicine Journal*);
- reviewing books or articles;
- updating knowledge through the internet or TV.

Other

- public service;
- voluntary work.

The CPD profile summary has four parts, which include:

- summary of practice history (up to 500 words);
- statement of how you met the standards (up to 1500 words);
- a dated list of the CPD activities you have carried out since you last renewed your registration;
- supporting evidence.

THE PURPOSE OF EACH PART OF THE PROFILE

The *summary of your practice history* should help to show the CPD assessors how your CPD activities are linked to your work. This part of the CPD profile should help you to show how your activities are *relevant to your current or future work*.

Your *statement* of how you have met the HCPC standards should clearly show how you believe you meet each of the standards, and should refer to all the CPD activities you have undertaken and the *evidence* you are sending in to support your statement.

Your *dated list* might be something you produce as a result of the audit, looking at your personal CPD record, or, it may be something you can produce automatically if you use an electronic record-keeping system.

The *evidence* you send in will reinforce the statements you make in your CPD profile. It should demonstrate that you have undertaken the CPD activities you have referred to, and should also show how they have improved the quality of your work and benefited service users. The evidence you provide should include a summary of all your CPD activities, as this will show that you meet Standard 1. From this, the CPD assessors should also be able to see how your CPD activities are a mixture of learning activities and are relevant to your work (and therefore meet Standard 2).

Writing the summary of your practice history

Your summary should describe your role and the type of work you do. The summary should identify the people you communicate with and work with most and identify the specialist areas you work in, including your main responsibilities, such as your job description if appropriate.

When you have written your statement about how you meet the HCPC standards for CPD, you may find it helpful to go back over your summary of work, to make sure that it clearly explains how your CPD activities are relevant to your future or current work.

Writing your statement

When you write your statement, the HCPC expect you to concentrate and focus on how you meet Standards 3 and 4 – how your CPD activities have improved the quality of your work and the benefits to service users. One way to complete your statement is to choose four to six CPD activities you have carried out and for each one you should describe:

- what the activity was;
- what you learnt; and
- how you think the activity improved the quality of your work and benefited your service users.

You can choose to tell the HCPC about the activities which you think benefited you the most and for which you have some supporting evidence. Writing your statement like this can be a clear and simple way of showing the HCPC how you have met the standards. However, there is more than one way of completing your statement, so this is only a suggestion. Other ways might include using your professional development plan or similar (if you have one) or structuring your statement around each of the CPD standards.

Not all paramedics have a PDP or review their role or performance – you may be self-employed, or your employer may not work in this way. But if you do have a personal development plan, you may find it helpful to use this as a starting point for writing your statement.

CPD and competence

There is no automatic link between your CPD and your competence. This is because it would be possible (although unlikely) for a competent paramedic not to undertake any CPD and yet still meet the HCPC standards for their skills and knowledge. Equally, it would be possible for a paramedic who was not competent to complete a lot of CPD activities but still not be fit to practise. Box 18.1 explains how the HCPC Standards 1–5 can be demonstrated in your CPD profile.

 Chapter 2 for more detail and advice regarding reflective writing.

Box 18.1 Explanation of how HCPC Standards 1–5 can be demonstrated within your CPD profile

Standard 1 – A registrant must maintain a continuous, up-to-date and accurate record of their CPD.

You can keep a record of your activities in whatever way is most convenient for you. However, the evidence you submit must include a summary page or sheet of all your CPD activities, which must be accurate, continuous and up to date, and concentrate on the CPD you have undertaken in the previous two years.

The simplest way to prove that you have kept a record of your CPD is to send the HCPC, as part of your evidence, a dated list of all of your CPD activities since your previous registration. This could be in any format you choose, but it is suggested that it might be a simple table which includes the date and *type* of each activity. See the HCPC website: http://www.hcpc-uk.org/registrants/cpd/

Standard 2 – A registrant must demonstrate that their CPD activities are a mixture of learning activities relevant to current or future practice.

You *do not* need to undertake or log a certain number of hours or days. This is because different people will be able to dedicate different amounts of time to CPD, and also because the time spent on an activity does not necessarily reflect the learning gained from it.

To comply with this standard, your CPD must include a mixture of learning activities – so you should include different types of learning activity in your CPD record. The CPD may be a mixture of what is relevant in your current job, and activities which are helping to prepare you for a future role. Or you may choose to concentrate most or all of your CPD on the new area of work you will be moving into. This means that your CPD may be very different from that which your colleagues undertake, even though you are from the same profession. For example, if you manage a team, your CPD may be based around your skills in appraising your team, supporting their development, and financial planning. *It might not even include dealing with patients.*

Standard 3 – A registrant must seek to ensure that their CPD has contributed to the quality of their practice and service delivery.

You should aim for your CPD to improve the way you work. Your learning activities should lead to you making changes to how you work, which improve the way you provide your service. This may mean that you continue to work as you did before, but you are more confident that you are working effectively.

You do not necessarily have to make drastic changes to how you work to improve the quality of your work and the way you provide your service. You may meet this standard by showing how your work has developed as your skills increase through your learning. In meeting this standard, you should be able to show that your CPD activities are part of your work, contribute to your work, and are not separate from it.

Standard 4 – A registrant must seek to ensure that their CPD benefits the service user.

You will meet this standard as long as you have demonstrated that your CPD has benefited your service users.

Where you work will dictate who your service users are; for many, this will be patients. However, if you work in education, your service users may be your students or the team of educationalists you oversee. Similarly, if you work in management, your service users may be your team, or other teams that you are part of. If you work in research, your service users may be the people who use your research. So, in this standard, 'service user' means anyone who is primarily affected by your work.

Standard 5 – A registrant must, upon request, present a written profile (which must be their own work and supported by evidence) explaining how they have met the standards for CPD.

If you are chosen for audit, the HCPC will send you a CPD profile. Under this standard, you must fill the profile in, with details of how you have met the standards for CPD. You must return the profile to them, with evidence to support it, by the deadline set.

CPD can and does take many forms; it does not, however, set down exactly how paramedics should learn. Paramedics may already be taking part in activities through which they learn, and which develops their work, but they may not call these activities CPD.

Many people think of CPD as only being formal education (for example, going on courses). The HCPC standards take account of the fact that a course may not be the most useful kind of CPD for all health professionals, and some health professionals may not have access to courses, or are unable to gain funding support or study time. Different registrants will have different development needs, and their CPD activities may be very different. However, the HCPC does stipulate that the CPD profile should be both the registrant's own work and a true reflection of their CPD activity.

The following are examples of CPD.

Paramedic registrant working in a clinical role

- attending a short course on new laws affecting your work;
- appraising an article with a group of colleagues;
- giving colleagues a presentation on a new technique.

Paramedic registrant working in education

- member of learning and teaching committee;
- review for a professional journal;
- studying for a formal teaching award.

Paramedic registrant working in management

- member of an occupational group for managers;
- studying management modules;
- supporting the development and introduction of a national or local policy.

Paramedic registrant involved in research

- presentation at a conference;
- member of a local ethics research committee;
- articles for scientific journals.

Two years' registration

The HCPC will only audit registrants who have been registered for more than two years (HCPC 2017b). They believe that all registrants should undertake CPD throughout their careers; they also believe that registrants should be allowed at least two years on the register to build up evidence of their CPD activities before they are audited.

This means that if you are a recent graduate, and you renew your registration for the first time, you will not be chosen for audit. Similarly, if you have had a break from work, and you have just come back onto the register, you will not be chosen for audit the first time you renew your registration.

WHAT HAPPENS TO YOUR COMPLETED CPD PROFILE?

The HCPC will ask CPD assessors to assess your CPD profile. At least one of these assessors will be a paramedic. While your profile is being assessed, and during any appeal that takes place, you will stay on the register and can continue to work. There are three possible outcomes at this point:

- Your profile meets the standards – you will stay on the register. The HCPC will write to you and let you know.
- More information is needed – the HCPC will write to you and let you know what information the assessors need to decide whether you meet the standards of CPD. You will stay on the register while you send more information to the assessors.
- Your profile does not meet the standards – the CPD assessors will then decide whether or not to offer you extra time (up to an extra three months) to meet the standards. The HCPC will normally ask you for more information before making this decision.

The CPD assessors will decide whether to offer you an extra three months by considering whether:

- you have made a reasonable attempt to provide a complete CPD profile;
- you have met some of the standards; and
- with extra time it would be possible for you to meet the standards.

If you do not meet the standards, the HCPC will remove you from the register. However, whatever decision they reach, they will advise you of their decision and the reasons for it.

Finding out more

Published example profiles can be seen on the HCPC website: www.hcpc-uk.org/. These profiles, which were put together in partnership with the College of Paramedics, are intended to show how health professionals can prove that their CPD activities have met these standards, and how they can write a statement that evidences this.

For even more information about the CPD audit, read the document *Continuing Professional Development and Your Registration* (HCPC 2017b). This is a helpful document, with more detail about continuing professional development, and about the audit process. You can download this document from the HCPC website or you can write to the HCPC to ask for a copy.

CONCLUSION

CPD is recognised as fundamental to the development of all health and social care practitioners, and registrants must seek to ensure that their CPD benefits the service user. Professional bodies and organisations campaign for greater support and recognition of your CPD activities, from your employers and other organisations. The College of Paramedics has regional groups which arrange and provide formal CPD events for members and non-members, and also provides e-learning CPD; these can be accessed via their website.

> ## Chapter key points:
>
> - The chapter has provided an explanation of the role and value of continuing professional development (CPD).
> - It has discussed the role of the HCPC CPD standards and discussed the associated documentation.
> - The chapter provides examples of CPD activity for inclusion in your profile.
> - Each of the relevant standards are discussed and ideas are provided about how you can meet the standards within your written profile.
> - An explanation of what will happen to your completed profile is given along with advice about how to obtain further information and guidance.

REFERENCES AND SUGGESTED READING

College of Paramedics (2017) *Paramedic Curriculum Guidance*, 4th edn. Bridgwater: College of Paramedics.

Health and Care Professions Council (2014) *Standards of Proficiency – Paramedics*. London: HCPC.

Health and Care Professions Council (2016a) *Guidance on Conduct and Ethics for Students*. London: HCPC.

Health and Care Professions Council (2016b) *Standards of Conduct, Performance and Ethics*. London: HCPC.

Health and Care Professions Council (2016c) *2013–15 Continuing Professional Development Audit Report*. London: HCPC.

Health and Care Professions Council (2017a) *Standards of Education and Training*. London: HCPC.

Health and Care Professions Council (2017b) *Continuing Professional Development and Your Registration*. London: HCPC.

Health and Care Professions Council (2017c) *How to Renew Your Registration*. London: HCPC.

Health and Care Professions Council (2017d) *Returning to Practice*. London: HCPC.

Health and Care Professions Council (2017e) *Confidentiality – Guidance for Registrants*. London: HCPC.

Quality Assurance Agency (QAA) (2016) *Subject Benchmark Statement – Paramedics*. Gloucester: The Quality Assurance Agency for Higher Education.

USEFUL WEBSITES

College of Paramedics: www.collegeofparamedics.co.uk
Department of Health: www.dh.gov.uk
Health and Care Professions Council: www.hcpc-uk.org/

Index

Page numbers in *italics* refer to figures and tables; those in **bold** indicate boxes.